Medical
Nutrition
A N D   D I S E A S E

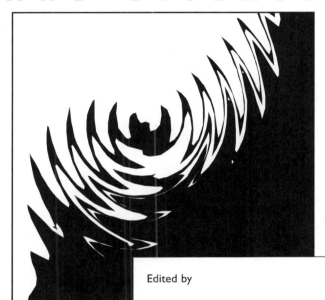

Edited by

Gail Morrison, MD
Vice Dean for Education
Director of Academic Programs
Professor of Medicine
University of Pennsylvania School of Medicine
Philadelphia, Pennsylvania

Lisa Hark, PhD, RD
Director, Nutrition Education and Prevention Program
University of Pennsylvania School of Medicine
Philadelphia, Pennsylvania

b
Blackwell
Science

Blackwell Science

Editorial offices: 238 Main Street, Cambridge, Massachusetts 02142, USA
Osney Mead, Oxford OX2 0El, England
25 John Street, London WC1N 2BL, England
23 Ainslie Place, Edinburgh EH3 6AJ, Scotland
54 University Street, Carlton, Victoria 3053, Australia
Arnette Blackwell SA, 1 rue de Lille, 75007 Paris, France
Blackwell Wissenschafts-Verlag GmbH Kurfürstendamm 57,
10707 Berlin, Germany Feldgasse 13, A-1238 Vienna, Austria

Distributors: *USA*

Blackwell Science
238 Main Street
Cambridge, Massachusetts 02142
(Telephone orders: 800-215-1000 or 617-876-7000)

Canada

Copp Clark, Ltd.
2775 Matheson Blvd. East
Mississauga, Ontario, Canada, L4W 4P7
(Telephone orders: 800-263-4374 or 905-238-6074)

Australia

Blackwell Science Pty Ltd
54 University Street
Carlton, Victoria 3053
(Telephone orders: 03-347-0300)

Outside North America and Australia

Blackwell Science, Ltd.
c/o Marston Book Services, Ltd., P.O. Box 87
Oxford OX2 0DT, England
(Telephone orders: 44-1865-791155)

Acquisitions: Joy Denomme
Development: Kathleen Broderick
Production: Heather Garrison
Manufacturing: Lisa Flanagan
Typeset by Leslie Haimes.
Printed and bound by Braun-Brumfield
©1996 by Blackwell Science, Inc.
Printed in the United States of America
96 97 98 99 5 4 3 2

Library of Congress Cataloging-in-Publication Data
Medical nutrition and disease / edited by Gail Morrison, Lisa Hark.
     p.   cm.
   Includes bibliographical references and index.
   ISBN 0-86542-491-8 (alk. paper)
   1. Dietetics. 2. Diet therapy. 3. Nutrition. I. Morrison,
Gail II. Hark, Lisa.
   [DNLM: 1. Nutrition. 2. Nutritional Support. 3. Diet Therapy.
WB 400 M4896 1996]
RM216.M456 1996
613.2--dc20
DNLM/DLC
for Library of Congress   96-26674
                                                     CIP

Dedication

We dedicate this book to Dr. William Darby and the Howard Heinz Endowment for making the development and implementation of a nutrition curriculum at the University of Pennsylvania School of Medicine a reality. On behalf of all of us involved in nutrition education, thank you Dr. Darby and the Howard Heinz Endowment.

Because this text has been student driven, we also dedicate the first edition to the students who have graduated and who will be graduating from the University of Pennsylvania School of Medicine since the inception of our nutrition education program. Thank you.

Contents

Consulting Editor

Lisa D. Unger, MD, FACP
Assistant Director, Home Nutrition Support
and Attending Physician, Nutrition Support
Service
Hospital of the University of Pennsylvania
Philadelphia, Pennsylvania

Section Editors

Frances Burke, MS, RD
Coordinator, Nutrition Education Program
University of Pennsylvania School of Medicine
Philadelphia, Pennsylvania

Lisa Hark, PhD, RD
Director, Nutrition Education and Prevention
Program
University of Pennsylvania School of Medicine
Philadelphia, Pennsylvania

Susan Ahlstrom Henderson, MS, RD
Research Associate, Program in Human
Nutrition
University of Michigan School of Public Health
Ann Arbor, Michigan

Carine M. Lenders, MD
Resident in Pediatrics
Massachusetts General Hospital
Boston, Massachusetts

Gary R. Lichtenstein, MD
Assistant Professor of Medicine
University of Pennsylvania School of Medicine
Director, Inflammatory Bowel Disease Program
Hospital of the University of Pennsylvania
Philadelphia, Pennsylvania

Scott Manaker, MD, PhD
Assistant Professor of Medicine
University of Pennsylvania School of Medicine
Director, Pulmonary Diagnostic Services
Hospital of the University of Pennsylvania
Philadelphia, Pennsylvania

Donna H. Mueller, PhD, RD, FADA
Associate Professor of Nutrition and Food
Sciences
Department of Bioscience and Biotechnology
Drexel University
Philadelphia, Pennsylvania

Gail Morrison, MD
Vice Dean for Education
Director of Academic Programs
Professor of Medicine
University of Pennsylvania School of Medicine
Philadelphia, Pennsylvania

Daniel J. Rader, MD
Assistant Professor of Medicine
University of Pennsylvania School of Medicine
Director, Lipid Referral Center
Hospital of the University of Pennsylvania
Philadelphia, Pennsylvania

Eugenia L. Siegler, MD
Associate Professor of Medicine
New York University School of Medicine
Chief, Section of Geriatrics
Brooklyn Hospital Center
New York, New York

Virginia A. Stallings, MD
Associate Professor of Pediatrics
University of Pennsylvania School of Medicine
Chief, Division of Gastroenterology and
Nutrition
Children's Hospital of Philadelphia
Philadelphia, Pennsylvania

Jean Stover, MS, RD
Out-patient Dialysis Center
Hospital of the University of Pennsylvania
Philadelphia, Pennsylvania

Melanie Stuart, MS, RD
Out-patient Dietitian, Ambulatory Nutrition
The Cambridge Hospital
Cambridge, Massachusetts

Scott Stuart, MS, RD
Medical Student, Class of 1997
Tufts University School of Medicine
Boston, Massachusetts

Andrew M. Tershakovec, MD
Assistant Professor of Pediatrics
University of Pennsylvania School of
   Medicine
Attending Physician, Division of
   Gastroenterology and Nutrition
Children's Hospital of Philadelphia
Philadelphia, Pennsylvania

Contributors

Margaret Barry, MS, RD, CS
Assistant Clinical Nutrition Manager
Children's Hospital of New Jersey
Newark, New Jersey

Diane Barsky, MD, FAAP, FACN
Assistant Professor of Pediatrics
Medical College of Pennsylvania and
   Hahnemann University
Director of Nutrition Support Service
St. Christopher's Hospital of Children
Philadelphia, Pennsylvania

Marcie Beck, MS, RD
Medical Student. Class of 1998
Hahnemann University
Philadelphia, Pennsylvania

Myhanh E.T. Bosse, MD
Assistant Physician
Gastrointestinal Associates
Abington Memorial Hospital
Abington, Pennsylvania

Seth Braunstein, MD, PhD
Associate Professor of Medicine
University of Pennsylvania School of
   Medicine
Division of Endocrinology
Hospital of the University of Pennsylvania
Philadelphia, Pennsylvania

Randi Cardonick, MS, RD
Out-patient Dietitian, Rodebaugh Diabetes
   Center
Hospital of the University of Pennsylvania
Philadelphia, Pennsylvania

Patricia Charlton, RD
Clinical Nutrition Support Service
Hospital of the University of Pennsylvania
Philadelphia, Pennsylvania

Kelly Davis, MD
Assistant Professor of Medicine
Division of Endocrinology and Metabolism
University of Pennsylvania School of Medicine
Philadelphia, Pennsylvania

Lisa K. Diewald, MS, RD
Instructor, Department of Nursing
Neumann College
Aston, Pennsylvania

Gregg J. Fromell, MD
Clinical Professor
University of Pennsylvania School of Medicine
Lipid Referral Center
Hospital of the University of Pennsylvania
Philadelphia, Pennsylvania

Anita Guevera, MS, RD
Director of Nutrition Services
General Clinical Research Center
Hospital of the University of Pennsylvania
Philadelphia, Pennsylvania

Lauren Hudson, MS, RD
Clinical Nutrition Support Service
Hospital of the University of Pennsylvania
Philadelphia, Pennsylvania

Mary Langan, MA, RD
Clinical Nutrition Support Service
Hospital of the University of Pennsylvania
Philadelphia, Pennsylvania

Rob Roy MacGregor, MD
Professor of Medicine
University of Pennsylvania School of
    Medicine
Director, AIDS Clinical Trials Unit
Hospital of the University of Pennsylvania
Philadelphia, Pennsylvania

Maria R. Mascarenhas, MD
Assistant Professor of Pediatrics
University of Pennsylvania School of
    Medicine
Director, Nutrition Support Service
Children's Hospital of Philadelphia
Philadelphia, Pennsylvania

Nancy Mathews, RD
Clinical Support Service
Hospital of the University of Pennsylvania
Philadelphia, Pennsylvania

Natalie McGuigan, MA, RD
Clinical Nutrition Support Service
Hospital of the University of Pennsylvania
Philadelphia, Pennsylvania

Eileen Smith, RD
Renal Dietician
Out-patient Dialysis Center
Hospital of the University of Pennsylvania
Philadelphia, Pennsylvania

Catherine B. Sullivan, MD
Associate Staff, Department of Pediatrics
Children's Hospital of Pennsylvania
Philadelphia, Pennsylvania

Preface

In 1990, the University of Pennsylvania School of Medicine Faculty unanimously approved the inclusion of a nutrition education experience in the medical school curriculum. Our only hurdle was that there was no time in the curriculum to incorporate nutrition topics, as is the problem with most medical schools. With this in mind, we wanted to offer students a unique experience using clinical cases which correlated basic science and clinical knowledge. Our goals were threefold: students should engage in active learning, nutrition would be integrated across the medical curriculum, and we would utilize an interdisciplinary faculty to develop the program.

To engage students in active learning, we used a self-instructional model, whereby students are required to read the material on their own which corresponded to existing courses such as Biochemistry, Physiology, Introduction to Clinical Medicine, and Pathophysiology as well as certain clinical clerkships. Because nutrition crosses over many disciplines, we felt it was very important to bring together an interdisciplinary group of physicians, registered dietitians, and nurses to develop the program. This group consisted primarily of faculty from the University of Pennsylvania Medical Center and the Children's Hospital of Philadelphia including the Departments of surgery, pediatrics, obstetrics, gynecology, nutrition, medicine including divisions of renal, pulmonary, gastroenterology, endocrine, and cardiology, and the Center for Aging. Every chapter and case has been co-written by these clinical faculty who have worked together to present a unique perspective, the medical as well as the nutritional implications of various clinical scenarios, hence the title *Medical Nutrition and Disease*. Therefore, *Medical Nutrition and Disease* represents a culmination of all these efforts over the past five years.

During implementation of this nutrition curriculum, it became apparent that the concepts and teaching methods that we were using were applicable to other disciplines. Registered dietitians who are teaching dietetic students, medical students, nursing students, dental students, medical residents, nurse practitioners, interns, residents, physicians, and other allied health professionals can easily use this book in a variety of courses or to develop lectures and case presentations. Nursing students and nurses who want to increase their nutrition knowledge can also benefit from using this text. Dietitians and nurses who desire to return to the clinical setting can use the text to update their nutrition knowledge base.

In addition to testing medical students' knowledge and skills, we were also interested in students' attitudes about incorporating nutrition into the curriculum. Ongoing focus groups with medical students indicate that students prefer nutrition cases that correspond to courses such as biochemistry, medical history, physical exam, and pathophysiology. During the clinical clerkships, students requested the opportunity to assess the nutritional status of their patients and present this information during rounds. We listened and developed a nutrition curriculum within the first, second, and third year of medical school.

The book format has been designed to introduce basic nutrition concepts including fundamentals of nutrition assessment and nutrition during the life-cycle, followed by the nutritional management of various diseases as well as the fundamentals of enteral and parenteral nutrition support. Students benefit because the book can be used for more than one course over several years. Lecture notes are given for each chapter as well as clinical cases which reinforce the material in the chapter while providing a practical approach to patient care. Each clinical case includes a list of questions; answers are then provided immediately following, offering the reader an opportunity to think through the questions and then read the answers.

Therefore, this text works very well for individuals teaching nutrition in a variety of settings including undergraduate and graduate dietetic, medical, and nursing education programs. The book also addresses the needs of the adult learner who desires to advance his/her knowledge and skills in nutrition on his/her own. In addition, we have developed and tested over 75 multiple-choice questions as a vehicle to review the material for a course exam, to use the text to prepare for a licensing or certifying exam depending on the reader's specialty, or simply to test the reader's knowledge about the concepts that were discussed in the chapters and case presentations.

We would also like to thank the following reviewers for their expert medical, nursing, nutritional, and editorial guidance in reviewing the entire text:

Shahab Aftahi, MD, Albany Medical College, Albany, New York

Mary Beth Arensberg, PhD, RD, Ross Products Division, Abbott Laboratories, Columbus, Ohio

Janet Z. Burson, EdD, RD, FADA, University of Southern Maine, Portland, Maine

Charlene Compher, MS, RD, Hospital of the University of Pennsylvania, Philadelphia, Pennsylvania

Kathleen M. Cornell, BA, University of Pennsylvania School of Medicine, Philadelphia, Pennsylvania

Larry Finkelstein, DO, Philadelphia College of Osteopathic Medicine, Philadelphia, Pennsylvania

Roseann Murphy Jones, PhD, University of Pennsylvania School of Medicine, Philadelphia, Pennsylvania

Anita Lasswell, PhD, RD, University of North Carolina School of Medicine, Chapel Hill, North Carolina

Kathleen Lindell, MSN, RN, University of Pennsylvania School of Medicine, Philadelphia, Pennsylvania

Gina McCleod, RN, BSN, Paoli Memorial Hospital, Paoli, Pennsylvania

Virginia Stallings, MD, University of Pennsylvania School of Medicine and Children's Hospital of Philadelphia, Philadelphia, Pennsylvania

Melanie Stuart, MS, RD, Cambridge Hospital, Cambridge, Massachusetts

Scott Stuart, MS, RD, Tufts University School of Medicine, Boston, Massachusetts

Lisa D. Unger, MD, Hospital of the University of Pennsylvania, Philadelphia, Pennsylvania

Jane White, PhD, RD, University of Tennessee College of Medicine, Memphis, Tennessee

For more information on how to successfully incorporate nutrition into your curriculm contact

Lisa Hark, PhD, RD
Director, Nutrition Education and Prevention
University of Pennsylvania School of Medicine
3450 Hamilton Walk
Philadelphia, Pennsylvania 19104-6087
Phone: 215-349-5795
Fax: 215-573-7075
Email: lhark@mail.med.upenn.edu

Contact our new home page at http://www.med.upenn.edu/~nutrimed

Gail Morrison, MD
Lisa Hark, PhD, RD

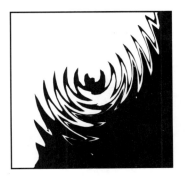

PART I

Fundamentals of
Clinical Nutrition

1

Nutrition Assessment in Medical Practice

Virginia A. Stallings and Lisa Hark

Objectives

- To recognize the prevalence of malnutrition in hospitalized and nonhospitalized patients.
- To identify the risk factors and usual physical findings associated with malnutrition.
- To interpret population reference data for the following nutritional measures: diet, weight, height, triceps skinfold, mid-arm circumference, and mid-arm muscle circumference.
- To assess a patient's nutritional status by integrating nutrition into the medical history, review of systems, physical examination, and laboratory evaluation.
- To develop a nutrition plan based on clinical findings.

Definition and Purpose of Nutrition Assessment

Nutrition assessment is the evaluation of an individual's nutritional status and nutrient requirements based on the interpretation of clinical information obtained from the medical history, review of systems, and physical examination, including anthropometric measurements and laboratory data. The purposes of nutrition assessment are: to accurately define individuals' nutritional status; to determine the level of nutritional support that individuals need; and to monitor changes in nutritional status and the effect of nutritional intervention during acute and chronic illnesses.

Nutrition assessment is important in clinical medicine because acute and chronic malnutrition—both under- and overnutrition—are common clinical findings. Malnutrition is a suboptimal (deficient or excessive) supply of nutrients that interferes with an individual's growth, development, and maintenance of health. Various examples of malnutrition are caloric, protein, vitamin, and mineral deficiencies. In this text, the term malnutrition refers to deficiency states observed in clinical medicine.

Obesity is a very common type of overnutrition in adults and children. In the United States, approximately 35 percent of women and 31 percent of men age 20 and older are obese, as are about 25 percent of children and adolescents. Obese individuals have an increased risk of certain types of cancer, diabetes, cardiovascular disease, hyperlipidemia, hypertension, osteoarthritis, respiratory diseases, orthopedic disorders, and biliary disease (gallstones). The hyperlipidemias (hypercholesterolemia and hypertriglyceridemia) are related to nutrition, although in these disorders as in obesity, non-nutritional contributing factors such as heredity, smoking, and the patient's age) must also be taken into account.

Prevalence of Malnutrition (Undernutrition) in the United States

Three groups in this population have been identified as particularly prone to malnutrition: hospitalized patients, the elderly, and out-patients. Malnutrition is thought to be present in

- 50 percent of patients in large urban surgical and medical hospital wards
- 35 to 55 percent of patients in children's hospitals
- 60 percent of hospitalized infants under three months of age

Among the elderly population, estimates of the percentage affected by malnutrition include

- 25 to 50 percent of nursing home patients
- 5 to 10 percent of older adults living in the community

The prevalence of malnutrition in the out-patient population is poorly documented. Risk factors for malnutrition among members of this group include

- chronic diseases
- multiple prescription medications
- poverty
- inadequate nutritional knowledge
- homebound and /or nonambulatory status

Population Guidelines and Individual Patient Nutrition Assessment

The goals of nutrition assessment are to recognize the nutritional status of your patients and to determine their nutritional requirements. Several important population guidelines support these goals, but care must be taken when translating these or any other group/population data or findings into specific recommendations for individual patients. The remainder of this section presents examples of reference data for specific age and gender groups developed from currently available population studies.

Recommended Dietary Allowances (1989)

The recommended dietary allowances (RDAs) establish adequate intake levels of essential nutrients required to meet the needs of healthy people under usual environmental stress. In the United States, the RDA's developed by the subcommittee of the Food and Nutrition Board of the National Academy of Sciences often exceed actual individual nutritional requirements because they are two standard deviations above the estimated mean requirements. For most people, meeting two thirds of the RDA is thus considered adequate (described in Chapter 2).

Healthy Weight Tables for Adults

The Metropolitan Life Insurance Ideal Weight Tables were used for many years as the standard against which to categorize people according to their height and weight. However, because these tables were developed from a limited sample that included only insurance policyholders between 25 and 59 years of age, they may not be appropriate for all individuals, especially older adults and non-Caucasians. Recently, the United States Department of Agriculture and the Department of Health and Human Services established an expert committee to develop the new, comprehensive Healthy Weight Tables (Table 1-1). The committee's recommendations encompass a wider range of acceptable body weights related to individuals' height.

National Center for Health Statistics Growth Charts for Infants and Children

Between 1962 and 1974, the United States Public Health Service performed a series of measurements on a large population of children from diverse racial, socioeconomic, and geographic backgrounds. Growth charts developed from this cross-section are used as reference standards to plot infant, child, and adolescent height (length), weight, and head circumference according to age and gender. The four available growth charts shown in Figures 1-1 to 1-4 are

Boys	Girls
Birth to 36 months	Birth to 36 months
2 to 18 years	2 to 18 years

Table 1-1   Healthy weights for adults.*

HEIGHT[a]	WEIGHT IN POUNDS[b]
4'10"	91–119
4'11"	94–124
5'0"	97–128
5'1"	101–132
5'2"	104–137
5'3"	107–141
5'4"	111–146
5'5"	114–150
5'6"	118–155
5'7"	121–160
5'8"	125–164
5'9"	129–169
5'10"	132–174
5'11"	136–179
6'0"	140–184
6'1"	144–189
6'2"	148–195
6'3"	152–200
6'4"	156–205
6'5"	160–211
6'6"	164–216

*Higher weights in the range generally apply to men, who tend to have more muscle mass and bone.
[a]Height without shoes.
[b]Weight without clothes.
Source: 1995 Dietary Guidelines for Americans. U.S. Department of Agriculture and the Department of Health and Human Services.

Anthropometric Standards for Nutritional Status

Using anthropometric standards to evaluate nutritional status allows classification of patients into categories ranging from undernourished to obese. Interpreting nutritional status from such measurements involves comparing the patient's measurements to these reference data, which are usually based on large numbers of healthy people from the general population. These measurements may be performed as part of the physical examination and reflect body composition (fat and muscle mass).

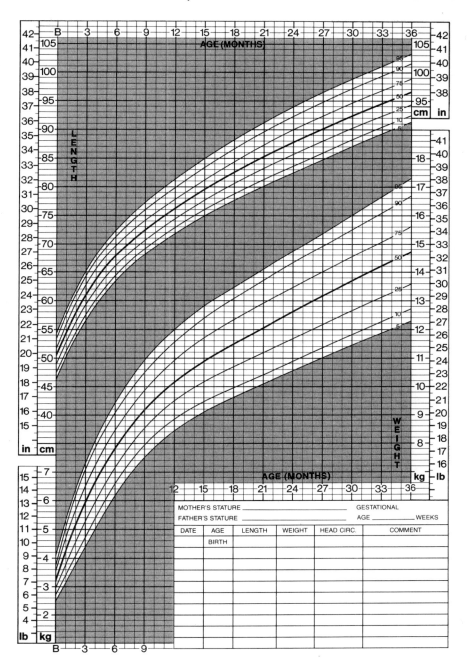

Figure 1-1 Physical Growth NCHS Percentiles: Boys, Birth to 36 Months (Length/Age and Weight/Age).

Source: Reprinted with permission from the American Society for Clinical Nutrition, from Hamill PVV. Physical Growth: National Center for Health Statistics. *Am J Clin Nutr* 1979;32: 607–629. Data from National Center for Health Statistics, Hyattsville, MD.

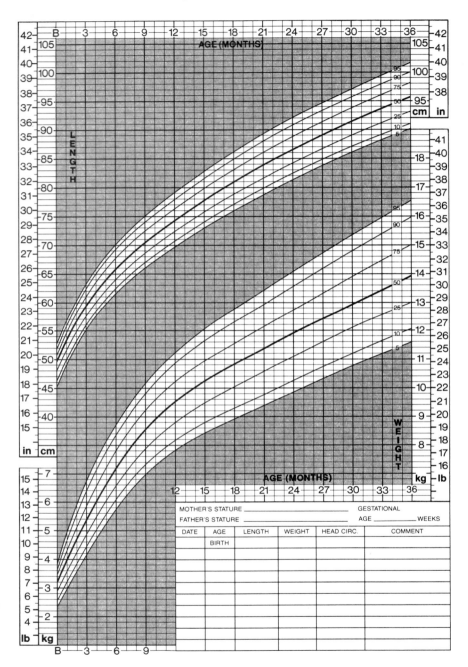

**Figure 1-2   Physical Growth NCHS Percentiles: Girls, Birth to 36 Months
(Length/Age and Weight/Age).**

Source: Reprinted with permission from the American Society for Clinical Nutrition, from
Hamill PVV. Physical Growth: National Center for Health Statistics. *Am J Clin Nutr* 1979;32:
607–629. Data from National Center for Health Statistics, Hyattsville, MD.

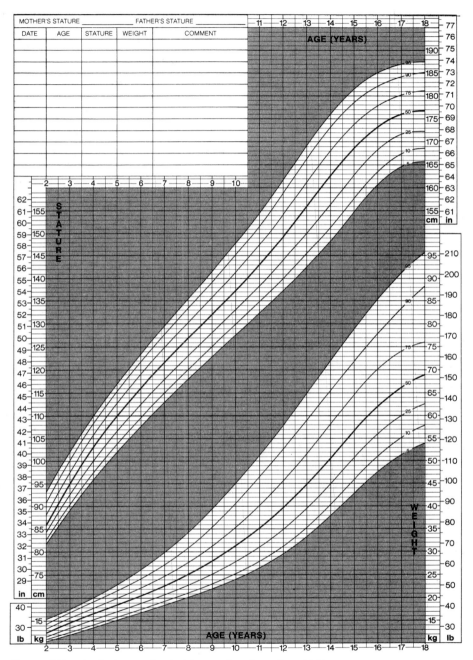

Figure 1-3   Physical Growth NCHS Percentiles: Boys, 2 to 18 Years (Stature/Age and Weight/Age).

Source: Reprinted with permission from the American Society for Clinical Nutrition, from Hamill PVV. Physical Growth: National Center for Health Statistics. *Am J Clin Nutr* 1979;32: 607–629. Data from National Center for Health Statistics, Hyattsville, MD.

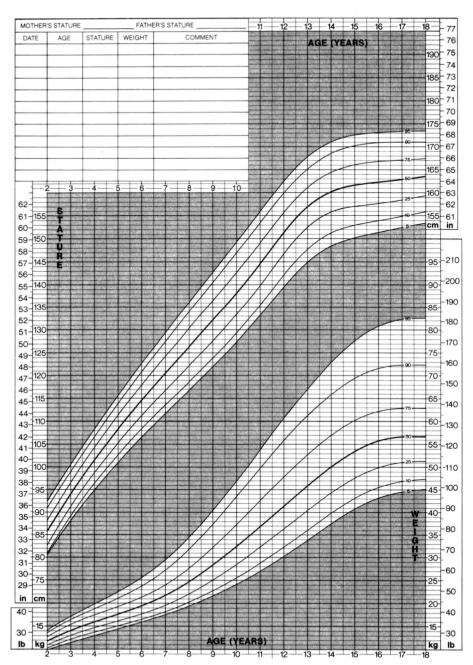

Figure 1-4 Physical Growth NCHS Percentiles: Girls, 2 to 18 Years (Stature/Age and Weight/Age).

Source: Reprinted with permission from the American Society for Clinical Nutrition, from Hamill PVV. Physical Growth: National Center for Health Statistics. *Am J Clin Nutr* 1979;32: 607–629. Data from National Center for Health Statistics, Hyattsville, MD.

Mid-Arm Circumference (MAC)

The MAC measurement of the circumference of the arm, which represents both muscle and fat stores, is taken with a metric tape measure at the midpoint between the acromion and the olecranon bones on the nondominant arm. The resulting value is used later in this section to calculate mid-arm muscle circumference (Table 1-2).

Triceps Skinfold Measurements (TSF)

The TSF measurement is also obtained on the nondominant arm at the same midpoint as the MAC by pulling the subcutaneous tissue on the underside of the arm away from the triceps muscle. A skinfold caliper may then be used to measure the amount of tissue which estimates the subcutaneous fat over the muscle. This value allows an estimation of dietary caloric adequacy and stored body fat (Table 1-3).

Mid-Arm Muscle Circumference (MAMC)

The MAMC estimates skeletal muscle mass based on the MAC and the TSF measurements. When using the following equation to determine the MAMC, be certain to keep the units used to express the MAC and the TSF consistent (in mm or cm).

$$\text{Calculated MAMC} = \text{MAC} - 3.14\,(\text{TSF})$$

Body Mass Index (BMI)

The BMI is a useful clinical calculation for diagnosing obesity because it is correlated with total body fat and is relatively unaffected by height (Figure 1-5). The normal range for the BMI is between 19.0 and 26.0. Patients with a BMI between 26.1 and 29.0 are considered overweight. Those with a BMI greater than 30 are obese. Note, however, that individuals with a BMI greater than 27.0 are thought to be at significantly increased health risk. The following formula is used to calculate the BMI.

$$\text{BMI} = \frac{\text{weight (kg)}}{\text{height (m}^2)}$$

Third National Health and Nutrition Examination Survey (NHANES III) (1989–1991)

NHANES III is the seventh in a series of national longitudinal studies conducted in the United States since 1960 by the Centers for Disease Control and Prevention (CDCP). In 1970 the basic design of the survey was updated to include a lengthy nutrition component. Nutrition assessments derived from individual interviews included food and nutrient consumption, alcohol intake, calcium intake, vitamin and mineral status, iron-deficiency anemia, overweight and obesity, osteoporosis, and findings from physical examinations. The goals of NHANES III are to

Table 1-2   Reference standards for mid-arm circumference (MAC) and mid-arm muscle circumference (MAMC). Percentiles of upper-arm circumference for Whites of the United States Health and Nutrition Examination Survey I of 1971 to 1974.

MALES

Age Group	Arm Circumferences (mm)							Arm Muscle Circumference (mm)						
(yrs)	5	10	25	50	75	90	95	5	10	25	50	75	90	95
1–1.9	142	146	150	159	170	176	183	110	113	119	127	135	144	147
2–2.9	141	145	153	162	170	178	185	111	114	122	130	140	146	150
3–3.9	150	153	160	167	175	184	190	117	123	131	137	143	148	153
4–4.9	149	154	162	171	180	186	192	123	126	133	141	148	156	159
5–5.9	153	160	167	175	185	195	204	128	133	140	147	154	162	169
6–6.9	155	159	167	179	188	209	228	131	135	142	151	161	170	177
7–7.9	162	167	177	187	201	223	230	137	139	151	160	168	177	190
8–8.9	162	170	177	190	202	220	245	140	145	154	162	170	182	187
9–9.9	175	178	187	200	217	249	257	151	154	161	170	183	196	202
10–10.9	181	184	196	210	231	262	274	156	160	166	180	191	209	221
11–11.9	186	190	202	223	244	261	280	159	165	173	183	195	205	230
12–12.9	193	200	214	232	254	282	303	167	171	182	195	210	223	241
13–13.9	194	211	228	247	263	286	301	172	179	196	211	226	238	245
14–14.9	220	226	237	253	283	303	322	189	199	212	223	240	260	264
15–15.9	222	229	244	264	284	311	320	199	204	218	237	254	266	272
16–16.9	244	248	262	278	303	324	343	213	225	234	249	269	287	296
17–17.9	246	253	267	285	308	336	347	224	231	245	258	273	294	312
18–18.9	245	260	276	297	321	353	379	226	237	252	264	283	298	324
19–24.9	262	272	288	308	331	355	372	238	245	257	273	289	309	321
25–34.9	271	282	300	319	342	362	375	243	250	264	279	298	314	326
35–44.9	278	287	305	326	345	363	374	247	255	269	286	302	318	327
45–54.9	267	281	301	322	342	362	376	239	249	265	281	300	315	326
55–64.9	258	273	296	317	336	355	369	236	245	260	278	295	310	320
65–74.9	248	263	285	307	325	344	355	223	235	251	268	284	298	306

FEMALES

Age Group	Arm Circumferences (mm)							Arm Muscle Circumference (mm)						
1–1.9	138	142	148	156	164	172	177	105	111	117	124	132	139	143
2–2.9	142	145	152	160	167	176	184	111	114	119	126	133	142	147
3–3.9	143	150	158	167	175	183	189	113	119	124	132	140	146	152
4–4.9	149	154	160	169	177	184	191	115	121	128	136	144	152	157
5–5.9	153	157	165	175	185	203	211	125	128	134	142	151	159	165
6–6.9	156	162	170	176	187	204	211	130	133	138	145	154	166	171
7–7.9	164	167	174	183	199	216	231	129	135	142	151	160	171	176
8–8.9	168	172	183	195	214	247	261	138	140	151	160	171	183	194
9–9.9	178	182	194	211	224	251	260	147	150	158	167	180	194	198
10–10.9	174	182	193	210	228	251	265	148	150	159	170	180	190	197
11–11.9	185	194	208	224	248	276	303	150	158	171	181	196	217	223
12–12.9	194	203	216	237	256	282	294	162	166	180	191	201	214	220
13–13.9	202	211	223	243	271	301	338	169	175	183	198	211	226	240
14–14.9	214	223	237	252	272	304	322	174	179	190	201	216	232	247
15–15.9	208	221	239	254	279	300	322	175	178	189	202	215	228	244
16–16.9	218	224	241	258	283	318	334	170	180	190	202	216	234	249
17–17.9	220	227	241	264	295	324	350	175	183	194	205	221	239	257
18–18.9	222	227	241	258	281	312	325	174	179	191	202	215	237	245
19–24.9	221	230	247	265	290	319	345	179	185	195	207	221	236	249
25–34.9	233	240	256	277	304	342	368	183	188	199	212	228	246	264
35–44.9	241	251	267	290	317	356	378	186	192	205	218	236	257	272
45–54.9	242	256	274	299	328	362	384	187	193	206	220	238	260	274
55–64.9	243	257	280	303	335	367	385	187	196	209	225	244	266	280
65–74.9	240	252	274	299	326	356	373	185	195	208	225	244	264	279

Source: Frisancho AR; New norms of upper limb fat and muscle areas for assessment of nutritional status. *Am J Clin Nutr* 34:2540–2545. © 1981, American Society for Clinical Nutrition.

- estimate the national prevalence of selected diseases and risk factors
- document national distributions of selected health parameters
- document and investigate reasons for trends of selected diseases
- contribute to an understanding of disease etiology
- investigate the natural history of selected diseases

Integrating Nutrition in the Medical History and Physical Examination

The following examples illustrate how to integrate nutrition assessment into all components of the medical work-up and nursing assessment, including the medical history, review of systems, physical examination, laboratory data assessment, and treatment plan.

Table 1-3   Triceps skinfold reference table for adult males and females. Percentiles for triceps skinfold for Whites of the United States Health and Nutrition Examination Survey I of 1971 to 1974.

TRICEPS SKINFOLD PERCENTILES (mm^2)

Age group (years)	0	5	10	25	50	75	90	95	0	5	10	25	50	75	90	95
1–1.9	228	6	7	8	10	12	14	16	204	6	7	8	10	12	14	16
2–2.9	223	6	7	8	10	12	14	15	208	6	8	9	10	12	15	16
3–3.9	220	6	7	8	10	11	14	15	208	7	8	9	11	12	14	15
4–4.9	230	6	6	8	9	11	12	14	208	7	8	8	10	12	14	16
5–5.9	214	6	6	8	9	11	14	15	219	6	7	8	10	12	15	18
6–6.9	117	6	6	7	8	10	13	16	118	6	6	8	10	12	14	16
7–7.9	122	6	6	7	9	12	15	17	126	6	7	9	11	13	16	18
8–8.9	117	5	6	7	8	10	13	16	118	6	8	9	12	15	18	24
9–9.9	121	5	6	7	10	13	17	18	125	8	8	10	13	16	20	22
10–10.9	146	5	6	8	10	14	18	21	152	7	8	10	12	17	23	27
11–11.9	122	6	6	8	11	16	20	24	117	7	8	10	13	18	24	28
12–12.9	153	6	6	8	11	14	22	28	129	8	9	11	14	18	23	27
13–13.9	134	5	5	7	10	14	22	26	151	8	8	12	15	21	26	30
14–14.9	131	4	6	7	9	14	21	24	141	9	10	13	16	21	26	28
15–15.9	128	4	6	6	8	11	18	24	117	8	10	12	17	21	25	32
16–16.9	131	4	6	6	8	12	16	22	142	10	12	15	18	22	26	31
17–17.9	133	5	6	6	8	12	16	19	114	10	12	13	19	24	30	37
18–18.9	91	4	6	6	9	13	20	24	109	10	12	15	18	22	26	30
19–19.9	531	4	6	7	10	15	20	22	1060	10	11	14	18	24	30	34
25–34.9	971	5	6	8	12	16	20	24	1987	10	12	16	21	27	34	37
35–44.9	806	5	6	8	12	16	20	23	1614	12	14	18	23	29	35	38
45–54.9	898	6	6	8	12	15	20	25	1047	12	16	20	25	30	36	40
55–64.9	734	5	6	8	11	14	19	22	809	12	16	20	25	31	36	38
65–74.9	1503	4	6	8	11	15	19	22	1670	12	14	18	24	29	34	36

Source: Reprinted with permission from Frisancho AR; New norms of upper limb fat and muscle areas for assessment of nutritional status. Am J Clin Nutr 34;2540–2545. ©1981, American Society for Clinical Nutrition.

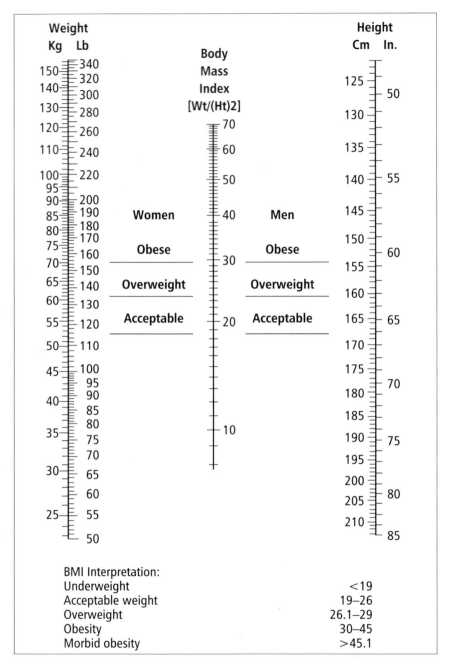

Figure 1-5   Body Mass Index (BMI) Nomogram and Interpretation. To determine BMI, draw a straight line from the person's weight to their height. Read the BMI from the point where it crosses the center.

Source: Reprinted by permission of Bray GA. The Classification and Evaluation of Obesity. In *Obesity.* Bjorntorp P and Brodoff BN, eds. Philadelphia: Lippincott 1992.

Medical History

Past Medical History

The patient is asked to describe and give the dates of immunizations, hospitalizations, operations, major injuries, chronic illnesses, and significant acute illnesses. Detailed information is requested about current or recent prescription medications and also about vitamins and minerals, laxatives, topical medications, other over-the-counter medications, and products such as nutritional supplements that patients frequently do not recognize as medications. Liquid nutritional supplements include any products that patients use to increase their caloric and protein intake. Information about all forms of medications is pertinent to nutrition assessment because of the possibility of drug-nutrient interactions such as those caused by potassium-wasting diuretics.

Examples of nutrition assessment questions to integrate in the past medical history

Is the patient taking vitamins, minerals, or nutritional supplements?
Does the patient have any known food allergies?
Does the patient suffer from milk (lactose) intolerance?

Family History

Patients are asked to identify their parents, siblings, children, and spouse, give their respective ages and health status, and indicate the cause of death of any deceased family members. Familial occurrences of disease also are recorded here. Nutrition assessment questions should probe for any family history of diabetes, heart disease, obesity, hypertension, and osteoporosis.

Social History

Pertinent nonmedical information recorded here includes the patient's occupation, daily exercise pattern, and marital and family status. Information is also solicited regarding the patient's education, economic status, residence, emotional response and adjustment to illness, and any other information that might influence the patient's understanding of his or her illness and adherence to a therapeutic program. Details concerning the duration and frequency of the patient's use of substances such as alcohol, tobacco, illegal drugs, and caffeine are also recorded here. These data can be extremely useful when formulating the nutrition assessment and treatment plan.

Appropriate methods for obtaining a diet history at this stage include the 24-hour recall approach, the usual food intake record, the food diary, and the food frequency questionnaire. These methods are the topic of the following section.

Examples of nutrition assessment questions to integrate in the social history

Has the patient been following a special diet (low salt, sugar-free, vegetarian)?

How successfully has the patient followed this special diet?

How many meals does the patient eat during the day? How many snacks?

Does the patient avoid any specific foods such as milk or meats?

If the patient has insulin-dependent diabetes, at what times are meals eaten?

If the patient has diabetes, does he or she self-monitor blood glucose levels? How often?

If the patient is obese, does he or she have a history of dieting?

If the patient is handicapped, does he or she require help when preparing and eating food? Is this help currently available to the patient?

Does the patient exercise on a regular basis? What type of exercise does the patient perform? How often? For how long?

Methods for Assessing Dietary Intake

The purpose of obtaining dietary information from your patients is to help you conduct the nutrition assessment and formulate a treatment plan. Dietary information may be obtained using any of the methods described in this section. Most of the suggested questions can be asked as part of the patient's social history. In addition, the patient's past and/or current patterns of food intake, other food-related behaviors, and cultural background should also be considered during the interview process.

Note that all three methods described here require gathering data and requesting information over different periods of time.

24-Hour Recall

Purpose This informal, qualitative, questioning method elicits all the foods and beverages the patient has consumed in the preceding 24 hours. In addition, you may also want to monitor hospitalized patients through calorie counts conducted by the nursing or dietary staff, who record the daily amounts of food and drink the patient consumes.

Questions Please describe everything that you ate and drank within the past 24 hours, including the quantities consumed and methods of preparation.

Begin with the last meal eaten or ask for a description of everything that the patient ate the day before. Family members are usually consulted if the patient is a child or unable to convey information.

Advantages Information is easily obtained using this method. The clinician may either conduct an oral interview or ask the patient to complete a questionnaire.

Patients generally can recall most of their dietary intake during the preceding 24 hours.

Disadvantages The limited, general information this method provides may not be sufficient or accurate enough to draw conclusions about an individual's usual intake. Furthermore, the patient's recollection may not reflect long-term dietary habits. For example, some patients may have difficulty remembering all the foods and beverages they consumed the day before. Patients who ate out on the previous day may be unable to estimate accurately the quantities of foods they consumed. Hidden fats in sauces and dressings may not be included in their responses. If the day in question was a weekend, birthday, or holiday, reported consumption, though accurate, may not reflect the patient's usual intake. Therefore, the 24-hour recall method, when used alone, may grossly underestimate or overestimate a person's usual, total fat and caloric intake.

Usual Intake/Diet History

Purpose Similar to the 24-hour recall, a usual intake/diet history is a retrospective means of obtaining dietary information by asking the patient to recall his or her normal daily intake pattern, including intake frequency and amounts of foods consumed.

Questions Describe your typical daily food and beverage intake, including meals and snacks.

As a busy clinician, this question may be all that you will have time to ask, but it can serve as a screening mechanism to identify patients who need further counseling with a registered dietitian.

Advantages This approach provides more information about intake patterns than the others and works well for people who do not vary their food intake a great deal. It also tends to reflect long-term dietary habits with greater accuracy.

Disadvantages Only limited information about the actual quantities of foods and beverages consumed is obtained using this method. Also, people who eat a wide variety of foods or are otherwise inconsistent in their intake find it difficult to describe their "usual" intake. Therefore, when using this approach it is important to be flexible. When you begin by asking patients to describe their usual intake you may learn that they do not have a usual diet. The best course of action in this case is to ask what the patient ate and drank the day before and switch quickly to the 24-hour recall method. Also bear in mind that some patients tend to report having eaten only those foods that they know are healthy.

Food Frequency Questionnaire

Purpose Another retrospective approach, the food frequency questionnaire is a technique used to determine trends in the patient's usual frequency of consumption of specific foods. Frequencies can be listed to identify daily, weekly, or monthly consumption patterns, or all three.

Questions The patient is usually asked to indicate on a standardized written checklist how often he or she eats a particular food or type of food. Up to 100 foods may be listed and organized into groups with similar nutrient content. Questions regarding the frequency of intake of a particular food can also be asked in the social history. Normally, these questions are geared toward the patient's existing medical conditions. For example, consider the following.

> What types of fats and oils do you use in cooking, on bread, and in salad dressings?
>
> What types of sweets, desserts, and snacks do you eat? How often?
>
> How often do you use dairy products? What type of milk do you drink?
>
> How often do you eat red meat? What type? How much? Do you normally trim off the fat?
>
> How many eggs do you eat in a week?
>
> How often do you eat out? How frequently do you eat in fast-food restaurants?
>
> How often do you eat fruits and vegetables?

Advantages Using this method identifies any food groups—fruits, vegetables, milk, or meats, for example—that a patient avoids and thus points out certain dietary deficiencies or excesses.

Disadvantages Patients may not remember exactly how frequently they consume various foods and may therefore overestimate their consumption of some and underestimate that of others. Also, little detail is obtained on cooking methods or on what combinations of foods the patient eats at mealtimes.

We recommend using a combination of these methods, particularly with patients who cannot remember what they ate or who have specific medical problems. For example, a patient with an elevated cholesterol level (hyperlipidemia) will benefit from a low-fat diet. Asking the usual intake questions as part of the social history will help you narrow your list of food frequency questions to identify only the high-fat foods: fried foods, nuts, chips, cheese, butter, margarine, cheeses, and so on.

Review of Systems

This subjective re-examination of the patient's history is organized by body systems. It differs from the past medical history by concentrating on symptoms, not diagnoses, and by emphasizing current as well as past information. All positive and negative findings are listed. Nutrition questions vary according to the patient's age. Example topics follow for each system that may have nutritional implications. One goal of this history is to determine whether any dietary changes have occurred in the patient's life, either voluntarily or as a consequence of illness, medication use, or psychological problems (see boxed list on p.19).

Physical Examination

The physical examination begins with the patient's general appearance: for example, "On examination, she is a well-developed, thin woman." When terms

---

Example topics with nutritional implications for the review of systems

General: appetite, weakness, fatigue, anorexia, clothes tighter or looser, weight change (how much and over what period of time?)

Skin: dry, rough, easy bruisability (ecchymosis), itching, rash

Hair: recent changes in texture, color, pluckability

Eyes: vision, blindness or blind spots, blurred vision

Nails: recent changes in texture, shape, brittleness, color

Mouth/throat: condition of teeth, gums, lips, tongue, dentures; decreased taste; painful swallowing

Cardiac: chest pain, palpitations, dyspnea on exertion

GI/abdomen: food intolerance, belching, vomiting, nausea, constipation, heartburn, diarrhea, stool changes, flatulence, indigestion

Female reproductive: amenorrhea

Endocrine: heat and cold intolerance, polydipsia, polyphagia, polyuria

Extremities: swelling, joint pain, ecchymosis, cold sensitivity

Neurological: seizures, tingling, headaches, decreased sensation, dizziness

Musculoskeletal: weakness, loss of muscle strength or atrophy

---

such as undernourished, thin, well-nourished, well-developed, or cachectic are used, they should be supported by findings in the physical exam and noted in the problem list.

Nutrition oriented aspects of the physical exam focus on the skin, head, hair, eyes, mouth, nails, abdomen, skeletal muscle, and fat stores. Areas to examine closely for muscle wasting include the temporal muscles and the interosseous muscles on the hands. The skeletal muscle of the extremities also serves as an indicator of malnutrition.

Subcutaneous fat stores should be examined for losses due to a sudden decrease in weight or for the excess accumulation that commonly occurs in obesity. Specific signs that are attributable to a vitamin or mineral deficiency are defined in the glossary. Isolated vitamin deficiencies such as scurvy and pellagra are rarely seen today in clinical practice. The most commonly encountered nutritional problem is malnutrition, due to inadequate calorie and protein intake, also known as marasmus. Marasmus is characterized by severe tissue wasting, loss of subcutaneous fat, and usually dehydration. Findings indicative of protein deficiency, or kwashiorkor, include growth retardation, changes in skin and hair pigmentation, edema, and pathologic changes in the liver. Additional clinical signs with nutritional implications appear in the boxed list on p. 20.

Clinical signs with nutritional implications on physical examination

Vital signs

temperature, heart rate, respiration, blood pressure

Anthropometric data

height, weight, percent ideal weight, percent weight change

General appearance: fatigue, obesity, edema, cachexia

Skin: rashes, xerosis, follicular hyperkeratosis, flaky dermatitis, pallor, dryness, ecchymosis, pressure ulcers, delayed healing, acanthosis nigricans, petechiae, purpura, pitting edema, xanthomas

Hair: dyspigmentation, easy pluckability, thinning, alopecia

Head: temporal muscle wasting, parotid enlargement, delayed closure of fontanelle

Eyes: pale, dull, thickened conjunctiva, scleral xerosis, ophthalmoplegia, arcus cornea, scleral icterus, Bitot's spots

Mouth: condition of teeth, dentures, and gums

Tongue: glossitis, edema, atrophic lingual papillae, fissuring

Lips: beefy red, cheilosis, angular stomatitis, fissures, scars

Cardiac: cardiomyopathy, arrhythmia, tachycardia, bradycardia

Pulmonary: barrel chest, tachypnea

Nails: brittle, pale, spoon-shaped, or thin in appearance; clubbing

GI/abdomen: ascites, hepatomegaly, wasting, splenomegaly, abdominal masses

Genital/urinary: Tanner staging for pubetal development in children and adolescents

Extremities: edema, excess or deficient subcutaneous fat, muscle wasting

Neurological: irritability, weakness, change in deep tendon reflex, sensory loss, asterixis

Musculoskeletal: muscle wasting , weakness or cramping, growth retardation, bone pain and tenderness, fractures, joint tenderness, epiphyseal swelling , rachitic rosary

---

Anthropometric Data for Adults

Anthropometric measurements included in the physical exam are described below. Interpretation of these measurements varies according to the patient's age and requires standardized methods, accurate equipment, and a well-trained observer. Note in particular that heights and weights reported by patients or family members are often inaccurate. Therefore you should obtain your own measurements during the medical examination to ensure reliability.

Ideal Body Weight

This value is estimated using the following rule-of-thumb method.

Males For a height of 5 feet, 106 lbs is considered ideal weight. For each additional inch over 5 feet, add 6 lbs ±10% for frame size.

Females For a height of 5 feet, 100 lbs is considered ideal weight. For each additional inch over 5 feet, add 5 lbs ±10% for frame size.

Percent Ideal Body Weight

The following equation calculates the percent ideal body weight (IBW) in adults.

$$\text{Percent ideal body weight} = \frac{\text{Current weight}}{\text{Ideal weight}} \times 100$$

Interpretations of percent ideal body weight are listed in Table 1-4.

Table 1-4   Interpretation of percent ideal body weight.

% IBW	DIAGNOSIS
> 200	Morbid obesity
150–200	Severe obesity
120–149	Obese
110–119	Overweight
90–109	Normal weight
80–89	Mild malnutrition
70–79	Moderate malnutrition
< 70	Severe malnutrition

Percent Weight Change

If weight loss was identified in review of systems, it is essential to determine the percent weight change as follows.

$$\text{Percent weight change} = \frac{\text{Usual weight} - \text{Current weight}}{\text{Usual weight}} \times 100$$

Interpretations of the significance of the percent weight loss appear in Table 1-5. When interpreting the severity of weight loss, it is important to consider the patient's current body weight and percent weight change.

Table 1-5   Interpretation of percent weight change.

TIME	SIGNIFICANT WEIGHT LOSS	SEVERE WEIGHT LOSS
1 week	1–2%	> 2%
1 month	5%	> 5%
3 months	7.5%	> 7.5%
6 months	10%	> 10%
1 year	20%	> 20%

Table 1-6   **Routine clinical measurements for obtaining anthropometric data on physical examination in pediatric patients**

MEASUREMENTS	UNITS/DEFINITIONS
Length	(cm) supine, children birth to 36 months
Height	(cm) standing, beginning at ages 2 to 3 years
Height for Age	Percentile on the growth chart
Current Weight	(kg) (1 kg = 2.2 lbs)
Head Circumference	(cm) plotted for children younger than 3 years
Weight for Age	Percentile on the growth chart

Interpreting Anthropometric Data for Infants, Children, and Adolescents

Growth charts are routinely used in clinical medicine to follow growth and development over time (see Figures 1-1, 1-2, 1-3, and 1-4). Their application to clinical findings is the topic of this section (see Table 1-6).

Ideal Weight for Height

To determine a patient's ideal weight for height, plot the patient's actual height/length on the appropriate growth chart for his or her age. Next, find the point where that height intersects the fiftieth percentile on the height/length chart by moving horizontally right or left. Draw a line down from this intersection on the height chart to the X-axis to find the age that corresponds to this fiftieth percentile height. Finally, find and record the fiftieth percentile weight for that age on the weight chart. This is the ideal weight for the patient's current height.

Example 1: The patient is a 12-year-old boy (see Figure 1-3)

His current height is 162 cm (90–95th percentile)

Weight = 75 kg (> 95th percentile)

Ideal weight for current height = 47 kg

Percent Ideal Weight for Height

Percent ideal weight for height is a number used to determine the degree of wasting or obesity in children and adolescents. Wasting is a term that describes the depletion of the body's fat and muscle stores. Endogenous fat and protein are the fuels the body uses for energy when an energy deficit exists due to inadequate food intake. Percent ideal weight for height describes the extent of any related changes in body composition resulting from intake deficits. This value is calculated by dividing the current weight by the ideal weight for height.

$$\text{Percent weight for height} = \frac{\text{Current weight}}{\text{Ideal weight for current height}} \times 100$$

Example 2: In the case of the 12-year-old boy from Example 1,

Weight = 75 kg

Ideal weight for current height = 47 kg

$$\frac{75 \text{ kg}}{47 \text{ kg}} \times 100 = 160\%$$

This patient's actual weight is 160% of his ideal weight based on his height, which leads to a diagnosis of obesity.

Ideal Height for Age

To determine the patient's ideal height for age, note the fiftieth percentile height measurement for the child's actual age on the growth chart.

Example 3: For the 12-year-old boy in the preceding examples,

Ideal height for age = 150 cm

Percent Ideal Height for Age

Percent ideal height for age evaluates linear growth patterns. This value is particularly useful in patients who exhibit stunting, a slowed rate of growth. Stunting occurs when a dietary deficit exists for a prolonged period of time, that is, in the presence of chronic malnutrition. To determine percent height for age, divide the current height by the ideal height for the patient's age.

$$\text{Percent height for age} = \frac{\text{Current height}}{\text{Ideal height for age}} \times 100$$

Example 4: In the case of the 12-year-old boy

Height = 162 cm (90–95th percentile)

Ideal height for age = 150 cm

$$\frac{162 \text{ cm}}{150 \text{ cm}} \times 100 = 108\% \text{ ideal height for age}$$

This slight departure from the expected value may be considered a normal variation in height.

Interpretations of the values for percent ideal weight for height and percent ideal height for age are listed in Table 1-7.

Table 1-7   **Interpretation of percent ideal weight for height and percent ideal height for age.**

% WEIGHT FOR HEIGHT	INTERPRETATION	% HEIGHT FOR AGE	INTERPRETATION
> 120	Obese		
110–120	Overweight		
90–109	Normal weight	95–105	Normal height
80–89	Mild wasting	90–94	Mild stunting
70–79	Moderate wasting	85–89	Moderate stunting
< 70	Severe wasting	< 85	Severe stunting

Laboratory Assessment

No single blood test or group of tests accurately measures nutritional status. Therefore clinical judgment is critical in deciding what tests to order based on the individual's history and physical findings. The following blood tests are useful for nutrition assessment and should be used when indicated by the physical exam and medical history results.

Electrolytes and Minerals Determining sodium, potassium, chloride, calcium, phosphorus, and magnesium status is an important part of nutrition assessment. The levels of these electrolytes and minerals are influenced by both dietary intake and clinical conditions.

Protein Status Visceral protein stores may be evaluated from blood tests such as blood urea nitrogen (BUN) and creatinine levels. Note, however, that these tests also are highly influenced by renal function. Clinically, visceral protein stores may be depleted by increased protein losses in the stool and urine, or as a result of wounds involving severe blood loss, as well as by poor dietary protein intake.

In addition, the following serum protein tests may prove useful in conjunction with other nutrition assessment parameters. Once again, however, each of these tests has limitations because serum protein levels are affected not only by nutritional and hydration status, but by disease states, surgery, and impaired functioning of the liver, where serum proteins are synthesized.

The half-life ($t^{1/2}$) of each protein test is given because knowing its duration allows the clinician to utilize these tests to diagnose short-term and chronic protein-calorie malnutrition. Remember, these measures of protein status are influenced by both calorie and protein intake, and no perfect laboratory test exists to distinguish the protein status from the calorie status.

Serum Albumin The serum albumin test has the longest half-life ($t^{1/2}$ = 18 to 21 days) and reflects nutritional status over the previous three weeks. Levels decrease with acute stress, overhydration, trauma, and surgery. However, false increases often occur with dehydration. This test is not a good indicator of recent dietary status or acute changes (less than three weeks) in nutritional status. Significantly reduced levels of serum albumin are associated with increased morbidity and mortality.

Serum Transferrin Serum transferrin has a half-life of $t^{1/2}$ = 8 to 9 days. Changes in serum transferrin levels are influenced by iron status, as well as by protein and calorie intake. Results of this test reflect intake over the preceding several weeks.

Serum Prealbumin With a half-life of $t^{1/2}$ = 2 to 3 days, serum prealbumin reflects nutritional status as well as protein and calorie intake over the previous week.

Serum Retinol Binding Protein Levels of this protein, which has a half-life of $t^{1/2}$ = 12 hours, reflect very recent changes in protein and calorie intake. Results of this test are also influenced by vitamin A status.

Other laboratory tests that are valuable in selected clinical conditions related to nutrition include iron and zinc status, cholesterol, tryglyceride, and vitamin levels, and measures of liver and renal function.

Problem List/Assessment

The physician develops a clinical assessment for the individual patient from the medical history, physical exam, and laboratory data. Active problems are listed in order of their importance. Inactive problems are also recorded here.

Evidence of a nutrition disorder should be considered primary if it occurs in an individual with no other etiology that explains signs and symptoms of malnutrition. A primary nutrition problem is usually the result of imbalances, inadequacies, or excesses in the patient's nutrient intake. Manifestations may include obesity, underweight, protein-energy malnutrition, or poor intake of iron, folate, or vitamin B_{12}.

Secondary nutrition problems occur when a primary pathological process results in inadequate food intake, impaired absorption and utilization of nutrients, increased losses or excretion of nutrients, or increased nutrient requirements. Common causes of secondary nutrition disorders include anorexia nervosa, malabsorption, diabetes, trauma, and surgery. Often malnutrition occurs as a result of critical illness or a chronic condition complicating the underlying illness.

Treatment Plan

After assessing each problem, the physician outlines a management plan that includes both a diagnostic component and a treatment plan. Patient education is an essential part of this management plan.

Examples of diagnostic plans related to nutrition

Recommend fasting test for total serum cholesterol, LDL, HDL, and triglycerides for a patient with a family history of heart disease.

Recommend hemoglobin A_1C tests to assess adherence to a diabetic diet.

Recommend albumin and prealbumin test for suspected protein malnutrition.

Recommend iron, ferritin, total iron binding capacity (TIBC) for a patient with microcytic anemia.

Recommend serum vitamin B_{12} and red blood cell folate tests for a patient with macrocytic anemia.

Recommend measuring triceps skinfold for a patient with malnutrition.

Examples of treatment plans and patient education related to nutrition

Recommend consultation with a registered dietitian for counseling on specific diets.

Recommend low-sodium diet for ascites, congestive heart failure, hypertension, or renal failure.

Recommend low-fat, low-saturated fat, low-cholesterol diet for a patient with heart disease.

Recommend maintaining a reasonable weight for a patient with diabetes.

Recommend high-calorie, high-protein diet for a malnourished patient.

Recommend vitamin D and calcium supplementation to treat rickets in children.

Protein-Energy Malnutrition (PEM)

Protein-energy malnutrition (PEM) results when the body's requirements for calories, protein, or both are not met by dietary intake. PEM is characterized by wasting and excessive loss of lean body tissue. Decreased protein intake usually is associated with decreased calorie intake, but it can occur independently. Regardless, if the protein deficiency is severe enough, one of two clinically different scenarios occurs: marasmus or kwashiorkor. The term marasmus is used to describe a deficiency of both protein and energy, whereas kwashiorkor describes a deficiency related predominantly to protein.

Causes of Protein-Energy Malnutrition

Decreased Oral Intake

Poor dentition, gastrointestinal obstruction or abdominal pain, anorexia, dysphasia, depression, social isolation, poverty, and pain from eating or swallowing are all possible causes of decreased oral intake.

Increased Nutrient Loss

Glucosuria, bleeding in the digestive tract, diarrhea, malabsorption, nephrosis, a draining fistula, and protein-losing enteropathy can all result in severe nutrient loss.

Increased Nutrient Requirements

Any hypermetabolic state or excessive catabolic process can result in increased nutrient requirements. Common examples of situations that can dramatically affect nutrient requirements include surgery, trauma, fever, infection, burns, and HIV/AIDS.

Clinical Manifestations of PEM

- Weight loss, anorexia, diarrhea, lassitude, glossitis, alopecia, dry and depigmented hair, desquamation of skin
- Progressive weakness, decreased muscle strength
- Stored fat utilization, protein depletion, loss of lean body mass
- Decline in functional status (increased difficulties associated with activities of daily life)
- Depressed immune function, increased susceptibility to infection
- Skin breakdown: pressure ulcers
- Decreased cardiopulmonary function
- Increased risk of morbidity and mortality

Laboratory Manifestations of PEM

- Fluid and electrolyte imbalances (sodium, magnesium, calcium, potassium, and phosphorus) depending on hydration status
- Iron-deficiency anemia (microcytic anemia on blood smear and CBC, decreased serum iron and ferritin, increased total iron binding capacity, and transferrin saturation)
- Macrocytic anemia (increased mean corpuscular hemoglobin-MCV, decreased red blood cell folate and serum vitamin B_{12} levels)
- Decreased serum albumin
- Decreased cholesterol and triglycerides
- Decreased urinary excretion of urea nitrogen and creatinine
- Decreased insulin and increased cortisol
- Low vitamin and mineral levels

Predicting Energy Requirements

Humans require energy to support normal metabolic functions, physical activity, and growth and repair of tissues. Energy is expressed in kilocalories (kcal) and is produced by the oxidation of dietary protein, fat, carbohydrate, and alcohol.

- One gram of protein yields approximately four kcal.
- One gram of carbohydrate yields approximately four kcal.
- One gram of fat yields approximately nine kcal.
- One gram of alcohol yields approximately seven kcal.

A calorie is the amount of heat required to raise the temperature of one gram of water by 1° Celsius. A kilocalorie is thus the amount of heat required to raise the temperature of one kilogram of water by 1° Celsius.

The amount of energy required to maintain vital organ function in a resting, fasting state is called the resting energy expenditure (REE). The basal metabolic rate (BMR) is the REE measured soon after an individual awakens in the morning, at least twelve hours after the most recent meal. Because the REE and the BMR differ in practice by less than ten percent, these two terms may be used interchangeably in clinical care. Equations developed to predict these values are the topic of this section.

Harris-Benedict Equations

The Harris-Benedict equations estimate the basal (resting) energy expenditure in adults.

REE equation for males

66 + [13.7· weight (kg)] + [5.0 · height (cm)]−[6.8 · age] = kcal/day

REE equation for females

655 + [9.6· weight (kg)] + [1.8 · height (cm)]−[4.7· age] = kcal/day

The Harris-Benedict equation should be modified for patients who are over 125 percent of their ideal body weight (IBW).

Adjusted Body Weight for Obese Patients

The Harris-Benedict equation is not accurate when assessing obese patients' energy requirements because only 25 percent of adipose tissue represents lean body mass, the tissue which is metabolically active. Using the Harris-Benedict equation would therefore overestimate the REE of an obese person. A more accurate determination can be made for the obese patient by using an adjusted body weight rather than current body weight when computing REE.

Adjusted body weight =

[(Current body weight − Ideal body weight) x 25%] + Ideal body weight

This adjustment assumes that 25 percent of fat tissue is metabolically active.

Example 5: Determine the adjusted body weight for a 188-pound female who is 5′1″ tall.

Step 1: Estimate the patient's ideal weight using the rule-of-thumb method.
5′1″ = 105 lbs

Step 2: 188 lbs − 105 lbs = 83 lbs x .25 = 20.8 lbs

Step 3: 20.8 lbs + 105 lbs = 125.8 lbs (57.2 kg)

This is the value that should be used to calculate the patient's REE.

Activity factors are added to the REE as necessary to calculate total daily caloric needs, which vary for hospitalized and non-hospitalized patients.

> ## Total daily caloric needs = REE x physical activity factor
>
> Physical activity factors
>   Hospitalized patients = 1.3
>   Nonhospitalized, active patients = 1.5

Estimation of Maintenance Calories

Caloric requirements for adults also can be estimated using the patient's activity level (see Table 1-8). In this approach, factors assigned to various activity levels are multiplied by the patient's ideal body weight (IBW) to estimate maintenance calorie requirements. Since the equation accounts for the activity level, no additional activity factors are added.

A summary of clinical signs and symptoms of nutritional inadequacy is given in Table 1-9.

Table 1-8   **Estimation of maintenance calorie requirements for adults.**

ACTIVITY	kcal/lb	kcal/kg
Bedrest[a]	11.5	25
Light[b]	13.5	30
Moderate[c]	16.0	35
Vigorous[d]	18.0	40

Examples

140 lb female with moderate activity requires: (140 lbs) (16 kcal/lb) = 2240 kcal/day

170 lb male with light activity requires: (170 lbs) (13.5 kcal/lb) = 2295 kcal/day

[a] Hospital patient, sedentary, weight maintenance.
[b] Daily routine activities.
[c] Regular exercise program in addition to daily activities.
[d] Heavy construction worker or athlete, multiple trauma, severe burns.

Table 1-9   Clinical signs and symptoms of nutritional inadequacy.

	CLINICAL SIGN OR SYMPTOM	NUTRIENT
General	Wasted, skinny	Calorie
	Loss of appetite	Protein-energy
Skin	Psoriasiform rash, eczematous scaling	Zinc
	Pallor	Folic acid, iron, vitamin B_{12}
	Follicular hyperkeratosis	Vitamin A
	Perifollicular petechiae	Vitamin C
	Flaking dermatitis	Protein-energy, niacin, riboflavin, zinc
	Bruising	Vitamin C, vitamin K
	Pigmentation changes	Niacin, protein-energy
	Scrotal dermatosis	Riboflavin
	Thickening and dryness of skin	Linoleic acid
Head	Temporal muscle wasting	Protein-energy
Hair	Sparse and thin, dyspigmentation, easy to pull out	Protein
Eyes	History of night blindness (also impaired visual recovery after glare)	Vitamin A
	Photophobia, blurring, conjunctival inflammation	Riboflavin, vitamin A
	Corneal vascularization	Riboflavin
	Xerosis, Bitot spots, keratomalacia	Vitamin A
Mouth	Glossitis	Riboflavin, niacin, folic acid, vitamin B_{12}, pyridoxine
	Bleeding gums	Vitamin C, riboflavin
	Cheilosis	Riboflavin
	Angular stomatitis	Riboflavin, iron
	Hypogeusia	Zinc
	Tongue fissuring	Niacin
	Tongue atrophy	Riboflavin, niacin, iron
	Scarlet and raw tongue	Niacin
	Nasolabial seborrhea	Pyridoxine
Neck	Goiter	Iodine
	Parotid enlargement	Protein
Thorax	Thoracic rosary	Vitamin D
Abdomen	Diarrhea	Niacin, folate, vitamin B_{12}
	Distention	Protein-energy
	Hepatomegaly	Protein-energy

Table 1-9 (continued)

	CLINICAL SIGN OR SYMPTOM	NUTRIENT
Extremities	Edema	Protein, thiamin
	Softening of bone	Vitamin D, calcium, phosphorus
	Bone tenderness	Vitamin D
	Bone ache, joint pain	Vitamin C
	Muscle wasting and weakness	Protein, calorie, vitamin D, selenium, sodium choride
	Hyporeflexia	Thiamin
	Ataxia	Vitamin B12
Nails	Spooning	Iron
	Transverse lines	Protein
Neurologic	Tetany	Calcium, magnesium
	Paresthesia	Thiamin, Vitamin B12
	Loss of reflexes, wrist drop, foot drop	Thiamin
	Dementia, disorientation	Niacin
Blood	Anemia	Vitamins E, B12, folic acid, iron, pyridoxine
	Hemolysis	Phosphorus

Source: Reprinted with permission from Wyngaarden JB, Smith LH, Bennett JC (eds.), *Cecil Textbook of Medicine*. 19th Edition. Philadelphia: WB Saunders, 1992.

Obesity

Kelly Davis and Randi Cardonick

Objectives

- To identify five methods used clinically to diagnose obesity in adults.
- To identify five chronic diseases associated with obesity.
- To understand the usefulness of determining body composition in clinical medicine.
- To assess the caloric and protein needs of an obese patient with a history of chronic dieting.
- To understand how and why some nutrient requirements change following an acute injury in an obese patient.

RS, a 37-year-old woman, consults her physician for advice about losing weight. She has a history of dieting, and this is the twelfth time she has begun a weight loss program in the past fifteen years. She states that her weight problems began when she had her children, because she never returned to her pre-pregnancy weight after the birth of any of her four children. RS has been thinking of starting the Quick Weight Loss Diet but wants her physician's input on the best diet for her. She gives the following information on the Quick Weight Loss diet.

1000 kcal/day
7 percent of the calories from carbohydrates (17 g/day)
45 percent of the calories from protein (112 g/day)
48 percent of the calories from fat (53 g/day)

Past Medical History

RS exhibits mild hyperglycemia (modest elevation in blood sugar without frank diabetes). Work-ups for other endocrine abnormalities have been negative in three previous evaluations. RS has been hospitalized four times for childbirth. She has no history of gallbladder disease, is not taking any medications or vitamins, and has no known allergies.

Family History

The family history is negative for diabetes, heart disease, and hypertension; positive for maternal obesity; and otherwise unremarkable.

Social History

The social history is negative for alcohol intake and tobacco use. RS drinks two cups of coffee daily. She has a history of dieting, eats three meals per day, and does not exercise. Although a number of the commercial weight loss diets she has followed resulted in weight loss, RS regained the lost weight after completing the diets.

Review of Systems

Skin: No history of rashes or unusual skin pigmentation; no stretch marks

Neurological: No headaches, tremors, seizures, or depression

Endocrine: Normal menstrual cycle; no abnormal heat or cold intolerances

Cardiovascular: No hypertension, heart disease, orthopnea, or dyspnea

Physical Examination

Vital signs

Temperature: 98.4° F

Heart rate: 88 BPM

Blood pressure: 130/80 mmHg

Anthropometric Data

Height: 5'1" (155 cm)

Current weight: 188 lbs (85.5 kg)

Triceps skinfold (TSF): 4 cm (40 mm)

Mid-arm muscle circumference (MAMC): 28 cm (280 mm)

General: Obese woman in no acute distress. No cushingoid features.

Exam: Nonpalpable thyroid; no hirsutism or striae; no dorsal, cervical, or supraclavicular fat; no acanthosis nigricans

Laboratory Data

All levels fall within normal limits, including a thyroid function test and serum glucose level.

Probable Diagnosis

The patient has essential (primary) obesity. No evidence exists to indicate medical causes of obesity or the presence of diseases that cause obesity. No further medical work-up is needed at this time.

Acute Injury in the Obese Patient

One month after visiting her physician, RS was involved in a car accident resulting in multiple fractures. She has been hospitalized for two weeks in the intensive care unit and is on a ventilator. While assessing RS and her hospital course, her physician notes that she has not eaten for ten days. Her serum albumin level is 2.7 g/dL (normal range: 3.5–5.0 g/dL).

Case Questions

1. Describe five methods that could be used to diagnose obesity in this patient.

2. What are the medical risks associated with obesity?

3. How does the Quick Weight Loss Diet compare with the recommended dietary guidelines for adults?

4. Describe the physiological consequences of the Quick Weight Loss Diet.

5. Using the Harris-Benedict equation, estimate RS's calorie needs for weight maintenance and weight loss. Is this method accurate in estimating an obese patient's calorie requirements?

6. How can food records help determine RS's dietary intake? What factors should be taken into consideration when patients are asked to complete a food diary?

7. What do the Weight Watchers, Jenny Craig, and Nutri/System diets have in common, and how do they differ?

8. The National Academy of Sciences recently established criteria for evaluating weight management programs. What are this committee's recommendations?

9. Assuming that RS decides not to join the Quick Weight Loss Diet or any other commercial weight-loss program, what advice can you offer her?

10. How could a consultation with a registered dietitian help RS lose weight?

11. RS returns with a question regarding obesity genes after having read an article in *The New York Times*. What is the *ob* gene and what are the implications for therapy of obese individuals?

12. On a subsequent follow-up visit, RS reports that her friend has consulted an obesity specialist and is taking diet pills to help with her weight loss. How do these medications work? Are they effective?

13. What physiological and metabolic changes have occurred in the past two weeks due to an acute injury that RS sustained?

14. What nutritional problems should be of concern because of RS's acute injury and her low serum albumin?

Answers begin on the following page.

Answers to Questions: Case 1

Part 1: Diagnosis

1. Describe five methods that could be used to diagnose obesity in this patient.

   ### 1. Percent Ideal Body Weight (% IBW)

   Obesity is defined as a body weight greater than 120 percent of ideal weight. To calculate the percentage of ideal body weight relative to their current body weight, first determine the patient's ideal body weight (IBW).

   Step 1: Calculate RS's ideal body weight using the rule-of-thumb estimation.

   Male = 106 lbs for 5 feet in height plus 6 lbs for each additional inch

   Female = 100 lbs for 5 feet in height plus 5 lbs for each additional inch

   RS's IBW = 100 lbs + 5 lbs (1 inch) = 105 lbs

   Step 2: Calculate the percent ideal body weight.

   $$\% \text{ IBW} = \frac{\text{Current weight}}{\text{Ideal weight}} \times 100$$

   For RS, the result is

   $$\% \text{ IBW} = \frac{188}{105} \times 100 = 179\%$$

   Because RS's percent ideal body weight is greater than 120%, she is clinically obese.

   ### 2. Triceps Skinfold (TSF) Measurement

   TSF is performed with a caliper that measures the thickness of the skin and fat at the middle of the upper arm over the triceps muscle. It estimates the amount of excess energy (calories) stored as subcutaneous fat. The result of this measurement is compared to reference tables for the population of the United States. Obesity is suspected when TSF is greater than the ninety-fifth percentile in the table. Note: Although a weight greater than 120 percent of ideal weight is usually indicative of obesity, the seemingly excessive weight may reflect extra muscle mass rather than body fat. The TSF measurement allows a distinction to be made between extra fat and muscle.

   RS's TSF, 4 cm (40 mm), is greater than the ninety-fifth percentile. For a female at age 37, the fiftieth percentile = 23 mm, and a measurement greater than 38 mm indicates obesity. Coupled with her percent ideal body weight, the TSF measurement supports a diagnosis of obesity.

   ### 3. Mid-Arm Muscle Circumference (MAMC) Estimation

   The mid-arm circumference (MAC) is measured at the same site as the TSF. Next, the MAMC is calculated from the MAC and the TSF. This value is useful for differentiating body fat and muscle. Obesity can be suspected if the MAMC exceeds the ninetieth percentile in the reference table.

Calculated MAMC = MAC − 3.14(TSF)

For a female at age 37, the fiftieth percentile = 218 mm. A value greater than 260 mm (ninetieth percentile) indicates obesity.

RS's MAMC was calculated at 280 mm, again greater than the ninety-fifth percentile in the reference tables. The fact that both the TSF and the MAMC were greater than the ninety-fifth percentile reflects increased fat stores.

4. Body Mass Index (BMI) Calculation

The body mass index (BMI) is a useful clinical calculation for diagnosing obesity because it correlates with total body fat and is relatively unaffected by height. The normal range for BMI is between 19.8 and 26.0. Individuals with a BMI between 26.1 and 29.0 are overweight, those who have a BMI greater than 30 are obese by definition.

$$BMI = \frac{Weight\ (kg)}{Height\ (m^2)}$$

In RS's case

$$BMI = \frac{Weight\ (kg)}{Height\ (m^2)} = \frac{85.5}{(1.55)^2} = 35.6\ kg/m^2$$

This result indicates significant obesity. (See also Figure 1.5.)

5. Healthy Weight Tables

According to the weight tables recently developed by the United States Department of Agriculture and the Department of Health and Human Services, RS's weight is not within the desired range. For a 37-year-old individual who is five feet, one inch tall, the desirable weight range is between 111 and 143 lbs. RS's weight is 188 lbs (see Table 1-1).

Part 2:   Medical Implications

2. **What are the medical risks associated with obesity?**

Obesity, a form of malnutrition (overnutrition), increases a person's risk of developing cardiovascular disease, hyperlipidemia, hypertension, osteoarthritis, gallstones, respiratory disease, cholecystitis, and certain types of cancer. Obesity also increases a patient's risk during surgical procedures because increased subcutaneous fat can prolong the surgical procedure and make it technically more difficult.

Ironically, despite America's preoccupation with diet over the past decade, the prevalence of obesity is increasing. In the population of the United States, 35 percent of women, 31 percent of men, and more than 25 percent of children and adolescents are considered obese. The benefits of weight loss are significant; recent clinical research has demonstrated that obese individuals who achieve and maintain a 10 percent reduction in weight for three years or more are likely to lower their blood pressure, serum glucose, and cholesterol and triglyceride levels, thereby reducing their risk of developing diabetes and heart disease, respectively. The incidence of other health problems associated with obesity, such as sleep apnea and osteoarthritis, also decreases with moderate weight loss.

3. **How does the Quick Weight Loss Diet compare with the recommended dietary guidelines for adults?**

Typically, the Quick Weight Loss Diet has a very high protein content, deriving 45 percent of the daily 1000 calories from protein sources (meat, chicken, or fish). In contrast, the United States Dietary Guidelines recommend that no more than 20 percent of the total calories come from protein. Clearly, the Quick Weight Loss Diet far exceeds these goals.

Furthermore, the protein that makes up 45 percent of the 1000 calories in the Quick Weight Loss Diet is equivalent to 450 calories. Because one gram of protein yields four calories, this means dieters in this program are eating a total of 112 grams of protein per day. The RDA for protein for an adult female is 0.8 g/kg adjusted body weight. RS's protein requirements are therefore 46 grams per day (0.8 x 57.2 kg) according to the guidelines—about half of the amount of protein provided by the Quick Weight Loss Diet.

Most foods with high protein content, such as meats and cheeses, are also high in fat. Consequently, a high-protein diet usually is also high in total fat and saturated fat. The diet described derives 48 percent of its total calories from fat, significantly exceeding the guidelines' recommendation of 30 percent. In addition, the Quick Weight Loss Diet derives only seven percent of its daily 1000 kcal from carbohydrates, compared to the United States Dietary Guidelines, which urge that carbohydrate intake be greater than 50 percent of total calories.

4. **Describe the physiological consequences of a Quick Weight Loss Diet.**

Low-calorie diets, particularly those that are high in protein and low in carbohydrates, are ketogenic. The liver produces ketones (acetoacetic acid and beta hydroxybutyric acid), which eventually are excreted in the urine as sodium or potassium salts, resulting in a net loss of sodium and potassium. High-protein diets also produce hyperuricemia (increased uric acid in the blood) and hyperuricosuria (increased excretion of uric acid), which increase the patient's risk of developing gout and uric-acid kidney stones. Stimulation of gluconeogenesis in the liver, from excess amino acids, leads to increased blood urea nitrogen.

Low-calorie diets that restrict carbohydrate intake also lead to rapid mobilization of protein and glycogen stores. Resulting decreases in plasma insulin levels can lead to reduced phosphorylation of regulatory enzymes used for anabolism. Because each gram of protein and glycogen is stored with three grams of water, rapid weight loss—equivalent to three to five percent of the body's weight—occurs for the first few days until labile protein and glycogen stores are depleted. Fat stores are lost much more slowly, however. A safe, healthy rate of weight loss that also reduces fat stores is one to two pounds per week.

Part 3:   Nutrition Assessment

5.   **Using the Harris-Benedict equation, estimate RS's calorie needs for weight maintenance and weight loss. Is this method accurate in estimating an obese patient's calorie requirements?**

The Harris-Benedict equation takes into account age, gender, weight, and height to calculate the amount of energy an individual needs at rest, referred to as basal or resting energy expenditure (BEE or REE). REE needs to be adjusted when assessing obese patients because adipose tissue is not as metabolically active as lean body mass, the REE would be overestimated if this factor were not taken into account. The equation for this adjustment is

[(Current body weight – Ideal body weight) x 25%] + Ideal body weight

Example: Determine RS's adjusted body weight.

Step 1: [(188 lbs – 105 lbs) x 0.25] = 20.8 lbs + IBW

Step 2: 20.8 lbs + 105 lbs = 125.8 lbs (57.2 kg)

This is the adjusted body weight.

Step 3: Calculate RS's REE using the Harris-Benedict equation for females.

655 + 9.6(57.2) + 1.8(155) – 4.7(37) = 1309 kcal/day

Step 4: Calculate RS's actual caloric requirements considering her activity level. Multiply the REE by a factor of 1.3 for a sedentary lifestyle and low physical activity.

1309 kcal x 1.3 = 1702 kcal/day

This value represents RS's calorie needs for weight maintenance.

Step 5: To estimate RS's caloric needs for weight reduction, subtract 500 calories from her daily needs (1702 – 500 = 1202 kcal/day). Reducing RS's daily caloric intake by 500 calories for seven days results in a total weekly deficit of 3500 calories. Maintaining her intake at this level should promote a weight loss of one pound per week, because there are 3500 calories in one pound of fat.

6.   **How can food records help determine RS's dietary intake? What factors should be taken into consideration when patients are asked to complete a food diary?**

A three-day food record should include two weekdays and one weekend day. Food records provide a good idea of usual intake, but may not

RS's Usual Daily Intake		
Breakfast (Home)	Apple juice	2 cups
	Brewed coffee	1 cup
	Powdered creamer	2 Tbs.
Lunch (Salad Bar)	Lettuce	2 cups
	Tomatoes (fresh, chopped)	4 oz.
	Carrot (raw, grated)	3 Tbs.
	Feta cheese	2 pieces
	Cottage cheese	3 Tbs.
	Potato salad	2 Tbs.
	Tuna salad	3 Tbs.
	Sunflower seeds	3 Tbs.
	Ranch dressing	6 Tbs.
Dinner: (Restaurant)	Split pea soup	1 cup
	Pasta/spaghetti	2 cups
	Meat sauce	1/4 cup
	Tea (unsweetened)	1 cup
	Italian bread	3 pieces
	Butter	1 Tbs.

Total calories: 2435 kcal/day
Protein: 14% of calories
Carbohydrate: 39% of calories
Fat: 47% of calories

represent the actual quantities ingested because individuals usually do not record their intake accurately, especially if they are asked to do so for more than three days.

When asking patients to complete a food diary, it is helpful to suggest that they record their intake immediately after eating so that they do not forget what they ate and drank. The longer patients wait to record their intake, the less they will remember. RS brought the following one-day food record with her when she returned for a follow-up visit.

RS's recorded dietary intake contained 2435 calories, 47 percent of which came from fat. Thus she exceeded her actual daily calorie requirements on that day by 725 calories. If she continues to exceed her requirements, she will gain weight. In addition, the percentage of RS's caloric intake that came from fat increases her risk of cardiovascular disease. The American Heart Association and many other national health organizations recommend a reduction in dietary calories from fat to less than 30 percent of the total daily caloric intake.

Part 4:   Nutrition Recommendations

RS also asks about the Weight Watchers, Jenny Craig, and Nutri/System diets. She wants to know if she should try one of these programs.

7. **What do the Weight Watchers, Jenny Craig, and Nutri/System diets have in common, and how do they differ?**

WEIGHT WATCHERS	JENNY CRAIG/NUTRI/SYSTEM
Balanced diet	Balanced diet
Eat your own food	Buy the company's foods and snacks
Foods available in supermarket	Food bought at centers
Peer support (meetings)	Peer support (meetings)
Weekly weight taken	Weekly weight taken
Relatively inexpensive	Expensive
Exercise component emphasized in all three programs.	

The main difference between these programs is that Jenny Craig and Nutri/System require clients to purchase all their foods at their centers, whereas Weight Watchers emphasizes selecting foods from grocery stores. The Jenny Craig and Nutri/System programs may help patients lose weight in the short term because they control portion sizes and limit decision making. However, the chance of regaining weight with all weight-loss programs is very high. Programs that encourage patients to make food choices and behavioral changes during the program rather than eat prepackaged foods may be a better choice in the long run.

Patients' lifestyle and financial situation should be considered when deciding on any diet program. Programs like Jenny Craig and Nutri/System, including the food, can cost about $100 per week. An additional consideration is where the patient eats. If a patient eats out all the time, complying with the diet may be very difficult.

Weight Watchers, on the other hand, provides participants with a written program based on selecting foods from the various food groups: breads, meats, fruits, dairy products, fats, and vegetables. Members learn about appropriate serving sizes within each food group and the number of servings they can have from each group in a given day without exceeding their recommended calorie requirement.

All three programs include nutrition education and exercise recommendations. Generally, their calorie allowances for women are 1200 kcal/day, and for men, 1800 kcal/day per day. In all of these regimens, more than 55 percent of the calorie intake comes from carbohydrates, about 15 percent comes from protein, and less than 30 percent comes from fat.

8. **The National Academy of Sciences recently established criteria for evaluating weight management programs. What are this committee's recommendations?**

Recently, the Food and Nutrition Board of the National Academy of

Sciences established a committee to develop criteria for evaluating the outcomes of approaches to preventing and treating obesity. Obesity experts from around the country evaluated the current literature and developed recommendations for health care professionals who treat obese individuals.

The most important emphasis from the report is that the definition of success that is applied in evaluating weight-loss programs be broadened and made more realistic based on the research findings that small weight losses can reduce the risk of developing chronic diseases. Speci-fically, the goal of obesity treatment should be refocused from weight loss alone, which is aimed at appearance, to weight management, achieving the best weight possible in the context of overall health.

The committee also recommended that weight-loss programs evolve into weight-management programs and be judged more by their emphasis on the overall health of participants than by their effect on weight alone.

9. **Assuming that RS decides not to join the Quick Weight Loss Diet or any other commercial weight-loss programs, what advice can you offer her?**

The first step in counseling RS regarding weight reduction is to establish a reasonable target weight that she feels she can achieve and maintain. This approach often leads to the discovery that some patients aspire to an unrealistic target weight, whereas others may not even see themselves as overweight.

RS's current weight is 188 pounds, and she is five feet, one inch tall. Using the rule-of-thumb estimation, her ideal weight is 105 pounds. Therefore she is 179 percent of her ideal weight. Using the newly revised Healthy Weight Tables, her weight also exceeds the normal range (122 lbs to 157 lbs) for a person over age 35.

The next logical step is to establish a reasonable time frame during which she can expect to lose the weight. She should be encouraged to lose one to two pounds per week to ensure a safe and steady weight loss. If RS loses weight quickly, she will probably be losing lean body tissue or fluid, and may become dehydrated if she does not consume adequate amounts of fluids.

A 24-hour dietary recall will be helpful to assess the general types of foods RS consumes. Determining how frequently she eats out is also important. Once you have this information, you can make appropriate recommendations, such as using low-calorie dressing, reducing consumption of cheese, skipping the butter, and eating more fruits and vegetables. Support from her friends, family, and spouse would be most helpful, as would a referral to a registered dietitian for assistance in developing an individualized meal plan.

Because exercise helps maintain muscle mass and thus the basal metabolic rate, RS should be encouraged to increase her physical activity. Advising her to begin walking or biking a few times per week is a reasonable exercise program and an attainable goal.

10. How could a consultation with a registered dietitian help RS lose weight?

Registered dietitians have more nutrition training than most physicians or nurses and can spend considerably more time with patients discussing their dietary habits. A registered dietitian could review RS's food diaries, assess her diet for nutritional adequacy, support the exercise and dietary prescription, and offer ideas for tasty, low-calorie foods that RS can prepare and serve to her family.

11. RS returns with a question regarding obesity genes after having read an article in *The New York Times*. What is the *ob* gene and what are the implications for therapy of obese individuals?

The autosomal recessive mutation, *ob/ob*, has been studied since the 1950s as a model for genetic obesity in mice. In 1994, the *ob* gene was identified, and its predicted product (leptin) is secreted by fat cells. Leptin is believed to interact with a receptor in the hypothalamus and to signal satiety. Potential therapies could include replacement of leptin in deficient patients or development of pharmacologic agents that interact with leptin receptors in the brain. Both would be expected to have an appetite-suppressing effect.

12. On a subsequent follow-up visit, RS reports that her friend has consulted an obesity specialist and is taking diet pills to help with her weight loss. How do these medications work? Are they effective?

Appetite suppressants fall into two broad pharmacologic categories—those that act on catecholamine neurotransmitters within the brain and those that increase CNS serotonin levels. Amphetamines, the first "diet drugs," were released more than 50 years ago but are no longer used for this purpose because their central stimulant and euphoriant properties and addictive potential made them popular drugs of abuse. In the past several years, however, there has been a resurgence of interest in appetite suppressants, primarily because of a large study which used a combination of amphetamine-like (but nonaddictive) phentermine and a newer drug, fenfluramine, that acts via serotonin pathways in the brain. This combination (known as Phen/Fen) is safe, well-tolerated, and when used with dietary restriction and exercise, subjects lost an average of 31 pounds (14 kg) in 34 weeks. Anorectic drugs should be reserved for patients who are clinically at risk from being overweight (>130 percent of IBW) and then only as a part of a comprehensive program including nutritional counseling, exercise, and behavior modification. These measures are essential if patients are to maintain the weight loss once the drugs are discontinued.

Part 5: Acute Injury in the Obese Patient

13. What physiological and metabolic changes have occurred in the past two weeks due to an acute injury that RS sustained?

Because RS is now in a hypermetabolic state, she has increased calorie requirements. To measure the degree of hypermetabolism, which helps establish calorie goals, the patient's resting energy expenditure can be assessed with indirect calorimetry. Indirect calorimetry measures resting energy expenditure based on oxygen consumed and carbon dioxide produced. She is also hypercatabolic, which means that her body exhibits increased breakdown of its stores of fat and protein. Therefore she also has increased protein needs. Both conditions are a result of her serious injuries.

14. **What nutritional problems should be of concern because of RS's acute injury and her low serum albumin?**

   RS's serum albumin level of 2.7 g/dL suggests moderately depleted visceral protein reserves, indicating that she is beginning to break down her body's muscle stores to attain her calorie and protein requirements. In a starved state, nutrients are mobilized from the patient's body stores if they are not provided exogenously. Glycogen stores only supply sufficient calories for approximately 24 hours, after which time lean body mass is catabolized to produce glucose and the amino acids needed for gluconeogenesis. Fat stores become the primary source of calories after the glycogen stores are depleted. Patients with acute injuries have an accelerated rate of catabolism related to the type and severity of their injury.

   Patients on ventilators cannot eat because the endotracheal tube in the oropharynx interferes with swallowing. Those who are mechanically ventilated for a period longer than seven to ten days require nutritional support to prevent weight loss and malnutrition. This support can be accomplished by feeding the patient liquids through a tube inserted into the nose that empties either into the stomach (nasogastric) or into the small intestine (nasoduodenal), a process called enteral feeding. (See Chapter 11 for an in-depth discussion of nutrition support.)

See Chapter Review Questions, pages A3–A4.

REFERENCES

Atkinson RL, Callaway CW, St Jean S, et al. A sane approach to weight loss. *Pat Care* 1995(11/15)152–169.

Brown ML. *Present Knowledge in Nutrition*, 6th ed. Washington, DC: International Life Sciences Institute Nutrition Foundation, 1990.

Buchsbaum DG. Quick effective screening for alcohol abuse. *Pat Care* 1995:(7/15)56–69.

Byers T. Body and weight mortality, editorial. *N Engl J Med* 1995;333:723–724.

Caltaldo C, Rolfes S, Whitney E. *Understanding Clinical Nutrition.* St. Paul: West, 1991.

Colditz GA, Willett WC, Rotnitzky A, et al. Weight gain as a risk factor for clinical diabetes mellitus in women. *Ann Intern Med* 1995;122:481–486.

Department of Health and Human Services. *Healthy People 2000.* National Health Promotion and Disease Prevention Objectives. Washington: DHHS Pub. no. (PHS) 91-50212, 1990.

Gibson R. 1990. *Principles of Nutrition Assessment.* New York: Oxford.

Kuczmarski RJ, Flegal KM, Campbell SM. Increasing prevalence of overweight among US adults: The National Health and Nutrition Examination Surveys, 1960 to 1991. *JAMA* 1994;272:205–211.

Kuczmarski RJ, Flegal KM, Campbell SM. Prevalence of overweight among adolescents—United States, 1988–1991. *MMWR* 1994;43:818–821.

Manson JE, Willett WC, Stampfer MJ, et al. Body weight and mortality among women. *N Engl J Med* 1995;333:677–685.

National Health and Nutrition Examination Survey (NHANES), National Center for Health Statistics, Centers for Disease Control. Public Health Service, U.S. Dept. of Health and Human Services, Hyattsville, MD.

National Research Council. 1990. *Diet and Health: Implications for Reducing Chronic Disease Risk.* Washington, DC: National Academy of Sciences Press.

Pate RR, Pratt M, Blair SN, et al. Physical activity and public health: A recommendation from the Centers for Disease Control and Prevention and the American College of Sports Medicine. *JAMA* 1995;273:402–407.

Rimm EB, Stampfer MJ, Giovannucci E, et al. Body size and fat distribution as predictors of coronary heart disease among middle-aged and older US men. *Am J Epidemiol* 1995;141:1117–1127.

Shils ME. 1993. *Modern Nutrition in Health and Disease*, 8th ed. Philadelphia: Lea and Febiger.

Troiano RP, Flegal KM, Kuczmarski RJ, et al. Overweight prevalence and trends for children and adolescents: The National Health and Nutrition Examination Surveys, 1963 to 1991. *Arch Pediatric Adolesc Med* 1995;149:1085–1091.

2

Vitamin and Mineral Therapy

Donna H. Mueller and Frances Burke

Objectives

- To identify the properties and sources of the vitamins and minerals.
- To define the role of vitamins and minerals in the promotion and maintenance of health.
- To recognize how vitamins and minerals affect medical therapies and how various disease states affect the body's ability to metabolize them.
- To evaluate current, investigative medical nutrition research on antioxidants.

Vitamins and minerals are classified as micronutrients: chemical substances required for normal growth and metabolism. Although micronutrients are found in all body tissues and fluids, they account for only a small percentage of body weight. Vitamins are organic compounds essential for hundreds of metabolic reactions within the body and help release energy from carbohydrates, fats, and proteins. Minerals are inorganic elements, and unlike carbohydrates, fats, and proteins, they do not furnish energy. For the most part, higher living organisms rely on intake from outside sources to supply their vitamin and mineral needs, because they are unable to produce or synthesize these compounds independently. Known exceptions to this rule of thumb are the production of vitamin K and biotin by certain intestinal microorganisms; the synthesis of vitamin D from its precursor, cholesterol; and the synthesis of niacin from its precursor, tryptophan.

Even though all of the vitamins and minerals and their major functions were known by nutritionists as far back as the 1950s, little attention was paid to their potential role in developing new medical therapies. Only recently have nutrition experts manifested renewed interest in research on micronutrient requirements and the benefits of using these substances for disease prevention and treatment. In the United States, the Food and Drug Administration (FDA) is the agency mandated to investigate and regulate the results of such research: the use of foods and dietary supplements for health and medical benefits.

Concurrently, public interest in and curiosity about vitamins and minerals has also heightened. Media headlines and widespread advertising by manufacturers of nutrient supplements emphasizing the role of vitamins and minerals in preventing or treating medical conditions by natural methods have led Americans to spend about three billion dollars annually on over-the-counter supplements. For advice on using these products, most consumers depend on salespeople in health food stores, mail-order dietary supplement companies, physical fitness magazines, or "health professionals" who sell vitamins and minerals as an integral component of their practice. Many supplement users regard them as an insurance policy, believing that if certain kinds and amounts are good, then more is better.

The ability to eradicate certain diseases now known to be caused by the lack of minuscule amounts of specific vitamins and minerals has been well documented as a major factor in promoting human health and prolonging life. Among the debilitating, often fatal diseases rarely seen in the West today thanks to improved levels of nutrition are

- scurvy, the scourge that took the lives of as many as half the sailors involved in the round-the-world voyages that took place from the fifteenth to the seventeenth centuries (due to vitamin C deficiency)

- beriberi, the paralyzing disease that plagued polished rice eaters in Asia (due to thiamin (vitamin B_1) deficiency)

- pellagra, the disease of the four Ds—dermatitis, diarrhea, dementia, and death—that claimed many lives, especially in the southern United States, at the beginning of the twentieth century (due to niacin(vitamin B_3) deficiency)

- goiter, the endemic, disfiguring disease of inland peoples that causes women to bear children who are severely mentally retarded (due to iodine deficiency)

Today, these diseases and many other micronutrient deficiencies still run rampant throughout many parts of the world. Perhaps, then, the most exciting aspect of this nutrition success story is that a varied diet of ordinary foods can prevent or cure these diseases.

Now, people are asking new questions. Will vitamin C promote longevity? Will vitamin E and folic acid protect against heart disease? Will the fluoride we use to prevent dental caries in children cause cancer when those children reach adulthood? Will megadoses of thiamin, niacin, and riboflavin protect the body from modern-day stress? Just as the use of iodized salt, a public health measure adopted in the 1920s, succeeded in preventing goiter, will a contemporary public health initiative to fortify breads and cereals with folate help pregnant women prevent their babies from being born with neural tube defects?

Fortunately, physicians and scientists continue to discover new information about the body's micronutrient requirements that helps people achieve optimal health, prevent acute and chronic diseases, and treat surgical and medical conditions. However, far too often patients self-prescribe vitamin or mineral doses ten times greater than the established recommended daily allowances (RDAs) because of claims that micronutrients prevent or cure colds, cancer, heart disease, impotence, stress, and other maladies common in modern times. Physicians and nurses educated in clinical nutrition can thus perform a much-needed service for their patients by helping them to examine the pros and cons of controversial medical nutrition issues, interpreting related information, diagnosing micronutrient abnormalities, and establishing appropriate therapy as needed. These issues are among the topics of the remainder of this chapter.

Properties and Sources of Vitamins

Vitamins occur in minute quantities in foods. Each vitamin has a specific chemical structure; some are simplistic (e.g., vitamin C), while others are more complex (e.g., vitamin B_{12}).

Vitamins are classified as either fat-soluble or water-soluble. Vitamins A (retinol, carotenes), D (cholecalciferol), E (tocopherols), and K (phylloquinone, menaquinone, and menadione) are fat-soluble (see Table 2-1). Vitamin C (ascorbic acid) and the B-complex: thiamin (vitamin B_1), riboflavin (vitamin B_2), niacin (vitamin B_3), pantothenic acid (vitamin B_5), pyridoxine (vitamin B_6), cobalamin (vitamin B_{12}), folate (folic acid), and biotin are water-soluble (see Table 2-2).

Individual vitamins differ in their chemical structure and functions, and produce characteristic symptoms of deficiency or toxicity (see Table 1-9, p. 30). Water-soluble vitamins are easily excreted in urine; excess levels of fat-soluble vitamins are readily stored in the liver and adipose tissue. Acute and chronic toxicities have been reported with both classes of vitamins, particularly vitamins A and D, niacin, pyridoxine, vitamin C, and folate.

Units of Measurement

Early methods for measuring the quantity and bioavailability of vitamins were often imprecise and soon gave way to the system of International Units (IU) commonly used to measure some vitamins until the 1980s. Although this designation is still seen in certain food composition tables and on some food/supplement labels such as vitamin D, the most current measurement units are milligrams (mg) or micrograms (µg).

Functions of Vitamins

Vitamins are essential contributors to the metabolic reactions within the body. Unlike the macronutrients, fat, protein, and carbohydrates, vitamins do not produce energy (kilocalories). Instead, most are involved in its release from carbohydrates, fats, and proteins by functioning as co-enzymes. Some vitamins function independently, while others are metabolically interrelated. In no event, however, can one vitamin substitute for another.

Table 2-1   Fat-soluble vitamin summary.

VITAMINS	METABOLISM/FUNCTION	DEFICIENCY OR EXCESS	FOOD SOURCES
Vitamin A:			
Retinol	Bile needed for absorption	Night blindness	
		Keratomalacia	
Retinal	Mineral oil prevents absorption	Lowered resistance to infection	
Retinoic acid	Stored in liver	Severe drying and scaling	Liver, kidney
		of skin; eye infections; blindness	
Provitamin A:	Bone and tooth structure	Overdoses are toxic: skin, hair,	Egg yolk, butter, fortified
Carotenes	Healthy skin and mucous	and bone changes, petechiae	margarine
	membranes		Milk, cream, cheese,
	Vision in dim light		Dark-green leafy and
			deep-yellow vegetables
			Deep-yellow fruits
Vitamin D	Some storage in liver	*Rickets*	*Fortified milk*
Precursors:	Liver synthesizes calcidiol	Soft bones	Concentrates: calciferol;
Ergosterol	Kidney converts calcidiol to	Enlarged joints	viosterol
in plants	*calcitriol*	Enlarged skull	Fish-liver oils
7-dehydro-	Functions as hormone in	Deformed chest	Exposure to ultraviolet
cholesterol;	absorption of calcium and	Spinal curvature	rays of sun
in skin	phosphorus; mobilization	Bowed leg	
	and mineralization of bone	*Osteomalacia*	
		Renal osteodystrophy	
		Even small excess is toxic	
Vitamin E	Prevents oxidation of	Deficiency not common	Salad oils, shortenings,
Tocopherols	vitamin A in intestine	Red cell hemolysis in	margarines
	Protects cell membranes	malnourished infants	Whole grains, legumes,
	against oxidation	Low toxicity	nuts, dark leafy
	Protects red blood cells		vegetables
	Limited stores in body		
	Polyunsaturated fats		
	increase need		
Vitamin K	Forms prothrombin for	Prolonged clotting time	Synthesized by
	normal blood clotting	Hemorrhage, especially in	intestinal bacteria
	Synthesized in intestines	newborn infants, and	Dark-green leafy
		biliary tract disease	vegetables
		Large amounts toxic	

Source: Robinson CH, Weigley ES, Mueller DH. *Basic Nutrition and Diet Therapy*, 7th ed. ©1993. Reprinted by permission of Prentice Hall, Upper Saddle River, New Jersey.

Table 2-2   Water-soluble vitamin summary.

VITAMINS	METABOLISM/FUNCTION	DEFICIENCY	FOOD SOURCES

Ascorbic acid
Vitamin C
	Form collagen
	Teeth firm in gums
	Hormone synthesis
	Resistance to infection
	Improve iron absorption
		Poor wound healing
		Poor bone, tooth development
		Scurvy
		  Bruising and hemorrhage
		  Bleeding gums
		  Loose teeth
			Citrus fruits
			Strawberries, cantaloupe
			Tomatoes, broccoli
			Raw green vegetables

Thiamin
Vitamin B$_1$
	Coenzyme for breakdown
	  of glucose for energy
	Healthy nerves
	Good digestion
	Normal appetite
	Good mental outlook
		Beriberi
		Fatigue
		Poor appetite
		Constipation
		Depression
		Neuropathy
		Angular stomatitis
		Polyneuritis
		Edema
		Heart failure
			Pork, liver, other meats,
			  poultry
			Dry beans and peas,
			  peanut butter
			Enriched and whole-grain
			  bread
			Milk, eggs

Riboflavin
Vitamin B$_2$
	Coenzymes for protein
	  and glucose metabolism
	Fatty acid synthesis
	Healthy skin
	Normal vision in bright light
		Cheilosis
		  Scaling skin
		Burning, itching, sensitive eyes
			Dairy products
			Meat, poultry, fish
			Dark-green leafy vegetables
			Enriched and whole-grain
			  breads, cereals

Niacin
Nicotinic acid
Niacinamide
	Coenzymes for energy
	  metabolism
	Normal digestion
	Healthy nervous system
	Healthy skin
	Tryptophan a precursor:
	  60 mg = 1 mg niacin
		Pellagra
		Dermatitis
		Angular stomatitis
		Diarrhea
		Depression
		Disorientation
		Delirium
			Meat, poultry, fish
			Dark-green leafy vegetables
			Whole-grain or enriched
			  breads, cereals

Vitamin B$_6$
Pyridoxine
Pyridoxal
Pyridoxamine
	Coenzymes for protein
	  metabolism
	Conversion of tryptophan
	  to niacin
	Formation of heme
		Cheilosis
		Gastrointestinal upsets
		Weak gait
		Irritability
		Neuropathy
		Convulsions
			Meat, whole-grain cereals,
			  dark-green leafy
			  vegetables, potatoes

Vitamin B$_{12}$	Formation of mature
	  red blood cells
	Synthesis of DNA, RNA
	Requires intrinsic factor
	  from stomach for absorption
		Pernicious anemia: lack of
		  intrinsic factor, or after
		  gastrectomy
		Macrocytic anemia: neurologic
		  degeneration, pallor
			Animal foods only: milk,
			  eggs, meat, poultry, fish

Folate
Folacin
Folic acid
	Maturation of red blood cells
	Synthesis of DNA, RNA
		Macrocytic anemia in
		  pregnancy, sprue,
		  pallor
			Dark-green leafy vegetables,
			  meat, fish, poultry, eggs,
			  whole-grain cereals

Biotin	Components of coenzymes in
	  energy metabolism
	Some synthesis in intestine
	Avidin, a protein in raw egg
	  white, interferes with
	  absorption
		Occurs only when large
		  amounts of raw egg whites
		  are eaten
		Dermatitis, loss of hair
			Organ meats, egg yolk,
			  legumes, nuts

**Pantothenic
  acid**
	Component of coenzyme A
	Synthesis of sterols,
	  fatty acids, heme
		Occurs rarely
		Neuritis of arms, legs;
		  burning sensation of feet
			Meat, poultry, fish, legumes,
			  whole-grain cereals
			Lesser amounts in milk,
			  fruits, and vegetables

Source: Robinson CH, Weigley ES, Mueller DH. *Basic Nutrition and Diet Therapy,* 7th ed.
©1993. Reprinted by permission of Prentice Hall, Upper Saddle River, New Jersey.

Sources of Vitamins

Not all vitamins come from external dietary sources. Some are the products of various conversions that take place within the body. For example, vitamin D, considered a hormone, is produced endogenously in a process whereby 7-dehydrocholesterol in the skin is transformed first into 25-hydroxycholecalciferol in the liver and ultimately into 1,25-dihydroxycholecalciferol in the kidney. Certain microorganisms commonly found in the body also have a role in the production of vitamins. For instance, bacteria residing in the large intestine synthesize vitamin K and biotin.

Although the primary source of vitamins is the food supply, no single food constitutes an ideal source of all vitamins. Consuming a wide variety of wholesome foods usually ensures an adequate and balanced vitamin intake. In evaluating the vitamin contribution of any one food, certain factors should be considered.

Quantity Parsley, an excellent source of vitamin A, is a case in point. Used frequently as a garnish, it is most often left on the plate. Furthermore, on the rare occasion when it actually is eaten, only a very small portion is consumed.

Frequency Cod liver oil, a fundamental source of vitamin D prior to the 1940s, is used only rarely today because of its taste and toxicity. Accessibility is another key consideration. For example, seafood, an important potential source of iodine, may not be readily available to people living inland.

Stability All foods are susceptible to vitamin reduction, most notably during processing or prolonged cooking. The most easily destroyed of all vitamins is vitamin C; its potency is reduced by oxidation, dehydration, and alkali. Also, because it is water-soluble, it rapidly migrates during cooking from food to its aqueous surroundings. Examples of various food processing methods and their negative effects on vitamin C content follow in ascending order.

Quick-frozen fruits and vegetables contain most of the vitamin C present in the fresh product.

Even when processed, low pH fruits and vegetables retain almost as much ascorbic acid as the fresh whole fruit. For instance, half of a medium grapefruit has 47 mg; one-half cup of canned juice provides 42 mg.

Cooked or canned, nonacidic fruits and vegetables lose more of their ascorbic acid. One medium raw pear contains 7 mg; one-half cup of canned juice has only 2 mg.

Dried foods contain only traces of vitamin C. Ten raw apricot halves provide 18 mg; ten dried halves contain 1 mg.

Some food manufacturers now add vitamin C to dehydrated potatoes, apple juice, and other foods; therefore, instructing patients to read labels for this information is a good practice.

Inadequate quantities of vitamins in food Natural whole and skim milk are very low in vitamin D. Thus vitamin D-fortified milk is a better dietary source of this vitamin. Exposure of the body's skin to the sun's ultraviolet rays is an excellent endogenous source of vitamin D. Refined grains (e.g., certain breads, crackers, and snack foods) contain negligible amounts of thiamin, niacin, and riboflavin, whereas enriched whole grains are fortified with these B vitamins.

Recommended Vitamin Intakes

Vitamins are crucial throughout life for proper growth, development, and metabolism. However, the required quantities of each vitamin change based on normal body changes at various stages of life. For example, the cellular requirements for vitamins are higher in infants, adolescents, and pregnant and lactating women than in fully grown, healthy, young adults.

In the United States, the Food and Nutrition Board of the National Research Council reviews the worldwide nutrition literature and, based on its findings, establishes recommended nutrient levels. For certain vitamins a considerable body of knowledge exists, and designated levels have been identified as recommended dietary allowances (RDAs) for various gender and age categories. These levels are set at two standard deviations above the mean to cover the needs of practically all healthy persons (Table 2-3). In the case of other vitamins for which only limited scientific data exist, the Food and Nutrition Board has set up a range of levels known as the estimated safe and adequate daily dietary intakes (ESADDIs).

Two caveats concerning these recommendations must be remembered: The suggested levels were established for groups of healthy people, not necessarily for particular individuals; and the requirements of individuals with special nutritional needs or medical conditions are not addressed by the Food and Nutrition Board.

The abundant food supply in the United States can adequately fulfill the vitamin needs of healthy individuals. Vitamin retention remains high with proper food handling and processing. As a whole, therefore, healthy individuals eating appropriate amounts of a wide variety of wholesome foods do not require vitamin supplements. The dilemma is that the people who do not need to take vitamin supplements are those most likely to take them, whereas the people who would benefit most from vitamin supplements often remain unidentified.

Vitamin Deficiency

In determining the adequacy of an individual's vitamin intake, several factors can be evaluated. As noted previously, certain processed foods are fortified or enriched with vitamins, whereas others are not; and food preparation can decrease vitamin content, as is the case, for example, when water-soluble vitamins are lost due to cooking, exposure to light or dehydration. Because the current RDAs and ESADDIs were established for healthy persons who consume

Table 2-3   1989 Recommended Dietary Allowances[a] (RDA) (Revised 1989)

Category	Age (yrs) or Condition	Weight[b] (kg)	Weight[b] (lb)	Height[b] (cm)	Height[b] (in)	Protein (g)	Vitamin A (μg RE)[c]	Vitamin D (μg)[d]	Vitamin E (mg TE)[e]	Vitamin K (μg)	Vitamin C (mg)	Thiamin (mg)	Riboflavin (mg)	Niacin (mg NE)[f]	Vitamin B6 (mg)	Folate (μg)	Vitamin B12 (μg)	Calcium (mg)	Phosphorus (mg)	Magnesium (mg)	Iron (mg)	Zinc (mg)	Iodine (μg)	Selenium (μg)
Infants	0.0–0.5	6	13	60	24	13	375	7.5	3	5	30	0.3	0.4	5	0.3	25	0.3	400	300	40	6	5	40	10
	0.5–1.0	9	20	71	28	14	375	10	4	10	35	0.4	0.5	6	0.6	35	0.5	600	500	60	10	5	50	15
Children	1–3	13	29	90	35	16	400	10	6	15	40	0.7	0.8	9	1.0	50	0.7	800	800	80	10	10	70	20
	4–6	20	44	112	44	24	500	10	7	20	45	0.9	1.1	12	1.1	75	1.0	800	800	120	10	10	90	20
	7–10	28	62	132	52	28	700	10	7	30	45	1.0	1.2	13	1.4	100	1.4	800	800	170	10	10	120	30
Males	11–14	45	99	157	62	45	1,000	10	10	45	50	1.3	1.5	17	1.7	150	2.0	1,200	1,200	270	12	15	150	40
	15–18	66	145	176	69	59	1,000	10	10	65	60	1.5	1.8	20	2.0	200	2.0	1,200	1,200	400	12	15	150	50
	19–24	72	160	177	70	58	1,000	10	10	70	60	1.5	1.7	19	2.0	200	2.0	1,200	1,200	350	10	15	150	70
	25–50	79	174	176	70	63	1,000	5	10	80	60	1.5	1.7	19	2.0	200	2.0	800	800	350	10	15	150	70
	51+	77	170	173	68	63	1,000	5	10	80	60	1.2	1.4	15	2.0	200	2.0	800	800	350	10	15	150	70
Females	11–14	46	101	157	62	46	800	10	8	45	50	1.1	1.3	15	1.4	150	2.0	1,200	1,200	280	15	12	150	45
	15–18	55	120	163	64	44	800	10	8	55	60	1.1	1.3	15	1.5	180	2.0	1,200	1,200	300	15	12	150	50
	19–24	58	128	164	65	46	800	10	8	60	60	1.1	1.3	15	1.6	180	2.0	1,200	1,200	280	15	12	150	55
	25–50	63	138	163	64	50	800	5	8	65	60	1.1	1.3	15	1.6	180	2.0	800	800	280	15	12	150	55
	51+	65	143	160	63	50	800	5	8	65	60	1.0	1.2	13	1.6	180	2.0	800	800	280	10	12	150	55
Pregnant						60	800	10	10	65	70	1.5	1.6	17	2.2	400	2.2	1,200	1,200	320	30	15	175	65
Lactating	1st 6 months					65	1,300	10	12	65	95	1.6	1.8	20	2.1	280	2.6	1,200	1,200	355	15	19	200	75
	2nd 6 months					62	1,200	10	11	65	90	1.6	1.7	20	2.1	260	2.6	1,200	1,200	340	15	16	200	75

a The allowances, expressed as average daily intakes over time, are intended to provide for individual variations among normal persons as they live in the United States under usual environmental stresses. Diets should be based on a variety of common foods in order to provide other nutrients for which human requirements have been less well defined. See text for detailed discussion of allowances and of nutrients not tabulated.

b Weights and heights of Reference Adults are actual medians for the U.S. population of the designated age, as reported by NHANES II. The median weights and heights of those under 19 years of age were taken from Hamill.* The use of these figures does not imply that the height-to-weight ratios are ideal.

c Retinol equivalents. 1 retinol equivalent = 1 μg retinol or 6 μg β-carotene.

d As cholecalciferol. 10 μg cholecalciferol = 400 IU of vitamin D.

e α-Tocopherol equivalents. 1 mg d-α tocopherol = 1 α-TE.

f 1 NE (niacin equivalent) is equal to 1 mg of niacin or 60 mg of dietary tryptophan.

* Hamill PVV, Drizd TA, Johnson CL, Reed RB, Roche AF, and Moore WM, 1979 Physical Growth: National Center for Health Statistics percentiles. Am J Clin Nutr. 32:607–629.

Source: Food and Nutrition Board, National Academy of Sciences—National Research Council, 1989.

a wide variety of nourishing foods, vitamin deficiency should be considered for people in the following circumstances.

Primary inadequate food intake Major factors contributing to inadequate vitamin intake due to insufficient food consumption include poverty, limited knowledge of nutrition, and substance abuse. A multivitamin supplement that furnishes 100 percent of the RDAs and ESADDIs may be necessary for people on low-calorie diets for extended periods of time; for the elderly, the physically or mentally challenged, people with oral anomalies, and others who may be unable to eat a varied diet; for individuals who choose to eat a restricted array of foods; and for those suffering from anorexia nervosa or other conditions considered high-risk from a nutritional standpoint, such as recovering chronic alcoholics who routinely receive thiamin, folate, and vitamin B_{12} supplements along with a multivitamin.

Increased nutrient requirements unmet by food selections Pregnant women may require folate and iron supplements if their food selections supply inadequate levels of these nutrients.

Increased metabolic demands Vitamin supplements may be required to meet increased cellular needs of patients under physiological stress due to infections, fevers, injury, burns and surgery.

Maldigestion and malabsorption Patients with chronic pancreatitis, prolonged diarrhea, surgical removal of a portion of the small intestine (short bowel syndrome), cystic fibrosis, sprue, bile duct obstruction, hepatitis, or cirrhosis usually require supplementation. This is especially the case with fat-soluble vitamins when bile acid production is impaired.

Drug-nutrient or medical treatment-nutrient interactions Medications and medical treatments should always be evaluated for food and nutrient interactions, and all patients receiving such therapies should be considered at risk for iatrogenic vitamin deficiences. Classic examples include GI tract side effects caused by radiation therapy (nausea and vomiting resulting in inadequate food intake) and antacid and cathartic overuse resulting in vitamin malabsorption. Patients with elevated serum cholesterol levels taking bile acid sequestrants may require fat-soluble vitamin supplementation. Some anticonvulsant medications interfere with liver synthesis of vitamin D. Antituberculous drugs may antagonize pyridoxine and thus inhibit the folate-dependent interconversion of glycine and serine.

Requirements for vitamins in pharmacologic doses Doses of niacin between 1 and 3 g/day have been shown to be effective in lowering serum cholesterol, but patients need to be counseled about possible side effects such as heartburn, esophageal reflux, facial flushing, and elevated liver enzymes.

Vitamin Toxicity

Toxic effects of vitamins usually result from food faddism, misuse of supplements, or dosage errors. Patients taking large doses of vitamins, whether self-prescribed or medically indicated, need education and close monitoring. Effects of excessive vitamin intake include the following.

Direct toxic effects Megavitamin therapy is a frequent cause of toxicity to which infants and children are the most vulnerable. Vitamins A and D are the most common agents involved in toxic reactions. Early symptoms include cracked lips, headaches, dry rough skin, and alopecia of eyebrows in the case of vitamin A; and anorexia, nausea, and vomiting in that of vitamin D. Large doses of B-complex vitamins can produce undesirable symptoms ranging from flushing, itching, and burning or tingling sensations (niacin) to progressive sensory ataxia and profound impairment of the lower-limb position and vibration senses (pyridoxine). Usually symptoms disappear when the megadose is withdrawn, but permanent organ damage can result depending on the dosage and duration of supplementation.

Dependency and withdrawal Newborn infants may exhibit signs of vitamin withdrawal. For example, when a pregnant woman ingests about 200 mg of vitamin C daily during her pregnancy, fetal tissue in utero may become dependent on the high levels supplied by the mother's intake. When the infant is born and receives an infant formula supplying the usual recommended allowance, withdrawal symptoms of a condition referred to as rebound scurvy appear. In adults, excessive doses of vitamin C have been reported to predispose individuals to oxalate urinary calculi and iron overload, as well as rebound scurvy.

Masking of concurrent diseases Both folate and vitamin B_{12} deficiencies can cause macrocytic anemia. Folate supplementation reverses the macrocytic anemia caused by vitamin B_{12} deficiency and pernicious anemia, but not the underlying nerve damage that only occurs secondary to vitamin B_{12} deficiency will progress. Therefore, arriving at a correct differential diagnosis requires checking both red blood cell folate and serum vitamin B_{12} blood levels before prescribing vitamin supplementation.

Drug-nutrient or medical treatment-nutrient interactions Intake of certain vitamins can cause erroneous interpretation of therapy outcomes. For instance, vitamin C can produce false-negative urine glucose test results in patients with diabetes mellitus. Vitamin supplements containing pyridoxine should be avoided by patients taking levodopa to treat Parkinson's disease, because together they form a vitamin-drug complex that makes the drug systemically unavailable.

Properties and Sources of Minerals

Mineral elements are inorganic substances that occur in simple forms such as NaCl or in combination with organic compounds such as the iron in hemoglobin and the sulfur in almost all proteins. (See Table 2-4 for a summary of macrominerals and microminerals.) Based on their percentages of the body's total content, minerals are classified as:

Macrominerals constituting more than 0.005% of the body's weight, or 50 parts

Table 2-4   Macromineral and micromineral summary

ELEMENT	FUNCTION	UTILIZATION/DEFICIENCY	FOOD SOURCES

Calcium	99% in bones, teeth
	Nervous stimulation
	Muscle contraction
	Blood clotting
	Activates enzymes
		10 to 40% absorbed
		Aided by vitamin D and
		  lactose; hindered by oxalic acid
		Parathyroid hormone regulates
		  blood levels
		Deficiency: fragile bones;
		  osteoporosis
			Dairy products
			Mustard and turnip greens
			Cabbage, broccoli
			Clams, oysters, salmon

Phosphorus	80–90% in bones, teeth
	Acid–balance
	Transport of fats
	Enzymes for energy
	  metabolism;
	  protein synthesis
		Vitamin D favors absorption
		  and use by bones
		Dietary deficiency unlikely
			Dairy products
			Meat, poultry, fish
			Whole-grain cereals, nuts, legumes

Magnesium	60% in bones, teeth
	Transmits nerve impulses
	Muscle contraction
	Enzymes for energy
	  metabolism
		Salts relatively insoluble
		Acid favors absorption
		Dietary deficiency unlikely;
		  occurs in alcoholism,
		  renal failure
			Milk, meat, green-leafy vegetables.
			  legumes, whole-grain cereals

Sodium	Extracellular fluid
	Water balance
	Acid–base balance
	Nervous stimulation
	Muscle contraction
		Almost completely absorbed
		Body levels regulated by
		  adrenal; excess excreted in
		  urine and by skin
		Deficiency: rare, occurs with
		  excessive perspiration
			Table salt
			Baking powder, baking soda
			Milk, meat, poultry, fish, eggs

Potassium	Intracellular fluid
	Protein and glycogen
	  synthesis
	Water balance
	Transmits nerve impulse
	Muscle contraction
		Almost completely absorbed
		Body levels regulated by
		  adrenal; excess excreted
		  in urine
		Deficiency: starvation, duiretic
		  therapy
			Ample amounts in meat, cereals,
			  fruits, fruit juices, vegetables

Iron	Mostly in hemoglobin
	Muscle myoglobin
	Oxidizing enzymes for
	  release of energy
		5–20% absorption
		Acid and vitamin C aid
		  absorption
		Daily losses in urine and feces
		Menstrual loss
		Deficiency: anemia, cheilosis,
		  pallor
			Organ meats, meat, fish, poultry
			Whole-grain and enriched cereal
			Green vegetables, dried fruits

Iodine	Forms thyroxine for energy metabolism	Chiefly in thyroid gland *Deficiency:* endemic goiter	Iodized salt Shellfish, saltwater fish
Fluoride	Prevents tooth decay	Storage in bones and teeth Excess leads to tooth mottling	Flouridated water

Copper	Utilization of iron for
	  hemoglobin formation
	Pigment formation
	Myelin sheath of nerves
		In form of ceruloplasmin in
		  blood
		Abnormal storage in Wilson's
		  disease
		Deficiency: rare
			Liver, shellfish, meats, nuts,
			  legumes, whole-grain cereals

Zinc	Enzymes for transfer
	  of carbon dioxide
	Taste, protein synthesis
		Deficiency: growth retardation;
		  altered taste
			Plant and animal proteins

Source: Robinson CH, Weigley ES, Mueller DH. *Basic Nutrition and Diet Therapy*, 7th ed.
©1993. Reprinted by permission of Prentice Hall, Upper Saddle River, New Jersey.

per million (ppm), such as calcium, chloride, phosphorus, potassium, magnesium, sodium, sulfur

Microminerals, which fall into two categories:

Minerals with identified roles in health maintenance, including chromium, cobalt, copper, fluoride, iodide, iron, manganese, molybdenum, selenium, and zinc

Minerals with unestablished roles in health maintenance, such as arsenic, boron, cadmium, lithium, nickel, silicone, tin, and vanadium

In foods, minerals occur as salts, such as sodium chloride. Because minerals are water-soluble, some loss occurs during cooking, especially when foods soak in water or marinate and when cooking liquids are discarded.

Units of Measurement

Minerals in foods are measured in milligrams (mg) or micrograms (µg), whereas mineral concentrations in body fluids are expressed in milliequivalents per liter (mEq/L), and as Système International units [SI].

Interrelated Mineral Functions

Within the body, minerals function together for tissue anabolism, catabolism, and in the regulation of body metabolism. Examples of their functions include

Bone formation Bone consists of a collagen matrix where minerals are deposited. Most of the body's calcium, phosphorus, and magnesium are deposited in the bones and teeth. Bones also store a reservoir of minerals to maintain proper cellular functioning in the event of an intake deficiency. Thus, although minerals are transported via the circulatory system, blood levels of minerals provide limited indication of the actual biochemical flux and body stores of minerals.

Tooth formation Tooth enamel and dentine (hydroxyapatite) contain appreciable amounts of calcium and phosphorus. When fluoride is incorporated into the structure, the resulting fluoroapatite is less soluble in an acid medium and therefore more resistant to the development of carrious lesions. Because enamel and dentine are not supplied with blood vessels, a decayed tooth cannot repair itself.

Soft tissue structure Like hard tissues, soft tissue structures contain many minerals, including potassium, sulfur, phosphorus, and iron.

Vitamin, enzyme, and hormone functions Minerals are constituents of various regulatory compounds. Sulfur is part of the thiamin molecule. Cobalt is present in the vitamin B12 molecule. Zinc forms part of carbonic anhydrase. Iodine is present in the thyroxine molecule.

Some minerals are cofactors; for example, calcium activates pancreatic lipase. In other instances, minerals catalyze reactions: copper is needed to incorporate iron into the hemoglobin molecule; zinc is necessary for the formation of insulin by the pancreas.

Nervous system response and muscle contraction Exact amounts of sodium, potassium, calcium, and magnesium are necessary to regulate the various cellular pumps and membrane ion channels. These elements control the passage in and out of cells of the materials that regulate the transmission of nerve impulses and muscle contractions.

Fluid and acid-base balances Fluid balance between the intracellular and extracellular spaces depends in large part on the correct concentrations of sodium (primarily in the extracellular fluid) and potassium (chiefly in the intracellular fluid). Acid-base regulation also involves minerals, especially as buffer salts such as phosphate and sulfate.

Sources of Minerals

As in the case of vitamins, no single food is the best source for all minerals. Consuming a wide variety of foods usually ensures adequate and balanced mineral intake. Eating processed foods can decrease or increase mineral intake. Some minerals are deleted in processing: iron and chromium, for example, are removed from whole grains during the refining process. Often, minerals are added in processing. Refined grains bearing the label "enriched" contain iron added to compensate for the amounts lost during processing. Sodium, mainly as sodium chloride, is added to numerous foods to enhance their taste and to serve as a preservative. Iodine is added routinely to table salt. Orange juice, cereals, and other foods are commonly fortified with calcium.

Undistilled water contains varying amounts of numerous minerals. Fluoride is present naturally in many water sources, and many municipal water supplies are fluoridated. Hard water contains calcium and magnesium. These minerals can be ion-exchanged with sodium to produce soft water. Water is also a source of iron in some geographic regions.

Recommended Mineral Intakes

In the United States, the Food and Nutrition Board of the National Research Council has established the following intake parameters with regard to minerals (see Table 2-3).

- Recommended dietary allowances for calcium, phosphorus, magnesium, iron, zinc, iodine, and selenium
- Estimated safe and adequate daily dietary intakes for copper, manganese, fluoride, chromium, and molybdenum
- Estimated minimum requirements of healthy persons for the electrolytes: sodium, chloride, and potassium

Mineral Adequacy

With proper selection from the abundant food and water supplies in the United

States, healthy individuals should be able to meet their needs for minerals. Because bioavailability of minerals varies, recognition of factors favoring or hindering absorption is important. Factors that influence individual needs and bioavailability of nutrients include the following.

Physiological need The amount of a mineral that the body absorbs depends on its needs. Pregnant women and growing children absorb a higher percentage of calcium and iron than adults. Likewise, iron-deficient individuals absorb a higher percentage of ingested iron.

Chemical forms of minerals The term bioavailability refers to the amount of an ingested nutrient that is digested and absorbed. Under normal conditions, individual nutrient bioavailability varies widely, principally for minerals, as follows.

Carbohydrate, lipid, and protein	> 90%
Sodium	± 100%
Calcium	± 30%
Iron	± 5 to 60%

Heme-iron, found in flesh foods, is more available than the non-heme iron found in eggs and plant foods. Thus the iron in meat is more readily absorbed than the iron in raisins.

Proper pH in the gastrointestinal tract Because an acid medium increases the solubility of calcium and iron salts in food, thereby improving their absorption, maintaining the stomach's normal pH is important. People suffering from achlorhydria or taking a strong, acid-suppressing medication may be at risk for malabsorption of calcium and iron. Absorption of minerals occurs at various pH levels, depending on where it takes place in the intestine. Inadequate secretion of bicarbonate to neutralize duodenal acidity, for example, can result in under- or overabsorption of minerals.

Presence of other nutrients in the gastrointestinal tract Vitamin C enhances the absorption of calcium, non-heme iron, and zinc. For instance, combining dark-green vegetables and orange juice in the diet converts the non-iron from the ferric to the more absorbable ferrous form.

Mineral Deficiency

In the United States, mineral deficiencies receiving the most attention are iron (iron-deficiency anemia), calcium (osteoporosis), iodine (goiter), and fluoride (dental carries). Because the body stores and reuses minerals, deficiencies may not be detected for years. Among the numerous factors that reduce mineral status, most relate to primary deficiency due to inadequate intake, decreased release from foods, malabsorption, or increased losses. Examples are

- *Chelating substances:* Dietary oxalic acid (spinach, green beans, tea), phytic acid (whole grains), tannins (tea, coffee), and some forms of fiber (wheat bran) bind minerals in such a way that they are poorly absorbed. Certain medications bind directly with minerals. For example, aluminum hydroxide antacids combine with food phosphates, and other antacids bind with bile salts. Hypocholesterolemic agents and aminogly-cosides also cause decreased absorption of iron, calcium, and electrolytes. Binding in these and other cases results in decreased absorption of minerals; for example, pregnant women who practice pica—the compulsive, persistent ingestion of nonfood substances such as dirt, clay, paint chips, and so on—may experience decreased iron and zinc absorption.

- *Intestinal motility:* Mineral oil, laxatives, and diarrhea increase motility, thereby decreasing both transit time and the time for absorption of certain minerals.

- *Increased intestinal loss:* Conditions affecting the intestines such as Crohn's disease, steatorrhea, or surgical interventions can seriously interfere with the absorption of minerals and other nutrients. Glucocorticoids decrease calcium absorption. In developing countries, intestinal parasites harbored by many children are a major cause of mineral malnutrition.

- *Increased urinary loss:* Excessive alcohol consumption can increase magnesium excretion. Numerous medications cause mineral wasting in the kidney. For example, digoxin increases urinary losses of calcium, magnesium, potassium, and zinc. While the desired effect of furosemide is to increase sodium and potassium excretion, it also increases excretion of calcium, magnesium, and zinc. Some medications increase both GI and urinary mineral losses. For instance, cholestyramine not only increases calcium excretion in the urine, but also promotes formation of a compound of calcium and unabsorbed fat in the GI tract.

- *Increased loss via perspiration:* High body and ambient temperatures commonly cause mineral loss in children and adults. The major minerals lost are sodium, chloride, potassium, and magnesium, and secondarily, calcium and iron. Classic examples include sick people with fevers, and healthy infants, older adults, athletes, and manual laborers exposed to excessive environmental heat.

Mineral Toxicity

Although mineral excesses do occur, their nuances may be indiscernible. This is frequently the case in mineral-mineral interference with absorption. Precautions must be taken to prevent excessive mineral intake. Unless they are medically indicated and monitored, megadoses of minerals—especially single doses—are to be avoided. The levels of minerals found in a mixed diet deemed sufficient to fulfill human requirements fall well below the levels of toxicity seen in cases of indiscriminate use of minerals in pill form.

Mineral toxicity has resulted from excessive intake of copper, fluoride, iodine, iron, manganese, and selenium. Examples of toxicity include

Supplements taken in excess Children have developed iron overload as a result of taking pills containing iron from an open bottle of supplements belonging to their parents. People treated for ulcers may develop milk-alkali syndrome caused by excessive intake of calcium and absorbable alkali. Toxic dosages of selenium have been fatal.

Vitamin-mineral interaction Excessive intake of vitamin D can cause over-absorption of calcium.

Exposure to toxic levels of minerals Lead poisoning may result from storing orange juice or other acidic juices in unglazed ceramic ware and wine in lead crystal carafes. Newer containers made from these materials carry warning labels to this effect. Natural mineral supplements, such as bone meal and dolomite, which often contain lead and other heavy metals, are another potential cause of mineral toxicity.

Allergic reactions Sulfite, used to prevent discoloration of salad bar vegetables and fruits and also as a reduction agent in some alcoholic beverages, can cause life-threatening pulmonary symptoms in people with asthma. Since 1987, by FDA mandate, sulfite use in the United States is restricted and must be listed on food labels.

Antioxidants

During the first half of the twentieth century, the role of vitamins and minerals as essential dietary components for proper body function was proven. Recent research on these substances has focused on their role in maintaining lifelong optimal health, preventing or delaying the onset of chronic diseases, and treating disease when it occurs. For example, increased intake of calcium has been studied as a treatment for hypertension and osteoporosis, and increased intake of vitamin C as a preventative and treatment for the common cold.

In the United States, the two diseases with the greatest morbidity and mortality rates continue to be cardiovascular disease and cancer. Recently, intense interest has proliferated among health professionals, scientists, and the public regarding the potential role of vitamins and minerals with antioxidant properties in the prevention and treatment of the various forms of these diseases.

Antioxidant Nomenclature

An antioxidant is a natural or synthetic compound that is oxidized very readily and thus spares another compound from being oxidized. There are an extensive number of antioxidants in the body which serve as a defense system to protect different sites and different types of oxidative processes. These include enzymes such as superoxide dismutase, catalase, and peroxidases; vitamins such as beta carotene, vitamin E, and vitamin C. Dietary sources of the antioxidant vitamins are listed in Table 2-5. Antioxidants are naturally present in foods, are added to processed foods, and are maintained in delicate balance by the body as a homeostatic mechanism.

Free Radicals

Atoms or molecules that have one or more unpaired electrons in their outer

Table 2-5   Dietary sources of antioxidant vitamins.

	SOURCE	SERVING SIZE	AMOUNT (IU)		SOURCE	SERVING SIZE	AMOUNT (mg)
Vitamin A	Apricots, dried	1/2 cup	7,085	**Vitamin C**	Acerola	1 cup	3,872
	Bran, wheat	1 cup	1,650		(Barbados cherry juice)		
	Broccoli, cooked	1 cup	3,800		Black currants	1 cup	200
	Cantaloupe	1/4	3,400		Broccoli, cooked	1 cup	140
	Carrots, cooked	1 cup	15,750		Brussels sprouts	1 cup	135
	Carrot, raw	1	11,000		Caulifower	1 cup	69
	Cornflakes	1 cup	1,180		Grapefruit	1	76
	Endive, raw	1 cup	1,650		Grapefruit juice	1 cup	95
	Mango	1	11,090		Guava	1	242
	Parsley, chopped	1 cup	5,100		Lettuce, loose	1 cup	75
	Peach	1	1,330		Mango	1	81
	Prunes, dried	1 cup	2,580		Mustard greens	1 cup	117
	Spinach, cooked	1 cup	14,580		Orange	1	66
	Squash, winter	1 cup	8,610		Orange juice	6-oz glass	124
	Tomato, raw	1	1,350		Parsley, chopped	1 cup	103
	Watermelon	1 slice	3,540		Peppers, green	1 cup	102
Vitamin E	Almonds	100 g	41		Strawberries	1 cup	88
	Margarine, hard	100 g	16		Tomato, raw	1	34
	Margarine, soft	100 g	21		Watermelon	1 slice	42
	Mayonnaise	100 g	19				
	Peanut oil	100 g	28				
	Safflower oil	100 g	59				
	Wheat germ oil	100 g	178				
	Soybean oil	100 g	12				
	Sunflower oil	100 g	73				
	Sunflower seeds	100 g	74				

orbital are referred to as free radicals. The imbalance alters the reactivity of the atom or molecule. Free radicals normally are produced in the body as by-products of normal metabolism and also by environmental pollutants. Examples are the superoxide anion, hydroperoxyl radical, hydroxyl radical, and peroxyl radical. All can be highly damaging to polyunsaturated fatty acids, DNA, and proteins. Ultimately, this can lead to such outcomes as cell membrane destruction or damage to nucleic acids and DNA.

Mechanisms of Action

The damage to nucleic acids, lipids, and proteins caused by the formation of free radicals can accumulate over time and may contribute to carcinogenesis and other degenerative diseases. Scientists have established the negative affects of oxidative processes on degenerative disease but what remains unclear is the preventative role of antioxidants. Antioxidants may prevent oxidative damage by trapping or scavenging these free radicals or by interrupting a free radical chain reaction as it occurs, for example, during lipid peroxidation. Lipid per-oxidation is defined as the autoxidation of polyunsaturated fatty acid side chains of lipids by a radical chain reaction.

As listed above, vitamin C, vitamin E, and beta-carotene are antioxidants. Because vitamin C is a water-soluble compound, it is able to scavenge many aqueous free radicals in both extracellular and intracellular fluids. Vitamin C very effectively prevents isolated LDL-cholesterol from being oxidized. Unoxidized LDL-cholesterol has little atherogenicity. However, when it is oxidized, the uptake of LDL-cholesterol by coronary arterial epithelium is increased.

Alpha-tocopherol is the most biologically active form of vitamin E. It is the most abundant lipid soluble antioxidant in the body. Lipid soluble antioxidants are present in cell membranes and lipoproteins. The primary role of alpha-tocopherol as an antioxidant is to inhibit lipid peroxidation and it may also prevent the oxidative modification of LDL-cholesterol which is beneficial for individuals at risk for heart disease. The role of antioxidants in the prevention of coronary artery disease appears to be better understood.

The first step in LDL-cholesterol oxidation is lipid peroxidation. Once lipid hydroperoxides are formed they break down to form reactive compounds which in turn leads to the modification of LDL-cholesterol. Macrophages take up the oxidized LDL-cholesterol particles and convert them into foam cells, which are thought to evolve into atherosclerotic plaque. This raises the possibility that antioxidant vitamins, which prevent or inhibit the oxidation of LDL-cholesterol, may reduce the risk of heart disease.

Increased dietary consumption of vitamin E is difficult to achieve because it is found only in a limited number of foods, namely margarine and oils. Individuals with elevated serum cholesterol levels are counseled to limit their intake of fats and therefore tend to have a low vitamin E intake.

Antioxidant Research

Reports in the scientific and lay literatures ascribe numerous attributes to the antioxidants, notably as anticancer, antiheart disease, antirespiratory disease, antiaging, and anticataract agents. Some investigators have studied the primary or the secondary prevention role of antioxidants, while others have investigated both.

Currently, laboratory animal and human studies are being conducted in the United States, Canada, Europe, and Japan. The scientific study designs mainly assess the relationships between dietary intake and targeted disease occurrence or progression; or dietary antioxidant intake and blood levels compared with markers of oxidant stress.

Evaluation of Published Results

Although a plethora of studies has been published, no definitive answers as to the effect of antioxidants on heart disease and cancer have emerged. Study

designs are beset by flaws such as
- failure to control for known confounding variables (including diet control);
- the short-term nature or limited number of animal subjects;
- overreliance on small statistical differences rather than large differences in actual outcomes;
- assignment of causality to statistical associations.

Some studies do disclose individual variability within aggregated data. Genetic markers rarely are ascertained. Dietary intake data are also weak, yet dietary intake is cited as the variable of interest. Even when dietary data are included, reported intake quantities stem from self-reported data unsubjected to computerized nutrient analysis. Primarily studied are those antioxidants known to have few toxic effects when consumed at levels above the RDAs, for example, beta carotene and vitamins C and E rather than selenium. In human subjects receiving concomitant drug therapies, drug-nutrient interactions are not addressed. Furthermore, in conflict with accepted scientific procedures for drug studies, most antioxidant studies lack laboratory analysis of the nutrients actually contained in the foods or supplements consumed, and of the subjects' absorption and excretion levels of these nutrients.

Consensus exists among scientists and public policy agencies around the world that some of the evidence from early studies is promising, but additional research is necessary to arrive at definitive answers regarding the therapeutic roles of antioxidants. To date, the American Heart Association, the American Cancer Society, and the National Cancer Institute do not recommend vitamin or mineral supplementation. Along with other dietary and lifestyle advice, they continue to recommend frequent consumption of fruits and vegetables. The Food and Drug Administration currently does not permit the inclusion of health claims pertaining to antioxidants on the labels of any food, beverage, or dietary or nutritional supplement.

Phytochemicals/Chemopreventors

There is some evidence which has shown that individuals who consume a diet rich in fruits and vegetables have a lower incidence of certain types of cancer. Recently, interest has focused on substances known as phytochemicals, which are present in plant foods, that may help to protect cells from mutagens and carcinogens through a variety of mechanisms listed Table 2-6.

The number of phytochemicals that have been identified to protect cells from injury is long. For example, ellagic acid found in grapes has been found to scavenge carcinogens and may render them unable to alter the cell's DNA. Cruciferous vegetables, such as broccoli, cauliflower, brussel sprouts, contain indoles which enhance the activites of enzymes that make the hormone estrogen less effective. Broccoli also contains dithiolthiones, which stimulate protective enzymes such as glutathione S-transferase, which also is reported to

Table 2-6   Phytochemicals: Mechanisms of action.

Extracellular

Reduce or inhibit the formation of mutagens and carcinogens during food preparation

Reduce the bioavailability of mutagens and carcinogens

Accelerate intestinal transit

Protect the intestinal mucosal barrier

Modify intestinal microbial flora

Inhibit the penetration of cells by mutagens and carcinogens

Intracellular

Enhance the activities of enzymes involved in detoxification of mutagens and carcinogens

Inhibit the activities of enzymes involved in formation of mutagenic and carcinogenic metabolites

Scavenge reactive oxygen species

Inhibit metabolic activation

Protect DNA

Inhibit the detrimental effects of procarcinogens on DNA

Source: Adapted with permission from Stavric B. Antimutagens and anticarcinogens in foods. *Food Chem Toxicol* 1994;32:79–90.

detoxify carcinogens. Soybeans contain the compound, genistein, which has antitumorigenic properties that specifically prevent the formation of new capillaries that are necessary for tumor growth and metastasis.

In conclusion, further research needs to be done in this quickly growing field because much of the evidence is based on animal studies and the anticarcinogenic activity of chemopreventers is poorly understood. In addition human studies need to be controlled for other variables, such as total fat consumption, alcohol use, and exercise. However, the best advice to give individuals is to eat a varied diet including the recommended three to five servings of fruits and vegetables daily.

See Chapter Review Questions, pages A4–A5.

REFERENCES

Alabaster O, Blumberg J, Stempfer MJ, et al. Do antioxidants really prevent disease. *Pat Care* 1995;18–44.

Anonymous. NIH Consensus Development and Panel on Optimal Calcium Intake. *JAMA* 1994;93(1):137–145.

Anonymous. The effect of vitamin E and beta carotene on the incidence of lung cancer and other cancers in male smokers. The Alpha-Tocopherol, Beta-Carotene Cancer Prevention Study Group. *N Engl J Med* 1994;330:1029–1035.

Berkow R, Fletcher AJ (eds). *The Merck Manual: Diagnosis and Therapy.* 16th ed. Rahway, NJ: Merck, 1992.

Daly LE, Kirke PN, Molloy A, et al. Folate levels and neural tube defects. Implications for prevention. *JAMA* 1995;274:1698–1702.

Food and Nutrition Board. National Research Council. *Recommended Dietary Allowances* (RDA). National Academy Press. 10th Edition.Washington, DC, 1989.

Groff JL, Gropper SS, Hunt SM. *Advanced Nutrition and Human Metabolism.* St. Paul: West, 1995.

Hodis HN, Mack WJ, LaBree L, et al. Serial coronary angiographic evidence that antioxidant vitamin intake reduces progression of coronary artery atherosclerosis. *JAMA* 1995;273:1849–1854.

Hoffman RM, Garewal HS. Antioxidants and the prevention of coronary heart disease. *Arch Int Med* 1995;155:241–246.

Hunter DJ, Manson JE, Colditz GA. A prospective study of the intake of vitamins C, E, and A and the risk of breast cancer. *N Engl J Med* 1993;329:234–240.

Jialal I, Fuller CJ, Huet BA. The effect of α-tocopherol supplementation on LDL oxidation. A dose-response study. *Arterioscler Thromb Vasc Biol* 1995;15:190–198.

Linder MC. *Nutritional Biochemistry and Metabolism with Clinical Application.* 2nd ed. New York: Elsevier, 1991.

Rimm EB, Stempfer MJ, Ascherio A, et al. Vitamin E consumption and the risk of coronary heart disease in men. *N Engl J Med* 1993;328:1450–1456.

Robinson CH, Weigley ES, Mueller DH. *Basic Nutrition and Diet Therapy.* 7th ed. New York: Macmillan, 1993.

Shils ME, Olson JA, Shike M (eds). *Modern Nutrition in Health and Disease.* 8th ed. Philadelphia: Lea and Febiger, 1994.

Stavric B. Role of Chemopreventers in Human Diet. *Clin Biochem* 1994;27: 319–326.

Stempfer MJ, Hennekens CH, Manson JE, et al. Vitamin E consumption and the risk of coronary disease in women. *N Engl J Med* 1993;328:1444–1449.

Symposium on antioxidant vitamins. *Amer J Med* 1994;97(Suppl 3A):1S–28S.

Zeman FJ. *Clinical Nutrition and Dietetics.* 2nd ed. New York: Macmillan, 1991.

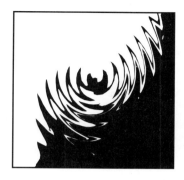

P A R T   I I

Nutritional Assessment Throughout the Life Cycle

3

Nutrition in Pregnancy and Lactation

Carine M. Lenders and Susan Ahlstrom Henderson

Objectives

- To determine the appropriate weight gain during pregnancy for normal weight, underweight, and overweight pregnant women.
- To understand the additional vitamin and mineral requirements for women during pregnancy.
- To counsel overweight and underweight pregnant women about appropriate dietary intake and weight gain during pregnancy.
- To recommend dietary modifications to help alleviate nausea, heartburn, and constipation during pregnancy.
- To identify pregnant women with special nutrient needs.

Nutrition plays a key role in normal as well as in high-risk pregnancies (e.g., twins and gestational diabetes). Pregnancy is an anabolic state resulting in an increased need for energy and nutrients. Pregnant women who are drug or alcohol abusers, vegetarians, smokers, anorexic or bulimic, underweight, or obese may have nutrition problems that can negatively affect the health of the fetus. Certain signs and symptoms such as hyperemesis (excessive vomiting), poor weight gain, weight loss, dehydration, and constipation during pregnancy also have nutritional implications. The goals of nutrition assessment in pregnancy are to

- identify conditions that could lead to a nutrition problem
- identify the nutrition problems that lead to specific conditions
- develop a management plan for nutrition problem(s)

Metabolic and Physiological Changes of Pregnancy

A woman's diet and nutritional status play a vital role in pregnancy. During pregnancy, metabolic and physiological changes occur in association with the growth and development of the fetus and maternal body composition. Changes include growth of the feto-placental unit, increased maternal blood volume, increased maternal fat stores, changes in GI motility, and breast development. An increase in feto-placental hormones associated with a corresponding increase in maternal insulin resistance favors glucose delivery to the fetus and the use of fatty acids by extrauterine tissues. However, additional energy and other nutrients required by the fetus must be supplied by the maternal diet, which is thus an important factor for optimal pregnancy outcome.

Integrating Nutrition into the Obstetrical History and Physical Exam

Prenatal Nutrition Assessment

Evaluation of a pregnant woman's nutritional status includes clinical, dietary, and laboratory components. The purpose of the nutrition assessment is to identify women with nutritional risk factors that could jeopardize their health and/or that of the fetus. Information obtained during the evaluation is used to develop a care plan and set goals jointly with the woman. Many women are especially receptive to nutrition counseling during pregnancy, making this an appropriate time to encourage the development of good nutritional practices. Pregnant women with nutritional risk factors should be referred to a registered dietitian for nutrition therapy.

Relevant Medical, Obstetrical, Lifestyle, and Psychosocial History

A major objective of the health care team is to collect sufficient information to identify pregnant women at nutritional risk. The medical history should include maternal risk factors such as infections, diabetes, phenylketonuria (PKU), sickle cell disease, hypertension, renal disease, anorexia, and bulimia. Young gynecological age (current age minus age at menarche), previous nutritional deficiencies, and caffeine, tobacco, drug, and alcohol use also should be identified.

The obstetrical history of previous pregnancies includes parity, weight-gain patterns, pregnancy intervals, nausea and vomiting, prior deliveries involving low birth weight, premature infants, or infants that were small for their gestational age, stillbirth, abortions, perinatal death, past history of gestational diabetes or pregnancy-induced hypertension, and contraceptive use. Additional questions regarding social, economic, and emotional stresses are important because they may influence a pregnant woman's nutritional status. Questions should address participation in medical and food assistance programs, help from family and the baby's father, the woman's feelings about the pregnancy, and her current workload.

Dietary Assessment

The format used to gather information about current and past dietary practices may be either an interview or a questionnaire. Pertinent information includes dietary habits such as appetite, meal patterns, skipping meals, snacks, cultural and religious practices or restrictions, vegetarianism, and food cravings and aversions. Information about abnormal eating practices such as following food fads and eating behaviors such as bingeing, purging, laxative or diuretic use, or pica (eating nonfood items: ice, detergent, starch, chalk, clay, rocks, and so on) is also essential. Other relevant information includes the habitual use of caffeinated beverages, sugar substitutes and other special "diet" foods, alcohol, tobacco, prescription and nonprescription drugs, vitamin and mineral supplements, and illicit drugs. A woman's current dietary practice can be assessed using a diet history or food frequency questionnaire. These methods are useful for identifying potential nutritional risks such as omission of food groups, poor total dietary intake, and excessive use of calorie-dense foods.

Physical Evaluation

An essential part of the clinical evaluation is assessing prepregnancy weight for height by calculating the body mass index (BMI = weight (kg)/height (m²)) or using BMI tables (see Figure 3-1). The BMI is used to evaluate weight status and to help the woman set appropriate weight-gain goals. Whenever possible,

Figure 3-1 **Directions: To find BMI category (e.g., obese), find the point where the woman's height and weight intersect. To estimate BMI, read the bold number on the dashed line that is closest to this point.**

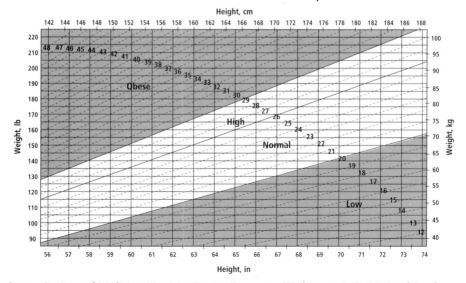

Source: Institute of Medicine. *Nutrition During Pregnancy.* Washington D.C.: National Academy Press, 1990.

prepregnancy weight should be ascertained from clinical records obtained just prior to pregnancy. Current weight should also be measured and assessed at each visit.

Laboratory Evaluation

Routine tests related to the nutritional status of pregnant women include evaluation for anemia (hemoglobin, hematocrit). When iron stores are questionable, as in the case of pregnant women with sickle cell disease, serum ferritin should also be tested. Routine tests for diabetes, including urinary ketones and glucose and serum glucose tests, should also be conducted.

Maternal Weight-Gain Recommendations

Maternal weight gain is attributable both to maternal weight and to feto-placental expansion during pregnancy. During the first half of pregnancy, weight gain reflects changes in maternal stores. In the second half of gestation, barring the development of maternal edema, weight gain is chiefly the result of the fetal growth. Because the relationship between maternal weight gain and infant birth weight has been clearly demonstrated, following the pattern of weight gain during pregnancy is important.

Low prepregnancy weight and low maternal weight gain are risk factors for intrauterine growth retardation, low birth weight, and increased incidence of perinatal death. Weight-gain goals vary depending on the prepregnancy BMI of the woman, the number of fetuses (twins, triplets, etc.), race, and the mother's age group. Current weight-gain recommendations set by the Institute of Medicine for a normal pregnancy are the same as those summarized by the American College of Obstetrics and Gynecologists (see Table 3-1).

Table 3-1   **Recommended total weight gain ranges* for pregnant women by prepregnancy body mass index (BMI).**

PREPREGNANT BMI CATEGORY	TOTAL WEIGHT (kg)	(kg)/ 4 WEEKS	TOTAL WEIGHT (lbs)	lbs/ 4 WEEKS
Underweight (BMI < 19.8)	12.7–18.2	2.3	28–40	5.0
Normal (BMI = 19.8 to 26.0)	11.4–15.9	1.8	25–35	4.0
Overweight (BMI = 26.1 to 29.0)	6.8–11.4	1.2	15–25	2.6
Obese (BMI > 29.0)	6.8	0.9	>15	2.0
Twin gestation	15.9–20.4	2.7	35–45	6.0

BMI = weight (kg)/height (m²).
*Applies to the second and third trimesters only.
Source: Institute of Medicine. *Nutrition During Pregnancy.* Washington, D.C.: National Academy Press, 1990.

Weight gain in short women (<157 cm) should fall toward the lower end of the recommended range for their BMI. Conversely, African-Americans and young adolescents (both groups at increased risk for low birth weight) should be encouraged to set weight-gain goals at the upper end of the recommended range based on their BMI. The younger the adolescent, the more weight she needs to gain to account for normal maternal growth during the nine months of gestation. Nonpregnant 13-year-olds who menstruated at age 12 tend on average to gain an additional 7 to 8 pounds. Because of this potential maternal growth and the competition for nutrients between the pregnant adolescent and her fetus, additional weight gain, especially among the most recently postmenarcheal, is advised.

Recommendations for Utilizing Maternal Weight-Gain Information

Prior to conception, consistent, reliable procedures should be used to measure and record the woman's weight and height (without shoes) accurately in the medical record. Based on this information, the following procedures may then be implemented readily during pregnancy.

- Determine the prepregnancy body mass index (BMI = weight (kg)/height (m^2)) or plot the woman's height and weight on the BMI chart (see Table 3-1).
- Measure height and weight at the first prenatal visit, using standardized procedures.

   Based on the prepregnancy BMI set a weight-gain goal, with the woman at the beginning of the initial comprehensive prenatal examination (see Table 3-1).

   Explain the importance of appropriate weight gain.

- At each subsequent prenatal visit, record and compare her weight gain to the recommended weight gain.

   Identify any abnormal weight-gain pattern that may indicate a need for nutrition intervention.

   Assess the actual rate of gain with respect to the established weight-gain goal.

- When weight gain is abnormal, talk with the woman about her usual intake, exercise level, and gastrointestinal symptoms such as nausea and vomiting.

Maternal Nutrient Needs

A woman's energy needs increase on average by 15 percent during the second and third trimesters of pregnancy. However, the most significant increases in nutrient needs are for protein, vitamins, and minerals. Protein needs increase by about 30 percent, folic acid needs by 200 percent, calcium and phosphorus needs by 50 percent, magnesium needs by 15 percent, and iron needs by at least 100 percent. Therefore, it is vital that pregnant women eat increased quantities of food. In addition, it is important to note that a deficiency or excess of selected nutrients during certain gestational periods may lead to poor pregnancy outcome. For example, early pregnancy is pivotal for organogenesis, mid-pregnancy for human brain growth, and late pregnancy for major increases in the number of fetal adipose tissue, muscle, and pancreas cells.

Note that incremental energy and nutrient intake recommendations for pregnancy generally do not consider age, resting metabolic rates, body size, physical activity, or pathological conditions. Much controversy exists over most nutrient recommendations for pregnant women because of lack of controlled studies, diverse individual nutritional needs and dietary backgrounds, diverse nutrient supplements and quantities used, duration of supplementation, patient compliance controls, physical activity, seasonality, and patient access to health care facilities.

Current Recommendations

The recommended dietary allowances (RDAs) and estimated safe and adequate daily dietary intakes (ESADDIs) for pregnant and lactating women are listed in Table 3-2. These recommendations are based on estimates derived from accretion rates of nutrients measured in fetuses, as well as from clinical and epidemiological data.

Energy Total energy needs during pregnancy are extrapolated from the average energy cost of pregnancy, estimated at more than 55,000 calories for a 40-week gestation. This figure represents approximately a 15 percent increase in energy needs compared to those of nonpregnant women. No additional energy is needed during the first trimester, except for those women with depleted bodily nutrient reserves due to conditions such as severe hyperemesis gravidarum or severe famine. Caloric intake requirements of pregnancy are estimated to be 300 kcal/day greater than normal during the second and third trimesters.

Protein The RDA for the pregnant woman is 60 grams per day, a 30 percent increase in the 46 grams per day recommended for non-pregnant women. This recommended increase in protein intake is intended to provide additional protein deposits in maternal (i.e., blood, uterine, and breast), fetal, and placental tissues.

Calcium Studies of maternal calcium supplementation with 1000 to 2000 mg/day tend to show a reduction of pregnancy-induced hypertension, preeclampsia, incidence of low birth weight, and premature delivery rates. Increased calcium intake is also recommended because of the potential risk of maternal bone demineralization during pregnancy. Therefore, the NIH Consensus Development and Panel on Optimal Calcium Intake recently recommended 1200–1500 mg/day for pregnant and lactating women. The best sources of calcium are found in dairy products. Women should be encouraged

Table 3-2 Recommended daily allowances (RDAs) and estimated safe and adequate daily dietary intakes (ESADDIs) for women of child-bearing age.

NUTRIENT	NONPREGNANT	PREGNANT	LACTATING
Protein (g)	46	60	65
Vitamin A (mcg RE)[a]	800	800	1300
Vitamin D (mcg)	10	10	10
Vitamin E (mcg)	8	10	12
Vitamin K (mcg)	55	55	65
Vitamin C (mg)	60	70	95
Thiamin (mg)	1.1	1.5	1.6
Riboflavin (mg)	1.3	1.6	1.8
Niacin (mg NE)[b]	15	17	20
Vitamin B_6 (mg)	1.6	2.2	2.1
Folic acid (mg)	0.18	0.4	0.28
Vitamin B_{12} (mcg)	2.0	2.2	2.6
Calcium (mg)	800	1200	1200
Phosphorus (mg)	800	1200	1200
Magnesium (mg)	280	300	355
Iron (elemental) (mg)	15	30	15
Zinc (mg)	12	15	19
Iodine (mcg)	150	175	200
Selenium (mcg)	55	65	75

[a] Retinol equivalents.
[b] Niacin equivalents.
Source: Institute of Medicine. *Nutrition During Pregnancy.* Washington, D.C.: National Academy Press, 1990.

Table 3-3 Recommended servings per day by food groups.

FOOD GROUP	SERVINGS/DAY
Bread and cereals	6 or more servings
Vegetables	3 to 5 servings
Fruits	2 to 4 servings
Low fat dairy products	3 to 5 (1 cup/serving)
Meat or meat substitutes	2 to 3 (3 to 4 oz./serving)
Alcohol	Contraindicated

to include three to five servings of yogurt, milk, hard cheeses, and green leafy vegetables in their daily diets. Use of lactase tablets or drops, lactose digested milk, or calcium supplements should be encouraged for women with lactose intolerance (see Table 3-3).

Magnesium Magnesium supplementation is controversial. Some studies indicate that magnesium supplementation (>320 mg/day) for pregnant women results in lower rates of preeclampsia, premature delivery, and fetal growth retardation, and fewer neonatal referrals to infant intensive care units. To increase magnesium intake, higher intakes of vegetables and unrefined grains are suggested during pregnancy.

Vitamin D Vitamin D supplementation (10 to 25 mcg/day) has been associated with higher serum values in women with vitamin D deficiency, increased fetal birth weight, and decreased incidences of neonatal hypocalcemia, neonatal seizures, and maternal osteomalacia. Sources of vitamin D include vitamin D fortified cow's milk or margarine, eggs, and butter. Most commercial yogurts are not fortified with vitamin D. Lack of exposure to the sun also contributes to low serum vitamin D levels.

Vitamin A In Western countries, vitamin A supplements are not required because of the adequate amounts found in the food supply. Vitamin A toxicity during pregnancy is associated with teratogenic effects on the fetus.

Folic Acid The hypothesis that folate supplementation in pregnant women decreases the risk of neural-tube defects in their offspring has been controversial for the past 30 years. However, a double blind, controlled, randomized clinical trial of pregnant women receiving vitamins with folic acid in Hungary (N = 4732) showed such a decrease in comparison with the expected occurrence of neonatal neural-tube defects. Recent studies have also confirmed these results.

To be most effective, folic acid supplementation must be started before conception. Folic acid supplementation during pregnancy is especially important during the first four weeks after conception, before the closure of the neural tube. Pregnant women are now supplemented with 0.4 mg/day of folic acid, the current RDA recommendation, throughout their pregnancy. Sources of folic acid include green leafy vegetables, potatoes, oranges and other fruits, and liver, but up to 50 percent of this nutrient is destroyed by usual food preparation, processing, and storage methods.

The recommended maximum daily intake of folic acid is 1 mg (1000 mcg) because higher doses may mask a vitamin B$_{12}$ deficiency. However, up to 4 mg of folic acid is suggested for women under the supervision of a physician who have a previous history of children born with neural-tube defects. Most current prenatal vitamin and mineral tablets contain at least 0.8 mg of folic acid, the normal RDA for folic acid for healthy adults in the United States.

Zinc Several studies have shown that high dietary intake of zinc is associated with decreased premature delivery and perinatal mortality rates and increased gestational duration. Major dietary sources of zinc in the United States include meat products, and to a lesser extent, whole-grain foods.

Iron Iron supplementation during pregnancy is important because low dietary iron has been associated with increased premature delivery rates and decreased birth weight. Controversy exists on the beneficial effects of iron supplements in nonanemic pregnant women. The best available iron sources contain heme iron, found in meat products. Iron in its less bioavailable form, nonheme iron, is found in vegetables and fortified cereals. Concurrent intake of vitamin C aids in the body's absorption of nonheme iron.

Ideally, iron supplements should be taken between meals because of their possible interaction with other nutrients, but doing so may produce gastrointestinal side effects such as constipation. Coated tablets may alleviate these symptoms but the amount of iron that the body absorbs from these tablets is much lower. The recommended elemental iron dose during pregnancy is 30 mg/day; therapeutic doses of 60 to 120 mg/day are prescribed for anemic pregnant women.

Fiber Fiber recommendations do not exist for pregnant women. Increased intake of high-fiber foods, such as fresh vegetables and fruits, is especially helpful to alleviate constipation, a common problem during pregnancy.

Fluids Fluids should be increased during pregnancy. Usual recommendations are to drink 8 to 10 glasses of water per day. Tap water consumption should be discouraged in areas where the water supply is suspected to contain lead because it may result in decreased stature and deficient neurocognitive development of the baby.

Mercury Mercury intoxication associated with contaminated grains and fish can lead to cerebral palsy, mental retardation, and multiple organ failure in newborns. Vegetables and fruits should be carefully washed and rinsed with soap or peeled. Eating raw fish (sushi, for example) or fish caught in contaminated waters should be avoided during pregnancy.

Alcohol Excessive consumption of alcohol, a potent teratogen, by pregnant women causes fetal alcohol syndrome (FAS). Although little evidence exists that drinking one alcoholic beverage can cause birth defects, even a small amount of alcohol may adversely affect a developing or growing fetal organ, especially during the first trimester. Therefore, alcohol intake should be avoided by pregnant women. Alcohol use, especially during pregnancy, can also result in decreased dietary intake, impaired metabolism and absorption of nutrients, and altered nutrient activation and utilization. Multivitamin and mineral supplementation is especially indicated for pregnant women who abuse alcohol. However, nutritional supplementation should not replace efforts to encourage women to avoid alcohol during pregnancy.

Caffeine Whether or not an acceptable level of caffeine intake during pregnancy exists is a somewhat controversial question. Recent studies indicate an association between excessive caffeine intake and increased risk of fetal loss, supporting the United States Food and Drug Administration's recommendation that pregnant women reduce their caffeine intake from coffee, tea, cocoa, and cola drinks.

Artificial Sweeteners The incidence of spontaneous abortion has not been associated with the use of any artificial sweetener. Because saccharine has been shown to be a weak teratogenic agent in rats, moderation of its use during childbearing years and especially during pregnancy and lactation is appropriate. Concerns have been raised about the use of aspartame (Nutrasweet) during pregnancy, because elevated serum phenylalanine in pregnant women with poorly controlled phenylketonuria (PKU) is known to cause fetal brain damage. However, individuals who do not suffer from PKU generally have sufficient liver phenylalanine hydroxylase activity to prevent a substantial increase in phenylalanine levels in the blood after consuming phenylalanine-rich foods.

Vitamin and Mineral Supplementation Guidelines

Routine vitamin/mineral supplementation for women reporting appropriate dietary intake and demonstrating adequate weight gain (without edema) is not mandatory. However, most obstetricians prescribe a prenatal vitamin and mineral supplement because many pregnant women do not consume enough food to meet their increased nutritional requirements, especially with regard to folic acid during the first trimester of pregnancy. The following summary characterizes conditions in pregnant woman who are at risk for nutrient deficiencies. In the presence of any of these factors, supplementation with a prenatal vitamin is advised.

- Pregnancy involving multiple gestations (twins, triplets)
- Frequent gestations (a pregnancy every year)
- Tobacco use
- Hyperemesis gravidarum
- Eating disorders, including anorexia, bulimia, and compulsive eating
- Obesity or underweight
- Adolescence
- Alcohol and drug abuse
- Strict vegetarianism (avoidance of all animal products, including dairy)

Pregnant women with the following medical conditions, as well as those of low socioeconomic status, may require special therapeutic diets and should be referred to a registered dietitian.

- Diabetes mellitus
- Sickle cell disease
- Phenylketonuria (PKU)
- Hypertension
- Chronic renal disease
- Malabsorptive disease

Common Nutritional Problems During Pregnancy

Discomforts of pregnancy such as nausea and vomiting, constipation, and heartburn may be alleviated by implementing the simple guidelines summarized below.

Nausea and Vomiting   Nausea and vomiting are associated with increased levels of the hormone human chorionic gonadotropin (HCG), which doubles every 48 hours early in pregnancy and peaks at 12 weeks, gestation. Nausea is experienced by 60 percent of pregnant women. Of these, 5 percent require hospitalization for hyperemesis gravidarum. Strategies for managing nausea and vomiting are:

- Eat small, low-fat meals and snacks, and eat slowly.
- Eat low-fat snacks such as fruits, pretzels, and nonfat yogurt.
- Drink fluids between meals, rather than with meals.
- Avoid citrus and tomato products, spearmint, peppermint, and caffeine.
- Avoid spicy and high-fat foods.
- Avoid eating or drinking for one to two hours before lying down and before bedtime.
- Take a walk after meals.
- Wear loose-fitting clothes.

Constipation Constipation during pregnancy is associated with increased progesterone levels and smooth-muscle relaxation of the GI tract. This results in GI discomfort, a bloated sensation, increased hemorrhoids, and decreased appetite. Strategies for managing constipation include the following.

- Drink two to three quarts of fluids a day, including water, juice, milk, and soup.
- Eat high-fiber cereals, whole grains, legumes, fruits, and vegetables daily.
- Participate in physical activity such as walking and swimming.

Heartburn or Indigestion Heartburn and indigestion are usually caused by gastric reflux after a large meal. Limited gastric capacity, secondary to a shift of organs to accommodate the growing fetus and support other organs, often contributes to these symptoms. Strategies for managing heartburn or indigestion are the same as those suggested previously for managing nausea.

Decreased Self-esteem Changes in hormonal levels may result in decreased self-esteem due to changes in body perception. Women with poor body images often limit their food intake, thus depriving the fetus of needed nourishment. Appropriate weight gain and proper nutrition are essential to produce a healthy baby and maintain the mother's health.

Lactation (Breast-Feeding)

Metabolic and Physiological Changes During Lactation

Breast enlargement begins early in pregnancy due to the hormones generated by the pituitary gland and the corpus luteum. The lacteal cells also differentiate in preparation for producing milk and releasing it when the infant is born. As the breast undergoes these preparatory changes, the areola (the brown-pigmented area surrounding the nipple) becomes darker and more prominent, and the skin over the nipple becomes harder and more erect to facilitate suckling.

Lactogenesis is believed to be initiated by the abrupt decrease in progesterone and estrogen following parturition. As the infant begins to suckle and thus stimulates the receptors in the nipple and areola, nerve impulses are sent to the hypothalamus. The hypothalamus stimulates the release of the hormones oxytocin and prolactin from the posterior pituitary gland. Prolactin stimulates milk production in the breast, and oxytocin stimulates the breast to contract and eject milk from the alveolus. Milk accumulates in the lactiferous sinuses under the areola and is released when the areola is compressed between the baby's tongue and palate. Factors that may influence milk production and composition include the following.

- Nutritional status of the mother, including fluid intake (recommended: 3 quarts per day)
- Breast-feeding schedule (frequent nursing increases milk supply)
- Breast care (after feeding, wash with water only and air dry)
- Infant weight and maturity
- Infant illness
- Maternal age and parity (number of children previously borne)
- Maternal stress
- Maternal use of cigarettes, alcohol, and oral contraceptives

Benefits of Breast-Feeding

Although breast-feeding has many advantages, studies from the 1970s showed that in the United States only 20 percent of women were breast-feeding their infants when they left the hospital following delivery. Less than 10 percent continued to breast-feed after six months. Aggressive national efforts to promote breast-feeding increased these statistics in the number of women who were breast-feeding on discharge from the hospital in 1988 to about 50 percent, but only 20 percent continue to breast-feed after six months. The current Healthy People 2000 Goals are to have 75 percent of mothers breast-feeding their infants. Specific benefits of breast-feeding include the following.

Immunological Benefits Breast milk contains over 100 substances with anti-infective properties. These include leukocytes (macrophages), immunoglobulins (secretory IgA, IgG, IgM, and antiviral antibodies), bifidus factor (to support GI *Lactobacillus bifidus*), lysozyme (promotes lysis of bacteria), interferon, and lactoferrin (binds whey protein and inhibits growth of *E.coli*).

Research has demonstrated that infants who are breast-fed exclusively during the first four months of life experience a decreased incidence of ear infections (acute otitis media), gastroenteritis, and respiratory illnesses during their first year of life as well as a decreased risk of otitis media for the first seven years of life. Breast-fed infants are also hospitalized less during their first six months of life.

Convenience Breast milk is ready to serve. Already at the proper temperature, it does not require heating, special preparation such as mixing with sterilized water, or storage. Except in certain cases where the mother has a communicable illness, breast milk is clean. Breast milk is a very economical food source that is adequate without supplementation until the baby is four to six months old.

Allergy Avoidance Feeding breast milk to a child significantly decreases the possibility of allergy or intolerance to cow's milk when it is introduced.

Reduced Incidence of Overfeeding Breast-fed infants are less likely to be overfed than their formula-fed counterparts.

Physiological and Social Benefits: Breast-feeding promotes good jaw and tooth development in the infant and also fosters mother-infant bonding.

Breast-feeding also has a number of mostly beneficial effects on maternal well-being including:

- delayed return of ovulation
- decreased accumulation of adipose tissue
- accelerated weight loss
- increased risk of osteoporosis
- decreased breast cancer rate

Table 3-4 lists several suggestions for the promotion of breast-feeding.

Table 3-4   What health professionals can do to promote breast-feeding.

- Encourage education on the benefits of breast-feeding at medical school, during residency, and in continuing medical education courses.
- Give patients preconception and prenatal guidance and preparation.
- Become familiar with how to initiate lactation and manage common problems.
- Give patients educational materials that promote breast-feeding.
- Help patients start breast-feeding within one hour of delivery.
- Give patients postpartum support.
- Support hospital initiatives to encourage breast-feeding.
- Work with hospitals to eliminate formula in discharge packs.
- Encourage hospital nursery policy that avoids all supplemental feedings and bottles, particularly at the initiation of lactation.
- Avoid medications that are unsafe during lactation, and choose alternatives with less distribution in the milk.

Source: Ackerman L. Breast-feeding. The primary care physician's role. *Family Practice Recertification.* 1995;17(8):32–53.

Types of Breast Milk

The human breast produces three distinct types of milk, depending on the age of the infant, the time of day, and whether it is early or late in a given nursing period. Colostrum, produced during the first few days of lactation, is high in protein, immunoglobulins, ß-carotene, sodium, potassium, chloride, fat-soluble vitamins and minerals. These substances encourage the growth of bifidus flora of the GI tract and the passage of the merconium or first stools. Transitional milk is produced during days six through fifteen and is higher in fat and lactose and lower in protein and minerals than colostrum. Mature milk, produced from day fifteen through weaning, provides 20 to 22 calories per ounce.

Breast Milk Composition

Breast milk is rich in all of the nutrients required to sustain the newborn during the first six months of life. Among the nutrients present in breast milk are the following components.

Fat The total amount of fat in breast milk is constant but its composition varies. Initially, breast milk is similar to skim milk, with a relatively low fat content. As the infant continues to suckle and a period of let down occurs, breast milk becomes higher in fat and calories. Encouraging the infant to suckle on each breast for at least ten minutes ensures adequate calorie consumption. The emptying time of breast milk from the infant's stomach is, on average, one and a half hours, compared to three hours for formula-fed infants. Therefore, breast-fed babies usually need to nurse every two hours for the first few months of life. The fat content of breast milk provides 50 percent of the infant's total energy requirements. The other 50 percent comes from protein and carbohydrates combined.

Protein Breast milk contains whey and casein. Whey protein accounts for 60 to 80 percent of the total protein in breast milk and is present mainly in the form of alpha-lactalbumin, lactoferrin and secretory IgA. Casein accounts for 20 to 40 percent of breast milk's total protein and forms micelles that enhance the infant's ability to absorb calcium, phosphorus, iron, zinc, and copper.

Carbohydrates The primary carbohydrate source in breast milk is lactose. Small amounts of glucose, oligosaccharides, and glycoproteins are also present.

Fluoride Breast-fed infants (and formula-fed infants whose formulas are prepared with nonfluoridated water) who do not receive fluoridated water require oral supplementation of fluoride for normal teeth development and to prevent cavities beginning at six months of age.

Vitamin D Breast-fed infants are at risk for rickets caused by vitamin D deficiency because breast milk contains only small quantities of this nutrient. Infants therefore benefit from vitamin D supplementation (400 IU/day), particularly if their bodies are always covered or they receive little exposure to sunlight during the winter months.

Vitamin K Breast milk contains a small amount of vitamin K, but supplementation after delivery generally is not necessary, provided that vitamin K is administered routinely via intramuscular injection in the newborn nursery.

Nutritional Recommendations for Lactating Women

Approximately 85 kcal are required to produce 100 ml of breast milk. Stored energy from maternal fat reserves provides 100 to 150 kcal/day. Current recommendations therefore advise that the daily caloric intake of lactating women be increased by 500 kcal/day. Consequently, maternal weight loss will be progressive throughout lactation, but should not exceed 4.5 pounds (2 kg) per month to ensure the baby's continued, adequate growth. If the amount of calcium in the mother's diet is inadequate, 2 to 8 percent of her body's calcium is lost in breast milk during lactation.

Iron requirements are lower during lactation than during pregnancy until menstruation resumes. In the United States, studies of lactating women consuming 2700 kcal/day suggest that they are not likely to meet the RDAs for calcium and zinc. Diets that contain under 2700 kcal/day may also be low in magnesium, vitamin B6, and folate. Adolescent mothers' diets may also be low in iron. Among adults of low socioeconomic status, diets are often low in calcium and vitamin A.

Prenatal vitamin supplements are routinely prescribed to lactating women to ensure adequate intake. However, lactating women should be encouraged to obtain their nutrients from a well-balanced, varied diet, rather than from a combined multivitamin and mineral supplement. They can achieve this goal by consuming at least three servings of dairy products and eating a wide variety of breads, cereals, grains, fruits, vegetables, and meats or meat alternatives daily. Eating one good food source of vitamin A (e.g., carrots, kale, or sweet potatoes) and vitamin C (e.g., orange juice, strawberries, or tomatoes) daily is recommended. Breast-feeding women should also continue to drink 2 to 3 quarts of fluids per day following delivery to prevent dehydration. Postpartum women should avoid diets and medications that promise rapid weight loss. Weight loss should always be gradual, and this is particularly true for lactating women, who burn more calories than nonlactating women to support breast milk production and may experience accelerated weight loss naturally as a consequence.

We know very little about the effect of the mother's diet and nutritional status on milk production and composition and even less about the effects of lactation on maternal health. The major indicator of the adequacy of the mother's diet during lactation is usually the health of the nursing infant rather than that of the mother. However, acute weight loss in a lactating woman is a warning for possible adverse effects on milk production and composition.

Common Problems Experienced While Breast-Feeding

Physicians can readily manage most of the more common problems associated with breast-feeding. Table 3-5 lists the most common problems and the suggested treatments. Breast-feeding is contraindicated in the following conditions:

Maternal Infections Tuberculosis, typhoid, herpes, rubella, mumps, HIV, and cytomegalovirus (CMV) are all contraindications for breast-feeding.

Medications Many medications and illegal substances, as well as nicotine, pass into breast milk when ingested by the mother and thus are indirectly administered to the child as well. This factor must be considered when treating any woman who is breast-feeding. Several drugs, including nicotine and estrogen-containing oral contraceptives, can decrease milk supply and interfere with milk production. Exposure of the nursing infant to medications may be minimized if the mother takes the medication after breast-feeding. Specific drugs that are contraindicated in the treatment of breast-feeding

Table 3-5   Common problems experienced while breast-feeding.

PROBLEMS	TREATMENT
Nipple	
Inverted nipples	Identify before delivery; recommend nipple shells.
Sore nipples	Advise patients to avoid soaps and ointments; recommend proper latch on and positioning of the infant.
Breast	
Abscess	Consider needle aspiration or incision and drainage.
Engorgement	Recommend hand expression or pumping; mild heat may soften the areolar mound.
Mastitis	Recommend rest, heat, massage, alternate feeding positions, frequent nursing; give antibiotics that cover *Staphylococcus aureus*.
Milk duct stasis	Recommend rest, heat, massage, alternate feeding positions, frequent nursing.
Infant	
Baby sleeps during feeding	Teach the mother to watch for facial movements indicating hunger; changing the diaper, massage, and visual stimulation may be helpful.
Hungry baby	Increase frequency or length of feedings for growth spurt; milk production will increase.
Jaundice	Identify cause; if it is breast-milk jaundice, continue feedings unless bilirubin is approaching 20 mg/dL (see Table 3-7)
Poor weight gain	Recommend frequent nursing (every two to three hours), adequate length of time for nursing; consider supplemental nursing system.
Other	
Inhibited let down	Warm shower, privacy, local heat, soft music, low lighting, relaxation techniques.
Medications	Assess need, choose drugs safe for lactation.
Monilial infections	Treat with topical antifungals on breast and oral nystatin for infant.
Work-related	Educate the patient about various breast pumps and devices; support and encourage using the pump at work.

Source: Ackerman L. Breast-feeding. The primary care physician's role. *Family Practice Recertification.* 1995;17(8):32–53.

women are bromocriptine, cyclophosphamide, cyclosporine, doxorubicin, ergotamine, lithium, methotrexate, phencyclidine (PCP), and phenindione. Commonly prescribed drugs that are compatible with breast-feeding are listed in Table 3-6. Women who are using illegal substances such as amphetamines, cocaine, heroin, or marijuana should be discouraged from breast-feeding.

Maternal Malnutrition In some cases, although the milk that a malnourished mother produces is inadequate in quantity or content, no better alternative is available to the child, especially in areas plagued by famine.

Jaundice Jaundice is a common problem seen in breast-fed infants, especially among Asians, Native Americans, and Alaskan Eskimos. See Table 3-7 for management of breast-feeding jaundice.

Table 3-6 **Commonly prescribed drugs compatible with breast-feeding.**

ANTIBIOTICS	ANTIHYPERTENSIVES	ANTICONVULSANTS
Ampicillin	Captopril	Carbamazapine
Cloxacillin	Hyperchlorothiazide	Phenobarbital
Dicloxacillin sodium	Methyldopa	Phenytoin
Penicillin		
Erythromycin	**ANALGESICS**	**OTHER**
Cefaclor	Acetaminophen	Digoxin
Cephradine	Aspirin	Heparin
Cephalexin	Codeine	Magnesium sulfate
Clindamycin	Ibuprofen	RhoGAM
		Rubella vaccine
		Warfarin sodium

Source: The transfer of drugs and other chemicals into human breast milk. *Pediatrics* 1994; 93: 137–150.

Table 3-7 **Managing breast-feeding jaundice.**

Early-onset (before five days postpartum)
- Encourage mothers to nurse frequently (at least eight times a day).
- Avoid formula supplementation unless milk production is inadequate.
- Do not give glucose water or sterile water supplementation.
- Monitor serum bilirubin concentrations daily on an outpatient basis.
- Advise mothers they may express milk after feedings to increase milk volume.

Late-onset (5–15 days postpartum)
- If bilirubin concentration reaches 17–20 mg/dL, breast-feeding should be interrupted for 24–48 hours as a diagnostic test.
- Instruct mothers to maintain milk production by regularly expressing their milk during the interruption.
- Monitor serum bilirubin levels every 12–24 hours.
- Resume breast-feeding after a decrease in serum bilirubin concentration confirms the diagnosis.

Source: Freed GL, Landers S, Schanler RJ. A practical guide to successful breast-feeding management. *AJDC* 1991;145:917–921. American Medical Association.

Summary Questions with Nutritional Implications
for the Obstetrical History and Physical Exam

Present Illness
General: Recent weight change, poor weight gain, edema, and dehydration

GI complaints: Diarrhea, nausea, vomiting, heartburn, and constipation

Medical History
Is the woman taking her prenatal vitamins? How often does she take them?

Does the woman take any additional iron supplements?

Does the woman have any food allergies? If yes, to what?

Does the woman have any nonfood cravings (pica: ice, dirt, cornstarch, clay, detergent)?

Social History
Does the woman drink alcohol? If so, type, quantity, frequency, duration?

Was the woman following any special diet prior to becoming pregnant?

How many meals does the woman eat daily? How many snacks?

Does the woman avoid any specific foods such as fruits, vegetables, milk or other dairy products, or meats?

What type of milk does the woman drink? (whole, 2%, 1%, skim, or none)

If the woman has diabetes, does she self-monitor her blood glucose levels?

Family History
Parents, siblings, children, and spouse are identified, and their ages and general health or cause of death are briefly noted. Familial occurrences of disease and any history of children with fetal anomalies are recorded.

Review of Systems
General: Fatigue, weight change (how much and over what period of time?)

Skin: Dryness, roughness

Hair: Recent changes in texture, color, or pluckability

Eyes: Pale conjunctiva

Mouth: Condition of teeth, gums, lips, tongue

Nails: Recent changes in texture, shape, brittleness

GI/Abdomen: Appetite, food intolerance, nausea, vomiting, constipation, or diarrhea

Musculoskeletal: Muscle wasting, excess fat (obesity)

Physical Examination for Pregnant Women

Vital signs *Temperature, heart rate, respiration, blood pressure*

General: Obesity, edema, cachectic appearance

Skin: Texture, color, rashes, xerosis, follicular hyperkeratosis, flaky dermatitis, pallor, ecchymoses, slow-healing wounds

Hair: Texture, color, dyspigmentation, easy pluckability

Head: Temporal wasting

Eyes: Pale conjunctiva, scleral xerosis

Mouth: Condition of teeth, gums

 Tongue: Glossitis, edema

 Lips: Cheilosis, angular stomatitis, atrophic lingual papillae

Nails: Texture, shape, brittleness

Extremities: Edema, subcutaneous fat

Neurological: Irritability, weakness, loss of deep tendon reflex, sensory loss, asterixis

Musculoskeletal: Muscle wasting

Anthropometric data

Height

Current weight

Prepregnancy weight

Weight gain during pregnancy so far? (pounds per week or month)

Ideal weight (estimated) or body mass index

Percent ideal weight (calculated)

Interpretation of percent IBW

Goal for appropriate weight gain during pregnancy

Laboratory Evaluation

Glucose: (normal = 70–110 mg/dL)

Hematocrit: (female normal = 36–46%)

Hemoglobin: (female normal = 11.8–15.5 mg/dL)

Assessment and Plan

Examples of diagnostic plans related to nutrition include the following.

Recommend fasting serum glucose and fructosamine tests for pregnant women with diabetes.

Recommend hemoglobin and hematocrit test for suspected anemia.

Examples of treatment plans related to nutrition and education include

Poor weight gain: Recommend high-calorie, high-protein diet with frequent snacks.

Excessive weight gain: Recommend calorie-controlled diet with moderate fat reduction.

Diabetes in pregnancy: Recommend calorie-specific American Diabetic Association meal plan.

Obese Pregnant Woman

Carine M. Lenders, Susan Ahlstrom Henderson, and Lauren Hudson

Objectives

- To determine appropriate total weight gain and rate of weight gain for an obese pregnant woman.
- To recommend dietary modifications to relieve common gastrointestinal discomforts of pregnancy.
- To assess the nutritional adequacy of an obese pregnant woman's diet.
- To recommend appropriate dietary modifications and vitamin and mineral supplementation for an obese pregnant woman.

PL is a 22-year-old woman who is pregnant for the fifth time (gravida 5). She is a para 3013. The term para *n* has four components related to the number of viable pregnancies: *n* full-term births; *n* preterm births; *n* abortions, including miscarriages; and *n* live children. Thus, as a para 3013, PL has had three full-term births, no preterm births, one abortion, and has three children. PL is a single woman, who presents for her first prenatal visit at 22 weeks of gestation (the normal gestation period is 40 weeks) complaining of constipation and heartburn.

Medical History

All of PL's newborns weighed more than 10 pounds at birth; however, she was never diagnosed with gestational diabetes. She has never had problems with high blood pressure during previous pregnancies. PL currently takes no medications.

Social History

PL is a single mother on welfare. She does not know about the WIC (Women, Infants and Children) Program.

Physical Examination

Anthropometric data

Height: 5'6" (168 cm)

Current weight: 259 lb (118 kg)

Estimated prepregnancy weight: 242 lb (110 kg)

General: Tired-looking, obese female; poor eye contact

Abdomen: Trunkal obesity

Extremities: Varicose veins, edema +1

Case Questions

1. What questions about PL's weight should be asked and why?

2. How much additional weight should PL gain throughout the remainder of her pregnancy?

3. What medical complications during pregnancy are associated with obesity?

4. What important questions about PL's present diet should be asked?

5. What dietary and lifestyle habits contribute to heartburn and constipation? What nutritional advice can be given to help the patient avoid these gastrointestinal discomforts?

6. What concerns do you have regarding PL's diet?

7. Based on the preceding assessment, what dietary modifications would you suggest?

8. Should a vitamin and mineral supplement be considered for this patient? Why or why not?

Answers begin on the following page.

Answers to Questions: Case 1

Part 1:   Appropriate Weight Gain

1. **What questions about PL's weight should be asked and why?**

    Information about the patient's weight history is needed to help identify when she first gained her excess weight. The following questions are appropriate to her situation.

    How much did she weigh prior to her first pregnancy?

    How much weight did she gain during each pregnancy?

    Did she lose the weight she gained after her previous pregnancies? How?

2. **How much additional weight should PL gain throughout the remainder of her pregnancy?**

    $$\text{Prepregnancy BMI} = \text{Weight (kg)}/\text{Height (m)}^2$$
    $$= 110 \text{ kg}/1.68 \text{ m}^2$$
    $$= 39.0 \text{ kg}/\text{m}^2$$

    The total desirable weight gain for an obese pregnant woman is about 15 pounds. During the first trimester (13 weeks) of pregnancy, weight gain should be kept to a minimum (0 to 3 pounds for the entire 13 weeks). Using PL's last confirmed weight as her prepregnancy weight (242 pounds), we can estimate her weight gain for the first 22 weeks of gestation to be 17 pounds. Most fetal growth and maternal weight gain occur during the second and third trimesters, so PL's weight should be expected to increase in the remaining 18 weeks of normal pregnancy. However, because she has already exceeded the recommended total weight gain for her size, an attempt should be made to control or slow her rate of weight gain during the second and third trimesters. Weight loss or maintenance to compensate for previous excessive weight gain should never be attempted during pregnancy.

3. **What medical complications during pregnancy are associated with obesity?**

    Pregnancy is considered a diabetogenic state, and 5 to 7 percent of pregnant women become overtly diabetic during pregnancy. Because adipose tissue is associated with insulin resistance, obese pregnant women are more likely to suffer from gestational diabetes mellitus (GDM). Other medical complications observed among obese pregnant women include leg varicosities, infant macrosomia (infant birth weight greater than 4500 grams, or 9.9 pounds), difficulty during delivery, and an increased rate of deliveries by cesarean section.

4. **What important questions about PL's present diet should be asked?**

> The first step is to ask the patient general questions such as
> What do you usually eat? Do you skip meals?
> Do you eat out in fast food restaurants? How often?

5. **What dietary and lifestyle habits contribute to heartburn and constipation? What nutritional advice can be given to help the patient avoid these gastrointestinal discomforts?**

> Heartburn frequently occurs after meals and usually results from the pressure exerted by the enlarged uterus against the stomach. Patients often show signs and symptoms of esophageal reflux after meals. Large, high-fat meals can precipitate heartburn. Eating low-fat foods in a relaxed atmosphere can help. Because foods and beverages with caffeine (colas, coffee, and tea) can cause increased gastric acid secretion, limiting or avoiding caffeine during pregnancy is also advised.

> Hormonal changes during pregnancy tend to relax the gastrointestinal muscles, contributing to constipation. Pressure from the enlarged uterus, especially during the latter part of pregnancy, is often associated with bowel movement difficulty. Also, many women complain that iron supplements cause constipation. Increased fluid intake (especially water) and use of natural laxatives, such as whole grains, bran cereals, fruits, and vegetables are usually needed. Patients should be encouraged to engage in some physical activity after eating, such as walking or moderate exercise, rather than reclining or sleeping.

Part 2:   Dietary Assessment

Because PL is obese and has already gained an excessive amount of weight, her diet should be evaluated prior to suggesting a nutrition plan. A frequently used evaluation tool is the 24-hour dietary recall (see box at top of p. 92).

6. **What concerns do you have regarding PL's diet?**

> The total number of calories in PL's diet is excessive, as is the amount of calories that come from fat, which represents 47 percent of her total caloric intake. Foods with a high-fat content that PL eats on a regular basis include fried foods, bacon, cheese, ice cream, and sweets. A larger percentage of her calories should come from complex carbohydrates rather than from fats. Her diet is also low in fiber, calcium, folate, vitamins A and D, and riboflavin because she does not eat many fruits, vegetables, or dairy products.

7. **Based on the preceding assessment, what dietary modifications would you suggest?**

> Encourage PL to increase her consumption of low-fat dairy products, fruits, and vegetables. She also should be advised to eat fewer high-fat foods. Recommendations for dietary changes are most readily accepted

PL's Diet from the Previous Day		
Breakfast (home)	Fried eggs	2
	Fried bacon	4 slices
	Orange juice	1 cup
	Toast/Margarine	2 slices/2 tsp.
Lunch (fast-food restaurant)	Cheeseburger	1/4 lb. size
	French fries	small
	Cola soda	12 oz.
	Apple pie	1 piece
Snack (while shopping)	Sticky bun/Margarine	1 small/1 Tbs.
Dinner (home)	Fried chicken breast	4 oz.
	Macaroni and cheese	1/2 cup
	Corn on the cob	1 ear
	Margarine	3 Tbs.
	Kool-Aid	16 oz.
Snack (home)	Ice cream	1 cup

Total calories: 2977 kcal/day
Protein: 13% of calories
Carbohydrate: 40% of calories
Fat: 47% of calories

when given gradually. Pregnancy is a good time to begin changing dietary habits, because patients are usually motivated and open to suggestions that will benefit their infants. In addition, referring PL to a dietitian for nutrition counseling to help her and her family implement these suggestions would be most beneficial.

8. **Should a vitamin and mineral supplement be considered for this patient? Why or why not?**

A standard, prenatal vitamin and mineral supplement that contains 100 percent of the RDA for pregnant women should be prescribed because PL's diet is deficient in key vitamins and minerals. Additional iron (above 30 mg ferrous iron) is needed only if her hemoglobin and hematocrit are below normal for a pregnant woman. Vitamins and minerals are absorbed best when taken on an empty stomach, but this approach may cause nausea and vomiting in pregnant women. However, prenatal vitamin and mineral supplements are usually tolerated with meals and with liquids. Women whose diets are well-balanced and varied may need only a low-dose iron supplement (30 mg), which is usually prescribed by the twelfth week of gestation.

Encouraging Breast-Feeding

Carine M. Lenders, Susan Ahlstrom Henderson, and Lauren Hudson

> **Objectives**
>
> - To understand the advantages of breast-feeding newborn infants.
> - To make appropriate dietary and vitamin and mineral supplement recommendations to lactating women.
> - To assist women in determining whether to breast-feed or bottle-feed their infants.
> - To assist women in initiating and continuing breast-feeding.

KH is a 26-year-old woman who is gravida 1, para 0, in her thirty-seventh week of gestation. She is 5'6" tall and weighed 130 pounds (59 kg) prior to becoming pregnant (prepregnancy BMI = 21.0). She now weighs 160 pounds (73 kg), and her pregnancy has been uncomplicated. KH questions her obstetrician about her life after the baby is born. She is considering breast-feeding, but is afraid that the baby may become too attached to her, making it difficult for her to return to work three months postpartum. She also plans to lose her pregnancy weight quickly and fears dieting will keep her from producing enough breast milk to feed the baby adequately.

Follow-up

KH, who has been breast-feeding her infant, returns at six weeks postpartum for her checkup. She weighs 140 pounds (BMI = 22.6). She complains that she is even hungrier than she was during her pregnancy, but cannot find time to eat. She is afraid that she is not producing enough milk because the baby always appears hungry and is not as chubby as her friends' formula-fed babies. Her mother told her that she should not eat vegetables or chocolate, because they will upset the baby's stomach and produce gas. KH is also concerned about how to feed the baby when she returns to work in two months. A 24-hour recall, obtained by her obstetrician, follows.

KH's Diet from the Previous Day

Breakfast (home)	Corn flakes	1 cup
	Skim milk	1/2 cup
Lunch (home)	Whole-wheat bread	2 slices
	Peanut butter	2 Tbs.
	Jelly	1 Tbs.
	Orange juice	8 oz.
Snack (home)	Snickers candy bar	1
	Water	1 cup
Dinner (home)	Baked chicken	2 thighs (6 oz.)
	Baked potato	1 medium
	Margarine	2 Tbs.
	Apple sauce	1/2 cup
	Diet cola	12 oz.
Snack (home)	Ice cream	1 cup

Total calories: 1848 kcal/day
Protein: 18% of calories
Carbohydrate: 46% of calories
Fat: 36% of calories

Case Questions

1. What advice can be given to KH to help her decide whether or not to breast-feed her baby?

2. How quickly can a postpartum woman expect to lose weight?

3. If KH decides to breast-feed her infant, what recommendations should be given to ensure that her baby will receive adequate nutrition?

4. Should nursing mothers avoid certain foods?

5. How often and for how long does a breast-fed baby eat? How does this pattern differ from a bottle-fed baby's?

6. How will KH know if her breast-fed baby is getting enough to eat? How do growth patterns differ for breast-fed and formula-fed infants?

7. What concerns should be addressed regarding KH's diet during lactation?

8. What dietary modifications could be suggested to KH at this time?

9. How can breast-feeding women prepare for returning to work?

Answers begin on the following page.

Answers to Questions: Case 2

Part 1:   Encouraging Breast-Feeding

1. **What advice can be given to KH to help her decide whether or not to breast-feed her baby?**

    According to the Subcommittee on Nutrition During Lactation, the Committee on Nutritional Status During Pregnancy and Lactation, the Food and Nutrition Board of the Institute of Medicine, and the National Academy of Sciences:

    Breast-feeding is recommended for all infants in the United States under ordinary circumstances. Exclusive breast-feeding is the preferred method for normal full-term infants from birth to four to six months. Breast-feeding, complemented by appropriate introduction of other foods, is recommended for the remainder of the first year, or longer if desired, but it may be difficult for some women to follow these recommendations for social or occupational reasons. In these situations, appropriate formula-feeding is an acceptable alternative.

    Breast-feeding is not best for everyone, especially when a mother does not receive social and emotional support for her decision to breast-feed. Women are most likely to succeed at breast-feeding when encouraged by their health care provider (see Table 3-5) and outside sources of assistance (lactation consultant, family, and support groups) are available during the first two weeks postpartum. When a mother is unable to breast-feed for medical or other reasons, commercial formulas provide the best alternative source of nourishment for infants.

2. **How quickly can a postpartum woman expect to lose weight?**

    A woman should not expect her body to return to its pre-pregnancy weight immediately after delivery. On average, a new mother loses 15 pounds within the first week after delivery. Many mothers are concerned about their weight gain during pregnancy and worry whether they will ever return to their prepregnancy weight. Lactating women eating self-selected diets typically lose weight at a rate of one to two pounds per month during the first four to six months of lactation. A weight loss of more than one and a half pounds per week, even in women with excess fat stores, can decrease breast milk production and jeopardize the nutritional status of both the mother and the baby. The best way to be sure that babies are receiving adequate amounts of breast milk is to monitor their growth and development. However, not all women lose weight during lactation. Some studies suggest that approximately 20 percent of women maintain or gain weight during this time.

3. **If KH decides to breast-feed her infant, what recommendations should be given to ensure that her baby will receive adequate nutrition?**

    Lactating women should be encouraged to obtain their nutrients from a well-balanced, varied diet. This group of women has an increased need for essentially all nutrients, especially protein, calcium, vitamin A, and vitamin C, compared to nonpregnant women. The specific needs of individual women vary depending on the volume of milk produced daily, their individual metabolism, and their postpartum nutritional status.

During pregnancy, most women store approximately two to four kilograms of body fat, which can be mobilized to supply a portion of the additional calories used for lactation. Body fat supplies an estimated 200 to 300 kcal/day during the first three months of lactation. The additional 500 to 600 kcal/day needed for lactation must come from the diet. The RDA for calories for a lactating woman is estimated to be 500 kcal/day greater than the RDA for a nonpregnant woman.

Food Group Recommendations for Lactating Women

FOOD GROUP	MINIMUM SERVINGS PER DAY
Breads and cereals	6
Vegetables	3 to 5
Fruits	2 to 4
Dairy products	4
Meat, poultry, or fish	3
Alcohol	Contraindicated

4. **Should nursing mothers avoid certain foods?**

   Foods that contain harmful substances should be avoided when breast-feeding. Examples are caffeine, alcohol, and any potentially harmful drugs or toxins (e.g., cocaine and marijuana) that enter the mother's bloodstream and are passed on to the infant through the breast milk.

   Some infants are sensitive to components of certain foods. Cow's milk, peanut butter, chocolate, egg whites, and nuts contain substances that enter the breast milk and cause allergy-prone infants to develop rashes, wheezing, or a runny nose. Onion and cruciferous vegetables (cabbage, cauliflower, and broccoli) are suspected to cause gas and cramps in some breast-fed infants. In general, breast-feeding women should experiment with small amounts of potentially offensive foods to see if the infant is sensitive. If this does not appear to be the case, these foods can be included in the diet. Elimination of major nutrient sources to treat allergy or colic in breast-fed infants is not recommended unless evidence from oral elimination-challenge studies determines that the mother is sensitive or intolerant to certain foods or that the breast-fed infant reacts to these foods when they are ingested by the mother.

5. **How often and for how long does a breast-fed baby eat? How does this pattern differ from a bottle-fed baby's?**

   Breast-feeding should be initiated as soon after delivery as possible. Feeding the baby on demand, frequent suckling, and completely emptying the breasts of milk help to increase the mother's milk supply. The duration of breast-feeding should not be limited during the first few days. In the beginning, it may take two to three minutes to establish letdown, the term for the moment when the milk begins to empty from the breast due to the contraction of myoepithelial cells or the letdown reflex.

Oxytocin stimulates the letdown reflex, while prolactin stimulates milk production. Removing the infant prior to letdown does not stimulate milk supply and may frustrate mother and infant alike. Allowing the infant to suckle for several minutes until the milk flows and to feed for five minutes on each breast during the first day, progressing to 15 minutes by the end of the first week, should work well since suckling is the key to establishing and maintaining lactation. However, the duration of feeding may vary among infants.

Once lactation is established, an infant who suckles vigorously usually empties the breast in seven to ten minutes after letdown has occurred. It is not necessary to continue feeding once the breasts are empty, especially if the nipples are tender.

Breast milk changes in composition and volume during each feeding. The milk provided when the breast is nearly empty is the richest in fat content. Babies need to nurse long enough to obtain sufficient calories from the breast milk for appropriate growth and satiety between feedings. Explain to mothers that the infant will get 90 percent of the milk volume in the first five minutes, but only 50 percent of the calories because breast milk becomes higher in fat and calories the longer letdown occurs.

If a newborn infant is being fed six to eight times during the day, it is not usually necessary to wake the infant to offer night feedings. However, most infants continue to demand a night feeding well beyond the first month. Most breast-fed infants adapt to the mother's schedule, feeding every three to four hours, with one or two nightly feedings by the age of three months.

6. **How will KH know if her breast-fed baby is getting enough to eat? How do growth patterns differ for breast-fed and formula-fed infants?**

Milk production generally works on the principle of supply and demand. That is, the more a baby feeds, the more milk is produced, unless the mother is not consuming enough calories to produce the milk. In the first few days of life, it is not uncommon for a newborn to feed every one to three hours during each 24-hour period; this helps to stimulate initial milk production. Once the milk supply is established, feeding frequency will diminish. A baby who has at least six wet diapers per day and is gaining weight appropriately (at least four to seven ounces weekly) is usually consuming enough milk. Breast-fed and formula-fed infants have slightly different growth patterns.

Breast-fed and formula-fed infants gain weight at about the same rate during the first two to three months postpartum, though breast-fed infants consume less milk and have a lower energy intake. After the first few months, breast-fed infants gain weight more slowly than those fed with formula.

Part 2: Follow-up

7. **What concerns should be addressed regarding KH's diet during lactation?**

   KH's weight loss may have been too quick (total weight loss of 20 pounds in the first four weeks postpartum). According to the diet history, she is not consuming adequate calories to maintain her weight and simultaneously produce adequate amounts of breast milk to feed her baby. Her calorie requirements for lactation are 2700 kcal/day, calculated on the basis of 30 kcal/kg/day plus an additional 500 kcal/day for lactation. Her diet is also deficient in iron, calcium, vitamin A, vitamin B12, folate, and zinc.

8. **What dietary modifications could be suggested to KH at this time?**

   KH needs to take in more calories. She should be encouraged to eat when she is hungry and follow the food group recommendations discussed in the answer to question 3. As a reminder to eat, she may find it helpful to make a point of eating or drinking something whenever she feeds the baby. For example, she could drink a glass of milk or eat yogurt, and a piece of fruit, or eat a slice of toast with cheese or peanut butter while breast-feeding the baby. Snacks will also increase her energy level after the baby is finished feeding. Suggesting simple foods that require little or no preparation is a useful strategy in such cases.

   KH could also be encouraged to get help from a relative or friend with household duties such as grocery shopping or housecleaning, so that she will not feel so overwhelmed by her new responsibilities. If KH continues to limit her food intake and is not already taking a vitamin/mineral supplement, one should be prescribed to ensure that she receives adequate vitamins and minerals during lactation. Most obstetricians make it a policy to recommend that breast-feeding women continue to take their prenatal vitamins.

9. **How can breast-feeding women prepare for returning to work?**

   A mother returning to work can continue to breast-feed if she chooses. She may rent or purchase a breast pump to remove milk during the day whenever her breasts feel engorged. The advantages of pumping the breast are to ensure that the baby will receive breast milk when the mother is at work and to promote the continued supply of breast milk even though the baby is not feeding during the day. If possible, breast-feeding exclusively on weekends or whenever the mother is not working will help milk production to continue. Breast milk can be stored in the freezer for three months or more, or in the refrigerator for up to two days.

   If the mother decides to wean her infant from breast-feeding, she can begin to prepare her infant two to three weeks in advance by offering a bottle of breast milk or formula. This is best done when the baby is awake and alert, but not overly hungry or full. Expressed breast milk or commercial infant formula can be used. The father or a caretaker should offer the bottle because the baby may expect to breast-feed when the mother is present. Offering one bottle every day will help the infant to learn how to suckle from a bottle, a procedure different from breast-feeding. Once the mother returns to work, the baby should be given either expressed breast milk or formula from the bottle during the day. When the mother is home, she can continue to breast-feed if she chooses.

See Chapter Review Questions, pages A5–A7.

REFERENCES

Ackerman L. Breast-feeding: The primary care physician's role. *Family Practice Recertification* 1995;17(8):32–53.

American College of Obstetrics and Gynecology (A.C.O.G.). Nutrition during pregnancy. *A.C.O.G Technical Bulletin* 1993;179:1–7.

Anonymous. Routine iron supplementation during pregnancy. US Preventive Services Task Force. *JAMA* 1993;270(23):2848–2854.

Anonymous. NIH Consensus Development and Panel on Optimum Calcium Intake. *JAMA* 1994;272(24):1942–1948.

Committee on Drugs. The transfer of drugs and other chemicals into human milk. *Pediatrics* 1994;93(1):137–145.

Czeizel AE, Dudas I. Prevention of the first occurrence of neural-tube defects by periconceptional vitamin supplementation. *N Engl J Med* 1992;327:1832–1835.

Daly LE, Kirke PN, Molloy A, et al. Folate levels and neural tube defects: implications for prevention. *JAMA* 1995;274:1698–1702.

Dewy KG, McCrory MM. Effects of dieting and physical activity on pregnancy and lactation. *Am J Clin Nutr* 1994;59(suppl):446S–453S.

Gartner LM. On the question of the relationship between breastfeeding and jaundice in the first five days of life. *Seminars in Perinatology* 1994;18(6):502–509.

Institute of Medicine (I.O.M.). *Nutrition During Pregnancy and Lactation. An Implementation Guide.* Washington, DC, National Academy Press, 1990.

Institute of Medicine (I.O.M.). Nutrition during pregnancy. Washington, DC, National Academy Press, 1990.

King JC, Butte NF, Bronstein MN, et al. Energy metabolism during pregnancy: influence of maternal energy status. *Am J Clin Nutr* 1994;59(suppl):439S–445S.

Lawrence RA. *Breast Feeding: A Guide for the Medical Profession.* 4th ed. St. Louis: Mosby, 1994.

Lenders CM, Hediger ML, Scholl TO, et al. Effect of high-sugar intake by low-income pregnant adolescents on infant birth weight. *J Adol Health* 1994;15(7): 596–602.

National Research Council. *Recommended Dietary Allowances*. 10th ed. Washington, DC, National Academy Press, 1989.

Nehlig A, Debry G. Potential teratogenic and developmental consequences of coffee and caffeine exposure: A review on human and animal data. *Neurotox Teratol* 1994;16(6):531–543.

Oski FA. Infant nutrition, physical growth, breast feeding, and general nutrition. *Curr Opin Pediatr* 1994;6(3):361–364.

Rieder MJ. Prevention of neural-tube defects with periconceptional folic acid. *Clin Perinatol* 1994;21(3):483–503.

Rivard CI, Fernandez A, Gauthier R. Fetal loss associated with caffeine intake before and during pregnancy. *JAMA* 1993;27:2940–2943.

Rush D. Periconceptional folate and neural-tube defect. *Am J Clin Nutr* 1994;59 (2 suppl): 511S–515S.

Scholl TO, Hediger ML. Anemia and iron deficiency anemia: compilation of data on pregnancy outcome. *Am J Clin Nutr* Feb. 1994;59:492–500, discussion 500–501.

Scholl TO, Hediger ML, Schall JL, et al. Maternal growth during pregnancy and the competition for nutrients. *Am J Clin Nutr* 1994;60(2):183–188.

Scholl TO, Hediger ML, Schall JL, et al. Low zinc intake during pregnancy: its association with pre-term and very pre-term delivery. *Am J Epidem* 1993;137(10): 1115–1124.

Underwood BA. Maternal vitamin A status and its importance in infancy and early childhood. *Am J Clin Nutr* 1994;59(2 suppl):517–524.

US Department of Health and Human Services Public Health Service. *Healthy People 2000*. Washington, DC: US Government Printing Office. FHS 91 50212, 1990:379.

Villar J, Repke JT. Calcium supplementation during pregnancy may reduce preterm delivery in high-risk populations. *Am J Obstet Gynecol* 1990;163: 1124–1131.

Wada L, King JC. Trace element nutrition during pregnancy. *Clin Obstet Gynecol* 1994;37:574–586.

Wothington-Roberts BS, Williams SR. *Nutrition in Pregnancy and Lactation*. 5th ed. St. Louis: Mosby, 1993.

Zimmermann MB, Shane B. Supplemental folic acid. *Am J Clin Nutr* 1993;58: 127–128.

4

Infants, Children, and Adolescents

Andrew M. Tershakovec

Objectives

- To recognize the changing nutritional needs of developing children, from infancy to adolescence.

- To understand that nutritional recommendations for children vary by age and gender, and differ according to the expert groups who develop them.

- To perceive that nutritional and dietary behaviors learned in childhood can have significant impact on adult health concerns such as obesity and hypercholesterolemia.

- To differentiate the effects of acute versus chronic undernutrition on growth and development.

Childhood Growth and Development Patterns

Energy and nutrient requirements of children are proportional to their resting energy expenditure plus the energy needed for activity and normal growth. These requirements vary dramatically depending on the general stages of growth and on the child's individual development pattern. However, growth curves derived from observations of large numbers of normal, healthy children have been developed to establish expected ranges of weight, height, and head circumference growth for purposes of comparison. The most commonly utilized of these curves are age- and gender-specific.

Children undergo two rapid growth spurts: the first during infancy followed by a period of steady, slower growth; and the second in adolescence. Rapid body growth and brain development in the first stage, especially during the first three years of life, require a significant amount of calories and nutrients to support appropriate passage through all the developmental stages that characterize this period.

Individual Variability

When assessing the nutritional needs of children, considering individual differences is also important. Population growth curves may mask such differences because the population groups used to develop the normal values may not represent all children. Thus it is necessary to evaluate a child's stage of growth and development to assess that child's nutritional needs.

Mechanisms of Growth

Cell Division

In utero and early in life, much of an individual's growth is attributable to cell division. This consideration is important because malnutrition early in life may block cell division. When a cell loses the ability to divide, the total number of cells and the individual's potential growth are thereby diminished. Providing the optimal environment, including adequate nutrition, for dividing cells to achieve their growth potential is therefore crucial to prevent permanent stunting.

Differential Growth Patterns

Different organ systems develop at different times and at different rates (see Figure 4-1). The general growth pattern parallels the height growth curve, showing rapid early growth, a subsequent period of steady, slower growth, and the final growth spurt during adolescence. Key differences in specific organ systems that depart from that general pattern are the topic of this section.

Brain and Central Nervous System In the central nervous system (CNS) and the brain, rapid growth is seen in the first few years of life. The human brain reaches 70 percent of its adult size by age three years and 90 percent by age seven. Very little growth occurs after this time. Accordingly, the CNS of a malnourished child under age four may be very susceptible to permanent damage, and the consequences of famines may thus perpetuated for many years.

Lymphatic System The lymphatic system undergoes rapid growth until puberty, when it actually surpasses its ultimate adult size, and then regresses to that size.

Reproductive System The reproductive system is basically dormant until puberty, when it undergoes rapid growth. Malnutrition's profound effects on the reproductive system during adolescence are commonly demonstrated in anorexic girls with delayed sexual development or secondary amenorrhea.

Differences in Sexual Maturation

Evaluations of the rate of growth also define the differences in growth between boys and girls. Growth spurts occur earlier in girls than in boys for two reasons: girls begin puberty earlier than boys and undergo their growth spurts sooner in the pubertal period. Knowing the sequence of pubertal changes and their appropriate approximate timing, as outlined in the Tanner stages, is thus important in diagnosing pubertal delay and growth arrest (Table 4-1).

Table 4-1   Tanner stages of development of secondary sexual characteristics.

Boys: Genital (Penis) Development

	AGE	
Stage 1	11.0	Prepubertal: testes, scrotum, and penis of about same size and proportion as in early childhood
Stage 2	11.6	Enlargement of scrotum and testes. Skin of scrotum reddens and changes in texture
Stage 3	12.9	Enlargement of penis, at first mainly in length Further growth of testes and scrotum
Stage 4	13.8	Increased size of penis with growth in breadth and development of glans. Testes and scrotum larger; scrotal skin darkened
Stage 5	14.9	Genitalia adult in size and shape

Girls: Breast Development

Stage 1	11.1	Prepubertal: elevation of papilla only
Stage 2	11.1	Enlargement of areola diameter, breast bud stage: elevation of breast and papilla as small mound
Stage 3	12.2	Further enlargement and elevation of breast and areola, with no separation of their contours
Stage 4	13.1	Projection of areola and papilla to form a secondary mound above level of breast
Stage 5	15.3	Mature stage: projection of papilla only, due to recession of areola to general contour of breast

Both Sexes: Pubic Hair

Stage 1		Prepubertal: vellus over pubes is not further developed than over abdominal wall
Stage 2	m=11.7 f=13.4	Sparse growth of long, slightly pigmented downy hair, straight or slightly curled, chiefly at base of penis or along labia
Stage 3	m=12.4 f=13.9	Considerably darker, coarser, and more curled. Hair spreads sparsely over junction of pubes
Stage 4	m=13.0 f=14.4	Hair now adult in type, but area covered is still considerably smaller than in adult. No spread to medial surface of thighs
Stage 5	m=14.4 f=15.4	Adult in quantity and type with distribution of horizontal (or classically "feminine") pattern
Stage 6		Spread up linea alba (male-type pattern)

Source: Tanner JM. *Growth at Adolescence*, 2nd ed. Oxford: Blackwell Scientific, 1962.

Determining Pediatric Nutrient Requirements

As children grow, their body composition changes. The percentage of body weight attributable to fat, or fat mass, is high for infants and toddlers and decreases as children progress through their elementary school years. In puberty, the fat mass increases again until the developing adolescent finally reaches his or her adult body composition. The development of boys and girls,

Figure 4-1   **Yearly organ system growth chart**.

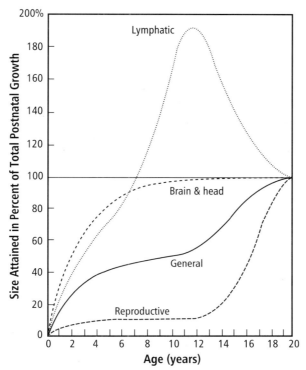

Source: Abraham M (ed). *Rudolph's Pediatrics*. 19th ed. Norwalk, CT: Appleton and Lange, 1991, 130.

from a body composition point of view, is basically parallel until puberty. At that point, boys lose some body fat as they become adults, whereas females deposit more body fat during adolescence and maintain this fat through adulthood. Differences between boys and girls also occur with respect to lean body mass (LBM). Again, the percentage of LBM is very similar in both sexes until puberty. Then, boys triple their LBM, while girls double theirs. As they enter adulthood, females manifest a higher percentage of total body fat and a lower percentage of muscle mass than males.

Normal Energy and Nutrient Requirements During Growth

Based on these body composition changes, various recommended energy and nutrient allowances have been formulated for growing children. In general, these recommended allowances are thought to fulfill children's energy and nutrient needs in proportion to the metabolically active tissue at various stages of development. As shown in Table 4-2, the basal metabolic rate (BMR) is the same for girls and boys until they enter puberty, when it increases more rapidly for boys to meet the demands of their higher percentage of muscle mass.

Table 4-2   Standard basal metabolic rate chart.

Weight (kg)	Male	Female
	kcal/24 hr	
3	140	140
5	270	270
7	400	400
9	500	500
11	600	600
13	650	650
15	710	710
17	780	780
19	830	830
21	880	880
25	1020	960
29	1120	1040
33	1210	1120
37	1300	1190
41	1350	1260
45	1410	1320
49	1470	1380
53	1530	1440
57	1590	1500
61	1640	1560

Source: Tsang RC, Nichols BL (eds). *Nutrition During Infancy.* Philadelphia:C.V. Mosby, 1988.

Adjustments for Activity and Illness

To estimate an individual's true energy needs, adjustments are necessary for special circumstances such as activity levels, illnesses, and other factors. For example, fever raises energy needs 12 percent for each degree above 37°C. Illness, trauma, recovery from malnutrition, and serious burns can almost double energy requirements. On the other hand, chronic malnutrition can decrease energy needs by 20 to 30 percent, and decreased growth and activity during severe illness can also decrease energy needs considerably.

Evaluating Dietary Adequacy in Children

Evaluating dietary intake is generally only necessary in the event of abnormal growth or development. When tracking a child's growth over time, it is important to pay attention to the percentile curve the infant follows in relation to the age- and gender-specific growth percentiles from one of the standard charts available for such monitoring purposes. In general, an infant who has been growing steadily and falls consistently in the fifth percentile for his or her age and sex is less of a concern than one who has placed consistently in the fiftieth percentile on the growth curve and subsequently drops to the fifth.

Infant Feeding: Breast Milk Versus Formula

Except for special formulas, manufacturers of infant formulas generally try to approximate the composition of human breast milk. The specifics of infant formulas are discussed in Case 1 at the end of this chapter and in Table 4-3. Table 4-4 compares the nutrient content of breast milk with that of infant formula. (Also see Chapter 3 for additional information on lactation.)

Weaning Babies from Breast Milk or Formulas

Most pediatricians feel that cow's milk (whole milk) is an important source of calories, protein, and calcium for most children over the age of one. The American Academy of Pediatrics recommends that cow's milk not be given to children under one year of age. When cow's milk is introduced earlier, it may cause the following disorders.

Table 4-3   Indications and types of infant formulas.

FORMULA	INDICATIONS	UNIQUE PROPERTIES	EXAMPLES
Milk-based	Breast milk substitute for term infants	+/- Iron Ready to feed, powder or liquid concentrate Variable whey: casein 20 kcals/ounce	Enfamil, Similac, Gerber, Good Start, Lactofree
Soy-based	Breast milk substitute for infants with lactose intolerance	Lactose-free, some sucrose, or corn-free 20 kcals/ounce May contain fiber	Prosobee, Isomil, Soyalac, I-Soyalac, Isomil-DF
Premature	Breast milk substitute for infants <38 weeks' gestation age	Low lactose Whey:casein 60:40 Higher Ca and Phos 24 kcals/ounce	Enfamil Premature Similac Special Care Similac Natural Care Enfamil HMF Similac Neocare
Older infant	Transition to whole milk	16 kcals/ounce	Advantage, Good Nature
Hypoallergenic	Milk or soy protein allergy	Hydrolyzed protein Sucrose-free Lactose-free	Nutramigen
Predigested	Malabsorption Short bowel syndrome	Lactose-free Hydrolyzed protein or free amino acids	Alimentum, Pregestamil, Neocate
Fat-modified	Defects in digestion, absorption, or transport of fat	Contains increased % of kcals as MCT	Portagen, Alimentum, Pregestamil
Carbohydrate-modified	Simple sugar intolerance	Requires addition of complex carbohydrate to be complete	RCF 3232 A
Amino acid-modified	Inborn errors of metabolism	Low or devoid of specific amino acids that cannot be metabolized	Multiple Products
Electrolyte-modified	Renal or cardiac disease or other disease state requiring low renal solute load	Decreased sodium content	Similac PM 60/40 SMA

Source: Department of Clinical Nutrition, Children's Hospital of Philadelphia.

Table 4-4   Comparison of breast milk and infant formulas (nutrients per 100 calories).

	Breast Milk	Similac	Enfamil	Isomil
Protein (g)	1.54	2.14	2.10	2.45
% of calories	6	9	8	11
Source	mature term human milk	cow's milk	reduced mineral/ whey/nonfat milk	soy protein isolate
Fat (g)	5.74	5.40	5.3	5.46
% of calories	52	48	47	49
Source	mature term human milk	soy and coconut oils	palm olean/soy coconut/sunflower	soy and coconut oils
Cholesterol (mg)	22	1.6	< 1	0
Carbohydrate (g)	10.6	10.7	10.9	10.3
% of calories	42	43	43	41
Source	Lactose	Lactose	Lactose	Corn syrup
Vitamins				
Vitamin D (IU)	3.0	60	60	60
Vitamin K (mcg)	0.3	8.0	8.0	15
Minerals				
Calcium (mg)	41	73	78	105
Phos. (mg)	21	56	53	75
Iron (mg)	0.04	1.8	1.8	1.8
Renal Solute Load				
(milliosmolar)	11.1	14.3	14.2	16.3

Source: Department of Clinical Nutrition, Children's Hospital of Philadelphia.

GI blood loss   The protein in cow's milk may induce a reaction with the small bowel mucosa, causing chronic gastrointestinal blood loss and subsequent iron deficiency anemia.

Iron deficiency   Infants who are fed cow's milk are at risk for iron deficiency due to the low iron content of the milk and its potential for inducing blood loss. Even though breast milk is lower in iron than cow's milk, the iron in breast milk is more bioavailable.

Excess renal solute load   Infants' kidneys are relatively immature and have difficulty handling the extra renal solute load occasioned by the somewhat concentrated protein and phosphorous content of cow's milk.

Introducing Solid Food

Recommendations concerning the introduction of solid food have changed considerably over the years. In the past, many children ate a wide variety of foods as early as the first month of life. Now, the consensus among pediatricians is to delay the introduction of solid foods at least for the child's first four months. At four months of age, the average infant consumes 32 ounces of formula or breast milk per day.

Introducing solid foods earlier in the infant's life may stimulate the development of food allergies. Furthermore, infants are not physiologically ready to accept solid foods from a spoon until approximately four months of age, when the oral extrusion reflex becomes extinguished. Other important considerations are the development of head and neck control and coordination of the oral musculature, both of which occur at roughly three to four months of age. Feeding solid food to a baby who cannot yet hold up his or her head or control the tongue's movements well enough to swallow it efficiently will be difficult at best.

The introduction of solid foods marks the beginning of a critical period during which the infant learns to master eating from a spoon and accept different tastes and textures. Not coincidentally, an infant's readiness for these experiences generally responds to a physiological need to supplement the amounts of calories and nutrients available from breast milk or formula. However, breast milk, formula, or a combination should still continue to be the major source of calories and nutrients during the remainder of the infant's first year. The common belief that solid food can help to "fatten up" or otherwise hasten the development of a baby is a misconception. As Table 4-5 shows, most solid foods are calorically less dense than breast milk or formula.

General Guidelines for Introducing Solid Foods

Although no real consensus exists among the experts regarding when and how to introduce solid foods, parents may find the following general guidelines helpful.

Introducing new foods New foods should not be introduced too often—generally not more frequently than every three days—nor should more than one new food be introduced at a time. Following this procedure allows detection of a child's inability to tolerate a newly introduced food.

Cereals The most common initial solid food is rice cereal. Generally offered first at four to six months of age, rice cereal is fortified with iron, nonallergenic, and usually well tolerated. Begin with one to two tablespoons per day, mixed with formula or breast milk. The cereal should be mixed to a consistency similar to that of applesauce. It may be thinned or thickened as preferred by the child. In general, cereal can be thickened as the child grows older. Feeding cereal from a spoon helps the baby learn this new skill, which takes a few weeks.

Table 4-5   Comparison of the relative caloric densities of common infant food sources.

Food	Caloric Density
Cow's milk	20 kcal/oz.
Infant formula	20 kcal/oz.
Human milk	20 kcal/oz.
Baby food vegetables	9–19 kcal/oz.
Baby food fruits	14–20 kcal/oz.

Fruits Infant apple and pear juice may be offered at four to six months of age, beginning with a few ounces per day. Cooked and strained or pureed fruits without added sugar are recommended for infants between six and eight months of age. Fresh, mashed bananas also may be introduced at this time because they are easy to swallow without chewing and are low in fiber. Peeled, soft fruits such as peaches and pears, cut into small pieces, may be offered at eight to ten months of age. Foods that are harder to chew, such as apples, should be deferred until the child is more able to chew food of greater consistency.

Vegetables Cooked, strained vegetables without added salt or spices are appropriate at six to eight months of age. The importance of avoiding salt and spices should be stressed. It has been suggested that acquiring a taste for salt in infancy can have health repercussions later in life. Young children often have difficulty tolerating spices. Raw vegetables such as cucumbers, tomatoes, and corn may be introduced at one year of age. Hard vegetables such as raw carrots should not be introduced until the child's top and bottom molars have erupted to prevent choking.

Eggs Egg yolks may be introduced to infants over the age of six months, but the introduction of egg whites should be delayed until they reach one year of age because of the potential risk of inducing an allergy to eggs in younger infants.

Meat Ground or finely chopped chicken, fish, and meats are generally introduced after age six to eight months. They should be well pureed to avoid the risk of choking.

Starch Children tend to like pasta, spaghetti, and noodles, and in general, pasta is a good source of calories. However, other essential foods with a higher nutrient density should be introduced first during the meal to ensure that the child's diet is complete and balanced.

Fat Children under age two years need a high-calorie diet to ensure normal brain development. Because fat is the most calorically dense food, limiting fat intake in young children's diets may jeopardize normal growth and brain development. Therefore, fat should not be limited before age two years. On the other hand, children need not eat high-fat foods such as hot dogs and ice cream every day.

Psychosocial and Behavioral Implications and Recommendations

Eating habits formed in the first two years of life are thought to persist for several years, if not for a lifetime. Therefore, healthy eating patterns should be established as early as possible. As their growth rate varies, so do children's appetites, which may fluctuate from day to day. Studies have shown that when children are allowed to determine on their own how much they eat, their intake may vary considerably from meal to meal, but over a period of days and weeks, it remains reasonably stable.

Potential Problems Children begin expressing personal preferences early and simultaneously develop mechanisms for self-control. Parents must therefore take care to strike a balance between limiting the child's food choices to develop healthy eating habits and providing sufficient opportunities for experimentation and control.

Rather than insisting that a child eat, parents need to focus on quality rather than quantity. In a basic sense, children who consume a variety of foods over time and demonstrate appropriate growth are likely consuming an adequately balanced diet. Parents who become frantic that their child is not eating enough and allow the child to eat anything simply to ensure that he or she eats something are probably succeeding in developing poor eating habits.

Problems also surface when parents get into prolonged power struggles with their children over eating issues. Two-year-old children often begin asserting their independence by insisting on eating the same food for days at a time. If their request is not totally unreasonable, meeting it may be a better response than turning mealtime into a battle. Left on their own, children eventually will tire of the same food, but if winning each mealtime struggle is in the balance, these episodes may worsen.

Confusion and rushing at mealtimes, especially common occurrences due to today's lifestyles, send children mixed messages about food. Rapid ingestion of food may also encourage overeating. Calm, quiet, unhurried meals eaten together as a family encourage good eating habits.

Children are keen observers and imitators, and their food preferences can be influenced by other family members. Parents who frequently eat junk food and sweets may have difficulty encouraging healthy eating habits in their children. Similarly, any dietary intervention must take into consideration the environment in the child's home and in other settings, such as day care, where the child spends considerable time.

Nutritional Recommendations for Adolescents

Adolescents undergo major physical and psychological changes that impact on their behavior and nutritional status. Issues of autonomy and rebellion, testing and searching behaviors, and the development of formal operational thought (logical reasoning) are all normal characteristics of adolescence that must be considered when addressing their nutritional needs and behavior.

Requirements for Growth

Adolescents' energy and nutrient needs increase as they enter their pubertal growth spurt. Though infants, children, and adolescents all grow rapidly, the energy needs of adolescents, on a per kilogram basis, are much lower than those of infants and children. Infants double their body weight over a few months, whereas older children and adolescents' may double their weight over a period of five to ten years.

Sexual Development

Previously described body composition changes that occur in adolescence also influence their energy and nutrient needs. Furthermore, these needs differ in men and women. As girls go through puberty and start menstruating, their iron and protein needs increase to replace their losses. As boys enter puberty, their percentage of lean body mass increases relative to girls, thus increasing their protein and calorie requirements greater than adolescent girls.

Nutritional Factors in Preventing Cardiovascular Disease

The association between elevated cholesterol levels and heart disease has been well documented in adults. Although no direct evidence exists to link elevated cholesterol levels with children's diets, several studies suggest that adult atherosclerosis has its roots in childhood. The epidemiology of childhood and adult hypercholesterolemia is described below:

War Victims   Some American soldiers killed in the Korean and Vietnamese wars were found to have significant atherosclerosis of their coronary arteries. Their young ages suggested the early onset of the atherosclerotic process.

Bogalusa Study   A large group of children living in Bogalusa, Louisiana, has been followed for over 20 years. Autopsy studies of those who have died of unrelated causes have shown a correlation between premorbid cholesterol levels and early atherosclerotic changes. Similar studies have demonstrated an association between atherosclerotic disease and other risk factors, such as smoking.

Tracking   Children with high cholesterol levels tend to become adults with high cholesterol levels. Because tracking is not perfect, some have argued that treating all hypercholesterolemic children is inappropriate, as not all the children will become hypercholesterolemic adults. Others feel that the initial dietary treatment is safe and healthy for all children and therefore will not harm those who do not eventually become hypercholesterolemic adults.

Issues in Hypercholesterolemia Screening

Due to a number of concerns, the current recommendations for identifying hypercholesterolemic children suggest screening only those with a positive family history of early heart disease or hypercholesterolemia in first-degree relatives. A positive family history of early heart disease is defined as a father who had a heart attack before age 50 or a mother who had a heart attack before age 60. The following issues underlie these recommendations.

Inaccurate testing   Due to inherent biological and laboratory variability, measured cholesterol levels can vary significantly. Cholesterol tests completed without appropriate controls, such as those conducted in supermarkets and shopping malls, can be inaccurate. This potential inaccuracy could mislabel a child as hypercholesterolemic.

Failure to thrive Concern over the possibility of placing children inappropriately on low-fat diets and potential misdiagnosis have led many to question the safety of screening and intervention for hypercholesterolemia in children.

Problems with selective screening Multiple studies have shown that if only children with a positive family history are screened, half the hypercholesterolemic children will be missed. No direct association has been described between a positive family history and significant elevations in children's cholesterol levels.

Current Recommendations

An expert panel appointed by the National Heart, Lung and Blood Institute (NHLBI: 1993) issued recommendations concerning the identification and treatment of childhood hypercholesterolemia. A low-fat diet may help reduce cholesterol levels and potentially prevent heart disease as well as cancer and obesity. Thus, even if a child is not hypercholesterolemic, a low-fat diet should have a positive health impact.

However, dietary intervention must be viewed as only part of a program to reduce cardiovascular disease risk. Exercise, controlling elevated blood pressure, avoiding smoking, and moderating alcohol ingestion are all factors that should be recommended to adolescents.

The NHLBI guidelines opt for a population approach, recommending a low-fat diet, called the Step One or Prudent Diet, for all children over the age of two years (see Chapter 6).

Some have questioned the safety of dietary restrictions because of reports of failure to thrive among some children on very low-fat diets. In these cases, parents initiated dietary restrictions without professional guidance and fed their children diets that were very low in calories. Their experience suggests the need to offer families appropriate guidance to ensure that the children receive a balanced, complete diet.

Obesity in Childhood and Adolescence

According to the NHANES III (1988–1991), the prevalence of childhood obesity is rising among the population of the United States. The NHANES III indicated that 20 percent of boys and 22 percent of girls age 12 to 19 are overweight, based on the body mass index calculation. These figures represent a significant increase from the previous NHANES II (1976–1980), in which 15 percent of adolescent males and females alike were overweight. A rate of 15 percent is the nation's target goal according to the Healthy People 2000 report. Because the caloric intake of the general population does not seem to be rising, this increased incidence of childhood obesity may be due to a reduction of physical activity. Currently available information leads to the following conclusions.

Numerous tracking studies have demonstrated that an obese child runs an increased risk of becoming an obese adult. Also, early onset obesity may be more difficult to treat. Children with early onset obesity may be even more obese as adults than they would have been if they had become overweight in adulthood. Thus, preventing or treating childhood obesity should significantly decrease adult obesity and its accompanying medical problems.

Etiology: Genetics and Environment

According to current estimates, a child with two obese parents has an 80 percent chance of becoming obese, whereas the proportion drops to 40 percent of children with only one obese parent. Studies comparing the relative body weights of adopted children with their biological and adoptive parents suggest a major genetic component in the incidence of obesity.

However, despite this seemingly indisputable evidence of genetic influence on the development of obesity, environmental influences also have been well documented. A higher prevalence of obesity exists in only children, children of older parents, and children whose parents are separated. Children who watch many hours of television also have a greater chance of becoming obese. Decreased physical activity and increased snacking while watching TV most likely contribute to this phenomenon. The large number of food commercials aimed at children during children's shows may also be a factor.

Nutrition and Dental Health

Nutrition has an obvious impact on the development of teeth and ongoing dental health. To develop dental caries, cariogenic bacteria and an appropriate food source for the bacteria are necessary. Different foods have varying effects on the development of caries according to the food's sugar content and potential to adhere to the teeth. Eating frequently and consuming foods that adhere to the teeth provide the cariogenic bacteria with a readily available food source that promotes cavity formation.

As a result, nutritional recommendations are sometimes in conflict. Fruit leather—dried fruit rolled into sheets—has been described as a perfect snack food for children because of its low-fat content. However, its adherence characteristics and natural sugar content make it very cariogenic. Brushing children's teeth on a regular basis may help disturb the environment supportive of caries development. Thus it is essential to consider the overall impact of foods before making recommendations. Factors affecting dental health include

- tooth development and eruption
- cariogenic bacteria
- sugar intake (sucrose, maltose, lactose, and fructose)
- frequency of eating

- adherence of food
- fluoride

Fluoride, either in fluoridated water or in a supplement, helps prevent cavity formation. However, care must be taken to avoid administering too much fluoride because it may stain the teeth. Discoloration occurs most commonly in children who receive an inappropriately high fluoride supplement and also drink fluoridated water. The Committee on Nutrition of the American Academy of Pediatrics (AAP) has developed recommendations concerning fluoride supplementation based on the fluoride content of the local water supply. The Committe also suggests that infants under six months of age should not receive flouride supplements.

Calcium Requirements and Bone Density

Recent evidence suggests that bone mineral content is highest in young adults and then begins to decrease as a person ages. To minimize poor bone mineralization in the elderly, enhancing calcium intake in childhood and adolescence has been recommended. Studies have shown that calcium supplementation in children and adolescents increases the mineral content of bone. Surveys also show that many American children and adolescents have less than optimum calcium intakes. Dairy products are the most efficient source of calcium. Low-fat milk and cheese should be recommended to avoid excessive fat, saturated fat, and cholesterol intakes.

Optimal calcium requirements, as determined by the NIH Concensus Statement on Optimal Calcium Intake for Infants, Children, and Adolescents are listed in Table 4-6.

Table 4-6   Optimal calcium requirements for infants, children, and adolescents.

Group		Optimum Daily Intake (in mg of calcium)
Infants	Birth to 6 months	400
	6 months to 1 year	600
Children	1 to 5 years	800
	6 to 10 years	800–1200
Adolescents/Young Adults	11 to 24 years	1200–1500

Nutrition Questions for the Pediatric and Adolescent History and Physical Exam

Medical History

Is your child or teenager allergic to any food or drinks? Does he or she suffer from rashes or eczema?

Does your child or teenager take any vitamin and mineral, fluoride, iron, or food supplements?

If your child or teenager is not taking a fluoride supplement, does your water supply contain fluoride?

Has your child or teenager had any recent weight gain or loss? Reason?

Has your child or teenager tried to gain or lose weight by altering his or her diet or by taking medication? If yes, describe the results.

Has your child or teenager ever induced vomiting or taken diuretics or cathartics to lose weight or to keep from gaining weight?

Social History for Infants and Children

What type of milk (breast milk, formula, or cow's milk) are you feeding your child?

If you prepare formula, how much water and formula do you use?

How many ounces of formula or milk does your child drink per day?

What else does your child drink during the day? (Iced tea, soda, Kool-Aid, juice, punch, water)

Is your child put to bed with a bottle?

If your child is eating solid foods, when did you start to introduce them into his or her diet?

How many meals does your child eat daily? How many snacks?

Does your child usually eat the food that is prepared for the family?

Does your child avoid any specific foods or food groups such as milk or meats?

Does your child ever chew on any nonfood items such as dirt, clay, paint chips, woodwork, or plaster?

How old is your house? Do you have lead pipes? Has the water been tested for lead? Are you renovating your home?

Social History for Adolescents

Does the teenager drink alcohol? Type, quantity, frequency, duration?

Is the teenager following any special diet? How compliant is he or she with this special diet?

Over the past month, has the teenager observed any changes in his or her dietary intake?

What type of milk (whole, 2%, 1%, or skim) does the teenager drink? How many cups per day?

How many meals does the teenager eat daily?

How many meals away from home does the teenager eat every day?
Which meals?

How many snacks does the teenager eat during the day? Who prepares
meals and snacks at home?

Does the teenager skip meals? If so, which ones and why?

Does the teenager avoid any specific foods such as milk or meats?

Is the teenager physically active? How often does the teenager exercise
and in what type of exercise does he or she engage?

If the teenager has diabetes, does he or she self-monitor blood glucose
levels? When?

Does the teenager exhibit poor self-esteem or body image?

Review of Systems for Infants, Children, and Adolescents

General: Weight change, irritability, appetite changes

Skin: Rashes, lesions, eczema

Mouth: Lesions, appearance of teeth and gums

GI/Abdomen: Diarrhea, vomiting, spitting up, sucking or swallowing
problems

Endocrine: Polyuria, polydipsia, polyphagia, heat or cold intolerance

Physical Examination for Infants, Children, and Adolescents

Vital signs: *Temperature, heart rate, respiration, blood pressure*

Anthropometric data

Height (length): (cm or inches)	*Height for age:* (percentile)
Current weight: (kg or lb)	*Weight for age:* (percentile)
Ideal weight for height: (kg or lb)	*Ideal height for age:* (cm or inches)
Weight change	*Percent weight change*
Percent weight for height	*Percent height for age*
Head circumference (cm or inches):	(For children under 3 years of age)

General: Age and description of general appearance (well-developed,
well-nourished

Skin: Rashes, lesions, ecchymosis

HEENT: Open fontanelle (infants), temporal wasting, dentition,
cheilosis, glossitis

Lungs: Wheezing

Cardiac: Heart size, rhythm, murmurs

GI/Abdomen: Bowel sounds, hepatosplenomegaly, masses, obesity

Genitourinary: Tanner staging for pubertal development, gluteal wasting

Extremities: Subcutaneous wasting, metaphysical splaying (rickets)

Neurological: Reflexes, muscle tone, sensations

Musculoskeletal: Rachitic rosary, epiphyseal swelling, growth retardation

Iron Deficiency Anemia in Children

Andrew M. Tershakovec

Objectives

- To identify the risk factors associated with childhood iron deficiency anemia and the methods for diagnosing, preventing, and treating this disorder.
- To evaluate and interpret laboratory values needed to diagnose iron deficiency anemia in the pediatric patient.
- To differentiate iron deficiency from lead poisoning in the pediatric patient.

IR, a two-year-old boy, is brought to his family doctor for well-child care. His mother says that she has no specific complaints, but the child is inattentive, distracted, and seems unhappy. IR was born prematurely at 34 weeks by normal vaginal delivery (full term is 40 weeks). His past medical history is unremarkable. IR was breast-fed for three months and then changed to infant formula. At the age of seven months, he was switched to whole cow's milk.

On routine hematocrit screening at the age of two years, IR is found to be anemic. Also of note, his rate of growth is at the third percentile when corrected for prematurity. It is common practice to plot premature children on the growth curve at their chronological age (actual age since birth) minus the number of weeks they were born prematurely until the age of two years. Therefore, this child may be plotted at a point six weeks younger than his chronological age.

Past Medical History

IR was intubated for one week following his birth due to acute respiratory distress syndrome (ARDS). He was discharged at one month of age, when his weight reached two kilograms. His history shows no subsequent hospitalizations.

Review of Systems

Skin: Pale since birth; no history of easy bruisability

GI/Abdomen: No vomiting or diarrhea; dark stools for previous three months

Physical Examination

Vital signs

Temperature: 98.6°F

Heart rate: 110 BPM

Respiration: 26 BPM

Blood Pressure: 100/120 mmHg

Anthropometric Data

Length: 80 cm (31.5") 5th percentile

Current weight: 10.4 kg (23 lb) 5th percentile

General: Two-year-old child who appears weak and apathetic

HEENT: Facial pallor, pale conjunctiva

Cardiac: Systolic ejection murmur

Abdomen: Normal bowel sounds, no masses or hepatosplenomegaly

Rectal: Heme-positive stools

Extremities: Nail beds pale; no ecchymosis or purpura

Neurological: Development appropriate for age in gross and fine motor skills; mild delay in language acquisition; normal tone and deep tendon reflexes

Case Questions

1. Why might one suspect that this child is anemic?
2. How can the cause of the anemia be identified?
3. What is the interpretation of the lab results? What does the elevated erythrocyte protoporphyrin (EP) suggest?
4. What are the risk factors for lead poisoning?
5. Assuming that this child is iron-deficient, how could his anemia have been prevented?
6. The child is confirmed to be iron-deficient, and iron supplementation is prescribed. The parents note a significant change in their child's behavior shortly after he begins taking the iron supplement. What do they report?
7. The parents ask if their child may have suffered any long-lasting effects due to the iron deficiency.
8. This child's 15-year-old brother and sister are twins. The parents ask whether these siblings also should be screened for iron deficiency.

Answers begin on the following page.

Answers to Questions: Case 1

Part 1: Diagnosis

1. **Why might one suspect that this child is anemic?**

    Because the fetus gains large amounts of iron in the third trimester of gestation, premature infants are born with decreased iron stores. Thus, it is important to know if this child received iron supplementation or an iron-fortified formula during his first year of life. In addition, introducing cow's milk, which is low in iron, before age one may induce chronic gastrointestinal bleeding. This condition, evidenced by heme-positive stools, can cause iron deficiency. Folate and vitamin B12 deficiency leading to anemia is very unusual at this age, but must also be considered. Other causes of anemia include hemolysis, thalassemia, sickle cell disease, and chronic lead intoxication.

2. **How can the cause of the anemia be identified?**

    Obtain the following laboratory tests:

    Hemoglobin

    Mean corpuscular volume (MCV)

    Erythrocyte protoporphyrin (EP)

    Reticulocyte count

    Blood smear for microscopic examination

Part 2: Laboratory Data

Preliminary laboratory evaluation shows the following results.

Patient's Lab Values	Normal Values
Hemoglobin = 10 g/dL	11–14.5 g/dL
Mean corpuscular volume (MCV) = 68 fL	80–100 fL
Erythrocyte protoporphyrin (EP) = 42 mcg/dL	<35 mcg/dL
Reticulocyte count = 0.2%	0.8–2.8%

3. **What is the interpretation of the patient's lab results? What does the elevated erythrocyte protoporphyrin (EP) suggest?**

    The low hemoglobin level confirms the diagnosis of anemia. The low reticulocyte count suggests that the bone marrow is not producing a large number of red cells. The small size of the red cells, evidenced by low MCV, or microcytosis, suggests a problem of insufficient hemoglobin production for each red blood cell. A low reticulocyte count and microcytic red blood cells are consistent with iron deficiency anemia. However, because of the high incidence of lead intoxication in this age group, lead poisoning must be considered along with iron deficiency.

    The elevated EP is consistent with a blockage in hemoglobin production, commonly seen in both iron deficiency and lead intoxication. Thalassemia trait, a genetic hemoglobin trait, is also a possibility. Finally, children with viral illnesses can also be transiently anemic, but usually their cells are normochromic and normocytic, and their mean corpuscular volume also is normal. This type of anemia is not associated with iron deficiency and remits spontaneously. In this case, the low MCV is not consistent with anemia associated with a minor illness.

4. **What are the risk factors for lead poisoning?**

   Living in a house older than 50 years with lead paint or falling plaster chips, which an active toddler can ingest, is probably the most common cause of lead poisoning. Exposure to dust or fumes as paint and plaster are stripped away during home renovations must also be considered. Lead pipes and lead solder in older homes may also contaminate the water source. Less commonly observed sources of lead intoxication include ceramic dishes and industrial sources such as lead smelters. Questions that should be included in the pediatric social history include the following.

   How old is your house? Do you have lead pipes?

   Has the water been tested for lead?

   Has your child had his or her lead level evaluated?

   Does your child ever chew on paint chips, plaster or other debris?

5. **Assuming that this child is iron-deficient, how could his anemia have been prevented?**

   Because IR was born prematurely, he should have been receiving supplemental iron since birth. In addition, whole cow's milk should have been deferred until the age of 12 months to decrease the likelihood of the chronic blood loss and anemia often seen in younger children (IR was started on cow's milk at seven months). Encouraging consumption of iron-fortified solid foods or foods natu-rally high in iron would also have been helpful. Sources of dietary iron appropriate for infants and children include iron-fortified formula and infant cereals, red meats, dark green, leafy vegetables, and dried fruit such as raisins.

Part 3: Treatment

6. The child is confirmed to be iron-deficient, and iron supplementation is prescribed. The parents note a significant change in their child's behavior shortly after he begins taking the iron supplement. What do they report?

   Iron-deficient children who receive iron supplementation tend to become more interactive, attentive, and happier. They are also more active and energetic. These changes have been reported to occur before the anemia is corrected.

7. **The parents ask if their child may have suffered any long-lasting effects due to the iron deficiency.**

    Altered behavior and cognitive function have been reported in iron-deficient infants and toddlers. The data concerning the reversibility of these alterations are conflicting; however, an increasing body of evidence suggests that these differences may be long-term and possibly even permanent.

8. **This child's 15-year-old brother and sister are twins. The parents ask whether these siblings also should be screened for iron deficiency.**

    The prevalence of iron deficiency in the United States has decreased significantly over the last twenty years. Previously, the highest rates of iron deficiency were encountered in children under three years of age. This group was thought to be at risk for iron deficiency due to rapid growth rates, high iron requirements, and diets that were frequently low in iron. The current lower prevalence may be due to supplemental food programs for low-income families, such as the Women, Infants, and Children (WIC) Program, as well as increased iron supplementation in infant cereals and formulas.

    A few groups in the population of the United States are still at risk for iron deficiency, particularly adolescent female athletes. These girls have increased iron requirements once they begin menstruating, superimposed on the increased needs associated with the pubertal growth spurt. The association of iron deficiency with exercise is not well understood. It was postulated that runners may have chronic bleeding or hemolysis due to repeated heel and foot pounding, but an increased rate of iron deficiency has also been noted among swimmers. Thus, if the twins are athletes, possible iron deficiency also should be considered in their medical evaluation. (See also Case 3.)

Malnutrition and Refeeding Syndrome in Children

Catherine B. Sullivan and Marcie Beck

Objectives

- To describe the physiological adaptations that occur secondary to malnutrition in the pediatric population.
- To understand the correlation among basic biochemical adaptations to malnutrition.
- To identify the potential complications associated with refeeding the malnourished patient.
- To explain how the complications associated with refeeding syndrome can be minimized or prevented in the malnourished patient.

RD is an 11-year-old boy of Liberian descent who lives in the United States with his parents. In October RD and his family flew to Liberia to spend a few months with their extended family. Several weeks after his arrival, political unrest erupted. RD and his family were forced from their homes at gunpoint and taken to a university, where they were held against their will in overcrowded, unsanitary conditions. Medical and food supplies were scarce. Food was provided by soldiers outside the camp, who lowered buckets of rice and occasionally fish over the barbed wire fences. Daily tea was also provided. Many of the hostages died from starvation. RD and his family escaped after three months of captivity and fled to the United States Embassy. On the day they arrived, they were airlifted to a neighboring country. Shortly thereafter, RD returned to the United States. At the embassy, RD's vital signs were

Temperature: 97°F

Heart rate: 45 BPM

Respiratory rate: 18 BPM

Blood pressure: 100/80 mmHg

After these three months of virtual starvation, RD ate "everything he could get his hands on" for the four days before he arrived at The Children's Hospital of Philadelphia's (CHOP) emergency room.

Past Medical History

RD tested positive for malaria; no other problems were found. On admission, he was not taking any medications or vitamins. RD has no known food allergies.

Social/Diet History

Prior to his imprisonment in the refugee camp, RD's food supply met 100 percent of his needs. While in the refugee camp, his intake amounted to only 250 to 300 kcal/day, with 30 grams of protein per week. Four days after he escaped, his intake had risen to 2500 to 3000 kcal/day, with 80 to 90 grams of protein per day.

Further evaluation in the hospital produced the following clinical picture.

Physical Examination

Vital signs

Temperature: 101.8°F

Heart rate: 120 BPM

Respiratory rate: 30 BPM

Blood pressure: 80/50 mmHg

General: Eleven-year-old boy who appears apathetic and emaciated with temporal and interosseous muscle wasting

Skin: Dry, scaly dermatitis

Head: Alopecia, thinning hair lacking in luster

Abdomen: Mildly distended

Extremities: Bipedal edema

Anthropometric Data

Date	Height (cm)	Percentile	Weight (kg)	Percentile	%IBW (34.5 kg)	%UBW (39 kg)
1/7[a]	142	50	23.3	<5	68	60
1/10[b]	142	50	27.9	5–10	81	72

a At the embassy.
b At CHOP after eating.

Laboratory Data

Date	Ca (mg/dL)	PO$_4$ (mg/dL)	Mg (mg/dL)	K (mEq/L)	Albumin (g/dL)
1/7[a]	8.0	3.0	1.8	3.6	2.7
1/10[b]	6.3	1.0	0.9	2.0	2.4
Normal	(8.5–10.5)	(2.5–5.0)	(1.8–2.9)	(3.5–5.3)	(3.5–5.8)

a At the embassy.

Case Questions

1. From this history, it is obvious that RD's diet was very inadequate for three months and he was therefore malnourished. What physiological adaptations probably occurred in response to this period of malnutrition?

2. Based on the physical exam and laboratory data, what clinical and biochemical manifestations of malnutrition does RD exhibit?

3. What metabolic and physiological changes occur as RD begins to eat again (that is, when refeeding is initiated)? Why are his electrolyte abnormalities of primary concern?

4. Based on RD's physical exam and laboratory data, what complications of refeeding does he exhibit?

5. How could the complications of refeeding that RD experienced have been minimized or avoided?

6. Why is malnutrition a unique concern in the hospitalized pediatric patient?

Answers begin on the following page.

Answers to Questions: Case 2

Part 1:   Physiology

1. **From this history, it is obvious that RD's diet was very inadequate for three months and he was therefore malnourished. What physiological adaptations probably occurred in response to this period of malnutrition?**

    The body's systems adapt to calorie and protein deficits in a complex manner. Chronically malnourished patients progress gradually into a mildly catabolic state. The body's compensatory mechanisms involve changes in energy metabolism and hormone regulation. Fat and protein are mobilized and converted to energy via glucose and ketones. The basal metabolic rate (BMR) decreases to conserve energy; the body becomes hypothermic, hypotensive, and bradycardic, and physical activity decreases. Growth hormone and thyroid hormone regulation decreases or stops growth, which helps to lower the BMR. Production of insulin, which promotes anabolism of catecholamines, cortisol, and glucagon also decreases. The net effect facilitates survival by decreasing the BMR and promoting conservation of protein and organ function.

    Overall decreases in cellular mass may eventually result in functional loss in vital organs. Respiratory muscle loss may lessen respiratory efficiency. Myocardial atrophy may reduce cardiac output. Decreased intravascular fluid volume results in decreased cardiac output.

    GI atrophy slows motility and gastric acid secretion and also causes thinning of the mucosa, villous atrophy, and decreased production of digestive enzymes. These effects reduce GI function and can result in malabsorption and chronic diarrhea, further exacerbating the malnutrition and possibly increasing susceptibility to infection. Liver wasting also causes altered metabolism and decreased protein synthesis. Lastly, the kidney's ability to concentrate urine decreases, causing diuresis.

2. **Based on the physical exam and laboratory data, what clinical and biochemical manifestations of malnutrition does RD exhibit?**

    Specific manifestations include wasting and apparent emaciation secondary to depleted somatic protein and subcutaneous fat stores. Serum proteins may or may not be depleted in such patients. At initial presentation, serum albumin and protein values are normal due to the decreased blood volume. However, as the child is refed, the total blood volume increases, and albumin and protein concentrations decrease. Hypotension, bradycardia, hypothermia, and a decreased respiratory rate are common bodily defense mechanisms in malnutrition that result in decreased energy needs. Signs and symptoms of vitamin and mineral deficiencies, such as cheilosis (dry scaling of the lips), alopecia (hair loss), and scaly dermatitis are noted. Nonspecific manifestations include decreased growth rate and physical activity. The child generally appears apathetic and manifests flat effect.

apathetic and manifests flat effect.

RD's normal height, in the face of his very low weight and depleted body fat, suggests acute malnutrition, which is consistent with his history and presentation. If RD's starvation had been chronic, he would have manifested stunting, or slowed growth in terms of height. Adaptations and compensatory mechanisms manifested by RD include hypothermia, bradycardia, and a decreased respiratory rate. His low serum albumin level suggests depleted visceral protein stores as well. The changes in calcium, phosphate, magnesium, and potassium levels may be associated with his malnutrition or with rapid refeeding.

Part 2:   Initiating Refeeding

3.   **What metabolic and physiological changes occur as RD begins to eat again (that is, when refeeding is initiated)? Why are his electrolyte abnormalities of primary concern?**

Awareness of the physiological and metabolic changes of starvation and subsequent refeeding is of primary concern. It is important to note that these changes occur, to a greater or lesser degree, in every pediatric or adult patient who has been deprived of adequate nutrients. Refeeding syndrome is defined as the broad range of metabolic derangements that can occur due to rapid reinstitution of nutrients in a person with protein-energy malnutrition (PEM). These changes can lead to significant pathological consequences, including death.

When refeeding is initiated in the malnourished patient, anabolism begins almost immediately. A rapid alteration in hormonal levels, primarily insulin, occurs as glucose becomes the predominant fuel. At this time the basal metabolic rate increases, and the process of rebuilding lost tissue begins. A positive balance of nutrients, including minerals and electrolytes, occurs because of the shift to laying down new tissues. Anabolism requires energy and nutrients, in enzymes and as intermediate compounds, to act as building blocks for regrowth.

The cardiovascular adaptations of malnutrition, including myocardial atrophy and volume contraction, must also be considered when refeeding a malnourished patient. A rapid alteration in calories, fluid, and particularly sodium intake may cause fluid shifts and intravascular volume overload, causing the patient to go into congestive heart failure.

Increased requirements for anabolism may cause or unmask deficiencies, including life-threatening imbalances, thus inhibiting anabolism. The most common abnormalities encountered when refeeding malnourished patients are potassium, phosphate, magnesium, and calcium. The etiology of each of these abnormalities include the following:

Potassium   Insulin, secreted in response to the increased glucose load during refeeding, causes glucose and potassium to enter the intracellular space. Their presence results in a rapid fall in serum potassium that may alter nerve and muscle function.

Phosphate As anabolism increases, the need for phosphorylated intermediates also increases. Phosphate bound to these compounds is, in effect, "trapped" intracellularly. The resulting imbalance may cause severe hypophosphatemia, which may lead to cell damage and dysfunction resulting in organ failure.

Magnesium Magnesium is a cofactor for the enzyme ATPase. As the metabolic rate increases, magnesium requirements rise. Magnesium is also required for normal parathyroid function. Thus, hypomagnesemia may cause dysmetabolism by altering ATPase function and calcium and phosphate homeostasis.

Calcium As growth is initiated, calcium requirements increase. Maintenance of calcium levels may be affected if hypomagnesemia is present. Serum levels of calcium are maintained in such cases at the expense of bone deposits, resulting in osteoporosis in adults or rickets in children with chronic malnutrition. Hypocalcemia may alter muscle and myocardial function, causing tetany and cardiac arrhythmias.

4. **Based on RD's physical exam and laboratory data, what complications of refeeding does he exhibit?**

    RD exhibits fluid overload, as evidenced by the edema. This condition could be exacerbated by his low albumin level as fluid leaks from the capillaries because of decreased oncotic pressure. In addition, he may be in congestive heart failure because of his decreased cardiac output secondary to loss of heart muscle function from protein catabolism. Intake of a large volume of fluid and solutes could cause his weakened myocardium to decompensate. Furthermore, his myocardial function may be altered by electrolyte imbalances, putting him at greater risk for cardiac arrhythmia.

    RD lost weight during his first week of hospitalization as he mobilized the retained extracellular fluid and excreted the excess. In addition, RD demonstrated dangerously low serum calcium, phosphate, magnesium, and potassium levels secondary to rapid utilization of depleted stores of these minerals to initiate anabolic processes.

5. **How could the complications of refeeding that RD experienced have been minimized or avoided?**

    In patients who fall below 80 percent of their IBW or who have suffered a change from their usual weight greater than 10 percent in the preceding 1 to 2 months, consider the risk of refeeding syndrome. To avoid the complications of refeeding, adhere to the following treatment recommendations.

- Refeed slowly, beginning with approximately 75 percent of basal caloric needs.

- Provide electrolyte, vitamin, and mineral supplements.

- Increase calories by 10 to 25 percent per day, while closely monitoring lab values, specifically calcium, phosphate, sodium, potassium, and magnesium, and the patient's clinical state.

- Monitor fluid intake carefully to avoid stressing the malnourished cardiorespiratory system.

- Monitor vital signs closely during this process to detect changes in cardiorespiratory function early (EKG is also indicated).

- Monitor daily weight gain. Excessive weight gain suggests fluid retention.

6. **Why is malnutrition a unique concern in the hospitalized pediatric patient?**

   Surveys have suggested that the prevalence of protein-energy malnutrition (PEM) in pediatric wards in the United States approaches 50 to 60 percent of hospitalized patients. PEM can complicate the clinical presentation of the patient and confuse the diagnostic picture. Children have greater calorie and protein needs than adults, secondary to normal growth and development. Disease states may further increase children's nutritional requirements because of increased losses, diminished intake, and increased utilization.

   These factors make it difficult to meet the needs of hospitalized children, especially because their illness often interferes with nutritional intake. If PEM occurs, it can lead to delayed growth and development and significantly increased morbidity and mortality.

Case 3

Eating Disorders in Adolescent Athletes

Diane Barsky and Margaret Barry

Objectives

- To understand how rapid growth during puberty alters adolescents' nutritional requirements.
- To identify teenagers at risk for eating disorders and determine appropriate intervention.
- To assess the nutrient intake of adolescent athletes and their risk of developing nutritional deficiencies.
- To understand the time sequence of the adolescent growth spurt and the stages of pubertal development described by Tanner.

AN is a 15-year-old female who has been a member of her school's cross-country running team for the past two years. She presents to her family doctor complaining of an episode of fainting one week before while she was competing in a five-kilometer race. Prior to fainting she felt dizzy, but she has denied palpitations or visual changes. According to her records, AN was at 100 percent of her ideal body weight until last year. She has lost 15 pounds during the past year.

History of Present Illness

AN has experienced episodes of muscle cramping and headaches over the past two weeks. Six months ago she complained of abdominal pain and a burning sensation in her chest. Her symptoms subsequently improved with the use of antacids and a change in her eating pattern to consuming small, frequent meals.

Past Medical History

AN's history appears noncontributory—negative for heart disease, asthma, epilepsy, or diabetes. She has no previous history of fainting. AN takes antacids occasionally, but she is not taking any vitamins. She has no known food allergies.

Social/Development

AN is an above-average high achiever. Her current circle of friends includes mostly school athletes. Upon further questioning, AN expresses concern over recent changes in her body, such as breast development and widening hips. She wants to maintain a trim, muscular physique and fears excessive weight gain. She denies smoking, alcohol, drugs, or sexual activity.

Diet History

To prepare herself for the race, AN had been consuming a high-protein, low-fat, and low-carbohydrate diet for the past few weeks. Twenty-four hours prior to the race, she consumed two high-carbohydrate meals.

AN states that she enjoys eating, but follows a low-fat regimen to minimize weight gain. On occasion, she "indulges" in high-fat or high-sugar foods. She admits to small weight fluctuations during the past year, but she increases the intensity of her exercise routine to keep her weight at 90 pounds. She denies vomiting or taking laxatives or cathartics. AN frequently skips meals and compensates by snacking. During the interview, she frequently expresses concern that she is overweight and not muscular enough for long-distance running. Based on a 24-hour recall, AN consumes 1200 to 1500 kcal per day.

Menstrual History

Menses started when AN was 12 years of age. She reports a normal cycle every 30 days until 8 months ago, when menses abruptly ceased (a condition called secondary amenorrhea).

Physical Examination

Vital signs
   Temperature: 97°F
   Heart rate: 68 BPM
   Respiratory rate: 14 BPM
   Blood pressure: 90/62 mmHg

Anthropometric data
   Height: 162 cm (64 inches) (50th percentile for age)
   Current weight: 41kg (90 lb) (5th percentile for age)
   Ideal weight: 53 kg (117 lb) (50th percentile for age)
   Percent weight for height: 77 percent (41/53) (current weight/ideal weight for current height)
   Triceps skinfold (TSF): 1.0 cm (10 mm) (10th percentile for age)

Mid-arm muscle circumference (MAMC): 18 cm (180 mm) (10th to 25th percentile for age)

General: Thin, muscular female who appears sad, anxious, and younger than her age.

Skin: Dry

HEENT: Pale face, pale conjunctiva; no palpable goiter, dental erosions, gag reflex somewhat diminished

Cardiac: Normal rate and rhythm

Breasts: Elevation of breast mound with areola, Tanner 3

Genitalia: Coarse pubic hair with sparse distribution, Tanner 3

Neurological: Reflexes slightly decreased in upper and lower extremities

Laboratory Data

Patient's Lab Values	Normal Values
Sodium: 142 mEq/L	135–145 mEq/L
Potassium: 2.5 mEq/L	3.5–5.0 mEq/L
CO_2: 29 mEq/L	22–26 mEq/L
Calcium: 8.2 mg/dL	8.5–10.5 mg/dL
Phosphate: 4.2 mg/dL	2.5–5.0 mg/dL
Albumin: 3.5 g/L	3.5–5.0 g/L
Hemoglobin: 11.2 g/dL	12–16 g/dL

Case Questions

1. What clues in AN's medical history indicate that she may have an eating disorder?

2. Based on AN's laboratory values, what are the possible causes of her fainting spell, muscle cramps, and headaches?

3. Is AN's Tanner staging appropriate for her age?

4. Using AN's percent weight for height calculation based on the physical exam, is she well-nourished?

5. Is her present diet appropriate for her age and physical activity level?

6. What nutrient deficiencies is AN at risk for developing?

7. What recommendations are appropriate for AN?

Answers begin on the following page.

Answers to Questions: Case 3

Part 1: Diagnosis

1. **What clues in AN's medical history indicate that she may have an eating disorder?**

    The history of a burning sensation in her chest and abdominal pain that responded to antacids signals possible esophagitis, which may be secondary to self-induced vomiting, or purging. Purging behavior is associated with anorexia nervosa or bulimia. Bulimia is a severe disorder characterized by frequent episodes of binge eating followed by the ingestion of laxatives or cathartics to induce vomiting. Adolescents who binge and purge food also tend to demonstrate weight fluctuations. However, in anorexia nervosa, body weight is maintained significantly below normal weight for age (see Tables 4-7 and 4-8).

    Table 4-7   Diagnostic criteria for bulimia nervosa.

    - Recurrent episodes of binge eating. An episode of binge eating is characterized by both of the following:
        1. Eating, in a discrete period of time (e.g., within any 2-hour period), an amount of food that is definitely larger than most people would eat during a similar period of time in similar circumstances; and,
        2. A sense of lack of control over eating during the episode (e.g., a feeling that one cannot stop eating or control what or how much one is eating).
    - Recurrent inappropriate compensatory behavior in order to prevent weight gain, such as self-induced vomiting; misuse of laxatives, diuretics, or other medications; fasting; or excessive exercise.
    - The binge eating and inappropriate compensatory behaviors occur, on average, at least twice a week for three months.
    - Self-evaluation is unduly influenced by body shape and weight.
    - The disturbance does not occur exclusively during episodes of anorexia nervosa.

    SPECIFY TYPE:

    Purging type: The person regularly engages in self-induced vomiting or the misuse of laxatives or diuretics.

    Nonpurging type: The person uses other inappropriate compensatory behaviors, such as fasting or excessive exercise, but does not regularly engage in self-induced vomiting or the misuse of laxatives or diuretics.

    Source: American Psychiatric Association Committee on Nomenclature and Statistics: *Diagnostic and Statistical Manual of Mental Disorders*, 4th ed., Washington, DC: American Psychiatric Association, 1994.

Table 4-8 Diagnostic criteria for anorexia nervosa.

- Refusal to maintain body weight over a minimal normal weight for age and height (e.g., weight loss leading to maintenance of body weight 15 percent below that expected; or failure to make expected weight gain during period of growth, leading to body weight 15 percent below that expected.
- Intense fear of gaining weight or becoming fat, even though underweight.
- Disturbance in the way in which one's body weight, or shape is experienced, undue influence of body shape and weight on self-evaluation, or denial of the seriousness of current low body weight.
- In females, absence of at least three consecutive menstrual cycles when otherwise expected to occur (primary or secondary amenorrhea). (A woman is considered to have amenorrhea if her periods occur only following hormone, eg, estrogen, administration.)

SPECIFY TYPE:

Restricting type: During the episode of anorexia nervosa, the person does not regularly engage in binge eating or purging behavior (i.e., self-induced vomiting or the misuse of laxatives or diuretics).

Binge eating/purging type: During the episode of anorexia nervosa, the person regularly engages in binge eating or purging behavior (i.e., self-induced vomiting or the misuse of laxatives or diuretics).

Source: American Psychiatric Association Committee on Nomenclature and Statistics: *Diagnostic and Statistical Manual of Mental Disorders*, 4th ed., Washington, DC, American Psychiatric Association, 1994.

AN is expressing the characteristic preoccupation with her body image and fear of becoming overweight often seen in patients with eating disorders. Her insistence at maintaining her body weight at 23 percent below expected is consistent with the diagnosis of anorexia nervosa, purging type. She requires education and counseling to help her learn about the natural physical changes that occur during puberty, as well as to improve her self-image. Although treatment of eating disorders includes psychological counseling, these illnesses are very difficult to manage clinically. Patients with anorexia nervosa, characterized by chronic self-induced starvation and vigorous excercise to prevent weight gain, are relatively resistant to psychotherapy and many have abnormal eating behaviors throughout life, requiring long-term support (see Table 4-8).

Medical complications that occur in both anorexia and bulimia include acute gastric dilatation, abdominal pain, heart failure, pancreatitis, electrolyte disturbances, and amenorrhea. Amenorrhea is defined as an absence of menses for six months or for three usual cycle intervals following previous normal menstruation. Factors contributing to amenorrhea include excessive exercise, caloric restriction, and weight loss, all of which are often seen in patients with eating disorders. Amenorrhea is more common among female athletes than in the general population. Lower percentages of body weight, greater weight loss, and lower initial body weights have been documented among amenorrheic runners as opposed to runners with normal menses. Teenagers with eating disorders experience amenorrhea as well as irregular menstrual cycles.

Studies of athletes also have demonstrated decreased energy and protein intake in amenorrheic athletes as opposed to those with normal menses. Reportedly, at least 17 percent body fat is necessary for menarche to occur because fat cells are involved in hormone metabolism. Reducing exercise and increasing calories and fat intake may cause menses to resume.

2. **Based on AN's laboratory values, what are the possible causes of her fainting spell, muscle cramps, and headaches?**

   AN's low potassium level and metabolic alkalosis, indicated by an elevated carbon dioxide level (characteristic of base excess), may be due to losses of potassium and hydrogen ions during self-induced vomiting. Low serum potassium and/or low serum ionized calcium can lead to muscle cramps, headaches, dizziness, and abnormal heart rhythms. Dehydration may have precipitated the fainting episode.

   AN is at risk for dehydration if she has been inducing vomiting without orally replacing her fluid loss. During a race, she will lose additional free water and salt from sweating and will have no opportunity to replace this fluid. Also, depletion of glycogen reserves, due to inadequate consumption of energy and carbohydrates, may result in poor endurance. Iron deficiency anemia, indicated by this patient's low hemoglobin level, also may contribute to her early fatigue and muscle weakness (see Table 4-9).

3. **Is AN's Tanner staging appropriate for her age? (See Table 4-1.)**

   AN demonstrates an arrest of her pubertal development. Puberty starts in girls at an earlier age than in boys. Girls usually demonstrate acceleration of linear growth at the onset of puberty and reach peak growth velocity early, at Tanner stage two or three, whereas boys reach peak growth velocity when genital and pubic hair are at Tanner stage four or five. In normal girls, menarche usually occurs one year after their growth peak. Females typically reach their maximal growth velocity (a rate of 9.0 centimeters per year) at a mean age of 12.5 years. AN's height is already at the 90th percentile for her age, and she has experienced menarche. Therefore her Tanner stage should be more advanced.

Table 4-9   Medical complications of anorexia nervosa and bulimia nervosa.

ANOREXIA NERVOSA	BULIMIA NERVOSA
Physical Signs and Symptoms	
Cachexia, body fat depletion	Ulceration or scarring of knuckles (due to abrasions
Bradycardia, hypotension, hypothermia	received while inducing vomiting)
Salivary gland hypertrophy	Salivary gland hypertrophy
Lanugo hair	Dental enamel erosion, tooth decay
Amenorrhea	Oligomenorrhea or amenorrhea
Edema	Enlarged parotids
Constipation	Loss of gag reflex
Polyuria	Esophagitis
	Constipation/diarrhea
	Peripheral edema
	Irregular menses
Laboratory Findings	
Anemia, leukopenia	Electrolyte abnormalities (hypokalemic alkalosis)
Elevated liver enzymes	Elevated serum amylase
Hypoglycemia	Metabolic alkalosis/acidosis
Increased serum cholesterol	Hypoglycemia
Hypothalamic/pituitary/endocrine	Hypocalcemia
gland abnormalities	Dehydration
Delayed gastric emptying	
Cortical atrophy on computed tomography	
Complications	
Sudden death possibly related to the	Pancreatitis
presence of prolonged QT interval	Ipecac-induced cardiomyopathy
Acute gastric dilatation	Esophageal or gastric rupture
Osteoporosis	Pneumomediastinum
	"Cathartic colon"

Source: Reprinted from Devlin MJ and Walsh T. Anorexia Nervosa and Bulimia Nervosa. In *Obesity*. Bjorntorp P and Brodoff BN, eds. Philadelphia: Lippincott, 1992.

Part 2: Nutrition Assessment

4. **Using AN's percent weight for height calculation given on the physical exam, is she well-nourished?**

   According to the growth chart, AN's weight is 82 percent of the ideal weight for her height, a fact that supports the diagnosis of malnutrition. Her MAMC is between the 10th and 25th percentiles, and her TSF is at the 10th percentile, indicating that she has depleted subcutaneous fat stores.

5. **Is AN's present diet appropriate for her age and physical activity level?**

   No, AN's diet is inadequate to meet her needs, as she is consuming less than 1500 kcal per day and frequently skips meals. A sufficient diet would not normally maintain an adolescent at only 77 percent weight for height. Growing adolescents have increased energy requirements to support their rapid growth. In addition, vigorous exercise, such as running, further increases energy requirements 30 to 50 percent above basal needs.

It may be difficult for this patient to meet her high energy requirements while maintaining a very low fat intake. In addition, if AN avoids dairy products, she will be unable to meet her calcium requirement.

6.   **What nutrient deficiencies is AN at risk for developing?**

As mentioned in the preceding answer, AN is at risk for calcium deficiency. The highest requirements for calcium are during infancy and adolescence. Adolescents' high calcium requirement is due to increased bone modeling and skeletal consolidation as they reach their growth peak. Maximal bone mass during skeletal maturation is achieved by adolescence or early adulthood and provides the best protection against bone loss after menopause (osteoporosis). The time period between the ages of nine and twenty (possibly up to thirty) years is critical for developing peak bone mass. However, adolescents often do not consume enough dairy products to meet their RDA for calcium (1200 mg/day).

Females require an adequate percentage of body fat for menses to occur because adipose tissue provides an extragonadal source of estrogen. Adolescents who develop amenorrhea face an increased risk of osteoporosis because of their lower levels of estrogen. Estrogen promotes the maintenance of bone mineral density by favoring osteoblastic activity.

AN's low hemoglobin value is indicative of anemia, most likely iron deficiency anemia, another sign that her current diet is not meeting her macronutrient and micronutrient needs. Adolescents require increased dietary iron to support growth. Menstruating females have an even greater iron requirement due to monthly blood loss. Adolescents often do not consume foods rich in iron, which include liver, red meat, legumes, dried fruits, and green vegetables, especially when they skip meals.

Exercise can also increase iron needs due to hemolysis induced by trauma to the capillaries in the feet and increased body temperature. Additional losses of iron occur through sweating and muscle breakdown. GI bleeding has also been noted in runners. A study of high-school runners found increasing risk for iron depletion as training progressed. Female adolescents are also at greater risk for iron deficiency than males because of monthly menstrual losses. However, since AN has missed her periods, this is less of an issue. When her menstrual periods resume, her requirements will be even greater than normal, to allow restoration of her current deficiency and to keep up with her monthly blood loss.

7.   **What recommendations are appropriate for AN?**

Helping AN admit to and recognize that she has a problem is the first step in the management and treatment of an eating disorder. Although it may be awkward, questioning patients with this type of history whether they periodically induce vomiting and use laxatives is critical. Remember, eating disorders primarily occur in adolescents and college-aged women. Those especially at risk include dancers, long-distance runners, figure skaters, actors, models, wrestlers, and jockeys. The initial goal of therapy for AN should be to gain control over her purging and avoid periods of fasting becaus skipping meals will most likely contribute to her binging, purging, and fasting cycle. AN must also adopt a more realistic body image in order to accept a healthier weight goal.

Because of the associated complications, namely electrolyte imbalances and cardiovascular and GI symptoms, individuals with eating disorders need to be monitored medically and may need hospitalization. Those who are 25 to 30 percent below their ideal weight are often hospitalized. Since AN is currently at 77 percent of her ideal weight, she will require close monitoring by her physician and will need to be hospitalized if her weight does not increase in the next few weeks. She should be advised of the severity of her problem, and referred to a psychiatrist or psychologist specializing in eating disorders. Outpatient centers and programs are available for individual and group counseling.

AN requires nutrition counseling on a healthy diet that meets the energy and nutrient needs attributed to her vigorous exercise training and normal adolescent growth. By planning her own well-balanced meals with a registered dietitian experienced in treating patients with eating disorders, AN can meet these needs and prevent deficiencies. She should be advised to consume a well-balanced diet, avoid fad diets or skipping meals, and stop inducing vomiting. By consuming three well-rounded meals with an emphasis on complex carbohydrates, dairy products, fruits, vegetables, and meat, she will meet her needs. With the exception of organ meats, red meat is the best source of iron; therefore, AN should not eliminate red meat entirely from her diet. A vitamin and mineral supplement would also be beneficial, since it will take time to improve her diet. Moreover, such counseling should be completed carefully to not exacerbate AN's preoccupation with calorie counting.

See Chapter Review Question, pages A7–A9.

REFERENCES

Abraham M (ed). *Rudolph's Pediatrics*. 19th ed. Norwalk, CT: Appleton and Lange, 1991:130.

American Psychiatric Association: *Diagnostic and Statistical Manual of Mental Disorders*. 4th ed. (DSM IV). Washington, DC: American Psychiatric Association, 1994.

Anonymous. NIH consensus development and panel on optimum calcium intake. *JAMA* 1994;272(24):1942–1948.

Committee on Nutrition. *Pediatric Nutrition Handbook*. 3rd ed. Elk Grove Village, IL: American Academy of Pediatrics, 1993.

Fitzgerald FT. Bulimia: Recognizing a potentially deadly disorder for what it is. *Consultant* 1995;12:1765–1773.

Gallagher-Allred C, Gabel LL. Managing common adolescent nutritional problems. *Family Practice Recertification* 1995;17(7):21–37.

Halmi KA, Mitchell JE, Rigotti NA. Anorexia and bulimia: You can help. *Patient Care.* 1993;3:24–52.

Havala T, Shronts E. Managing the complications associated with refeeding. *Nutr Clin Prac* 1990;5:23–29.

Henderson RC. Bone health in adolescence: Anorexia and athletic amenorrhea. *Nut Tod* 1991;26:21.

Lauer RM, Clarke WR. Use of cholesterol measurements in childhood for the prediction of adult hypercholesterolemia. The Muscatine Study. *JAMA* 1990;264: 3034–3038.

Lozoff B, Jimenez E, Wolf AW. Long-term developmental outcome of infants with iron deficiency. *N Engl J Med* 1991;325:687–694.

Matkovic V, Fontana D, Goel P, Chestnut CH. Factors which influence peak bone mass formation: A study of calcium balance and the inheritance of bone mass in adolescent females. *Am J Clin Nutr* 1990;52:878–888.

Pathobiological Determinants of Atherosclerosis in Youth Research Group. Relationship of atherosclerosis in young men to serum lipoprotein cholesterol concentrations and smoking. A Preliminary Report From the Pathobiological Determinants of Atherosclerosis in Youth (PDAY) Research Group. *JAMA* 1990;264:3018–3024.

Rock CL, Zerbe KJ. Keeping eating disorders at bay. *Patient Care* 1995;11: 78–104.

Shils ME, Olson JA, Shike M (eds). Modern Nutrition in Health and Disease. 8th ed. Philadelphia: Lea and Febiger, 1994.

Snetselaar L, Lauer RM. Report of the Expert Panel on Blood Cholesterol in Children and Adolescents: The National Cholesterol Education Program. *Sem Pediat Gastroent Nutr* 1991;2:6–14.

Solomon SM, Kirby DF. The refeeding syndrome: a review. *J Parent Ent Nutr* 1990;14(1):90–97.

Stuhldreher WL, Orchard TJ, Donahue RP, et al. Cholesterol screening in childhood: Sixteen-year Beaver County Lipid Study experience. *J Pediat* 1991;119: 551–556.

Sullivan PF. Mortality in anorexia nervosa. *Am J Psychiatry* 1995;152: 1073–1074.

Thiel A, Broocks A, Ohlmeier M, et al. Obsessive compulsive disorder among patients with anorexia and bulimia nervosa. *Am J Psychiatry* 1995;152:72–75.

Wilson NW, Hamburger RN. Severe cow's milk induced colitis in an exclusively breast fed neonate. Case report and clinical review of cow's milk allergy. *Clin Pediat* 1990;29:77–80.

5

Older Adults

Eugenia Siegler and Lisa Hark

Objectives

- To understand the normal metabolic changes associated with aging and their influence on the nutritional requirements of older adults.
- To learn to assess the functional status of older adults and understand its relationship to nutritional status.
- To identify the most prevalent nutritional problems of older adults, such as malnutrition and osteoporosis.
- To identify common drug-nutrient interactions in older adults and to understand why this population is at risk for such interactions.

According to the United States Department of Health and Human Services report, *Healthy People 2000*, nutrition is one of the many factors affecting the health and longevity of older people. For many low-income and minority older adults, it may be the most important factor.

Working with older individuals can present many challenges, especially from a nutritional standpoint. Older people's nutritional status is related to a variety of circumstances, including social, economic, environmental, and physical changes normally associated with aging. An estimated 40 percent of older adults manifest nutritional problems such as protein energy malnutrition, obesity, or vitamin and mineral deficiencies.

Therefore, assessing and treating older adults successfully requires a basic understanding of the most commonly observed problems in this population. Although the nutritional assessment parameters described in Chapter 1 are applicable to older adults, little direct research has been done among this population.

In 1900, the average life expectancy was 48 years. By 1985, it had climbed to 75 years. As a result, in the United States the older adult population is rapidly expanding. Presently, 25 million Americans are over the age of 65. Furthermore, Americans 85 years of age and older are the fastest growing segment of the population. By the year 2050, an estimated 60 million Americans will be 65 or over, and one million Americans will be over 100.

Metabolic Changes Associated with Aging

Understanding the metabolic changes that usually occur with the aging process is helpful when assessing older adults. Among them are:

Decreased lean body mass (LBM) Lean body mass decreases 10 percent from age 25 to 60 years, another 10 percent from age 60 to 75 years, and 20 to 25 percent more after age 75. Moderate exercise preserves lean body mass and helps maintain healthy weight, thereby slowing down this process.

Decreased basal metabolic rate (BMR) The BMR decreases with age due to the body's decreased LBM and increased adipose tissue (see Table 5-1). Because older people's total energy expenditure decreases as a result of their declining activity level, they require fewer calories to maintain their weight. Therefore, older people who consume the same number of calories as always should increase their physical activity to prevent obesity. Once again, these metabolic changes can be prevented with exercise.

Table 5-1   Comparison of body composition in a 25-year-old and a 70-year-old.

TISSUE	25-YEAR-OLD	70-YEAR-OLD
Fat (%)	20–30	35–40
Lean body mass (%)	47	36

Nutritional Risk Factors for Malnutrition in Older Adults

Acute and Chronic Diseases

Eighty-five percent of older adults have one or more chronic disorders. Among the most common are obesity, diabetes, hypertension, arthritis, osteoporosis, cardiovascular disease, and malnutrition. Chronic diseases often require patients to follow a low-cholesterol, low-fat, low-salt, or low-protein diet. All of these special diets may offer less variety and result in decreased nutrient intake. Other conditions often associated with weight loss in older adults are: cancer, anemia, anorexia, pressure ulcers, dehydration, and hip fractures. Patients who present signs of malnutrition concurrently with acute or chronic illness should be monitored closely.

The American Dietetic Association, the American Academy of Family Physicians, and the National Council on Aging have jointly organized the Nutrition Screening Initiative and developed assessment protocols for nutrition screening of older adults. According to the Nutrition Screening Initiative, older adults with the following conditions or a history of these conditions have an increased risk of developing nutritional problems.

Nutritional Risk Factors for Older Adults

Alcoholism	Fecal impaction
Altered mental status/dementia	Fever/infections
Altered taste and smell/anorexia	Fractures
Anorexia	Gastrointestinal disorders
Burns	Hypertension
Cancer	Incontinence
Cardiovascular disease	Liver disease
Chronic obstructive pulmonary disease	Malabsorption
Congestive heart failure	Osteoporosis or osteomalacia
Degenerative bone or joint disease	Pressure ulcers
Dehydration	Renal disease (end-stage)
Depression	Stroke
Diabetes mellitus	Surgery
Diarrhea	Trauma
Dysphagia	Tube feeding

Source: The Nutrition Screening Initiative. 2626 Pennsylvania Ave. NW, Suite 301, Washington, DC 20037.

Risk Factors for Malnutrition

Dental Problems

Approximately 30 to 55 percent of older adults are edentulous by age 65. Patients who have loose, decaying, or missing teeth, difficulty chewing, or ill-fitting dentures, or who fail to wear their dentures, may be at risk for poor nutrition due to decreased intake.

Isolation/Depression

As many as one-third of all older adults live alone. Elderly patients experiencing loneliness, depression, apathy, physical disability, bereavement, and social isolation may have decreased food intake, appetite, and motivation to shop and prepare meals as a result. Loneliness, and in particular the lack of a companion at mealtimes, may have a negative impact on appetite. Depression is also a common precursor to weight loss.

Alcohol Abuse

Approximately 30 percent of individuals over the age of 75 drink alcohol, with 10 percent of those older than 65 diagnosed as alcoholics. The type of alcohol and the duration and frequency of alcohol consumption should be ascertained during the social history; although older adults drink smaller drinks, they tend to drink more drinks per day. Excessive alcohol consumption can lead to weight loss and cause primary vitamin A, B12, thiamin, and folate deficiencies, depending on the person's history of alcohol abuse.

"Determining Your Nutritional Health Checklist" is the basic Level I screening tool used to identify warning signs of poor nutrition (see box below). This checklist contains ten questions and addresses the number of meals eaten per day, medication use, and any weight change that has occurred over the previous six months—all potential identifiers of patients at increased nutritional risk.

Determine Your Nutritional Health Checklist

The warning signs of poor nutritional health are often overlooked. Use this checklist to find out if you or someone you know is at risk.

Read the statement below. Circle the number in the <u>Yes</u> column for those that apply to you or someone you know. For each <u>Yes</u> answer score the number in the box. Total your nutritional score.

	YES
I have an illness or condition that made me change the kind and/or amount of food I eat.	2
I eat fewer than two meals per day.	3
I eat few fruits, vegetables, or milk products.	2
I have three or more drinks of beer, liquor, or wine almost every day.	2
I have tooth or mouth problems that make it hard for me to eat.	2
I don't always have enough money to buy the food I need.	4
I eat alone most of the time.	1
I take three or more different prescribed or over-the-counter drugs a day.	1
Without wanting to, I have lost or gained 10 lbs. in the last six months.	2
I am not always physically able to shop, cook, and/or feed myself.	2
	TOTAL

0–2   Good! Recheck your score in six months.

3–5   You are at moderate nutritional risk. See what can be done to improve your eating habits and lifestyle. Your local office on aging, senior nutrition program, senior citizens center, or health department can help. Recheck your nutritional score in three months.

6+   You are at high nutritional risk. Bring this checklist the next time you see your doctor, dietitian, or other qualified health or social service professional. Talk with them about any problems you have. Ask for help to improve your nutritional health.

Source: Nutrition Screening Initiative. 2626 Pennsylvania Ave. NW, Suite 301, Washington, DC 20037.

Financial Constraints

Poverty is estimated to be twice as common among older adults than among the general population. As many as 40 percent of older adults have annual incomes under $6000. Consequently, older persons may have difficulty purchasing food or participating in food programs that require transportation. Both of these factors can significantly reduce their food intake. In a recent survey of almost 6000 adults over 65, 16 percent felt that they could not afford to feed themselves adequately. Therefore, considering the patient's socioeconomic status and consulting available social services are essential to selecting the best treatment option.

Medication Side Effects

In the United States, older adults represent just 12 percent of the population, yet they consume 30 percent of all prescribed and over-the-counter drugs sold annually. Twenty percent of older men and women take at least one medication daily, and 23 percent take at least five. Because aging is associated with decreased total body water and increased body fat, older adults maintain higher serum drug levels than younger people given the same dosage.

Medications affect nutritional status by

- altering food intake, absorption, metabolism, and excretion of nutrients
- decreasing appetite, taste, and smell, thereby contributing to weight loss
- causing GI disturbances such as constipation or diarrhea

The following examples are typical drug-nutrient interactions:

Psychotherapeutic agents Antidepressants, antipsychotics, and sedatives may cause dry mouth, anorexia, alter appetite, diminish awareness of mealtimes, and exacerbate constipation.

Diuretics Used to treat hypertension and edema, diuretics can affect mineral excretion and deplete the body's store of sodium, potassium, magnesium, calcium, or zinc.

H-2 blockers and antacids Used to treat gastric ulcers, heartburn, and gastritis, these medications may impair absorption of calcium, iron, zinc, and vitamins B_{12}, C, and D.

Laxatives Excessive use of agents intended to relieve constipation may ultimately contribute to constipation. Overuse of mineral oil, which can trap the fat-soluble vitamins A, D, E, and K, may decrease the body's ability to absorb them. Laxatives of all types may also cause potassium depletion.

Phenytoin use in tube-fed patients Tube feedings inhibit the absorption of phenytoin. Patients receiving enteral nutritional support (tube feeding) who take phenytoin must therefore receive the drug apart from the feeding. The recommended separation between tube feeding and administration of a scheduled dose of phenytoin (before or after the feeding) is two hours.

In addition, the following medications can interfere with the normal metabolism of certain vitamins and minerals.

Antibiotics: vitamin K

Barbiturates: vitamin D and folate

Colchicine: vitamin B_{12}

Digitalis preparations: zinc

Dilantin or phenobarbital: vitamins D, K, B_6, and folate

Isoniazid (INH): vitamin B_6

Methotrexate: folate and calcium

Bile acid resins: vitamins A, B_{12}, E, and K, and folate

Assessing the Nutritional Status of Older Adults

Functional Status

The medical history of an older adult should include an assessment of his or her functional status. Older adults with limited functional capacity are clearly at risk for nutritional problems if their deficits are not properly identified and addressed. Functional capacity is defined as the ability to perform a number of routine daily living activities required for general well-being. For each of the activities, the patient can be described as independent, dependent, or in need of assistance.

Activities of Daily Living (ADLs) measure functional disability in older adults. Individuals who are bedridden or are unable for other reasons to perform these activities are considered frail and are more likely to be undernourished. In a recent Medicare survey, 19 percent of noninstitutionalized older adults reported limitations in the following activities of daily living.

- Toileting
- Dressing
- Bathing
- Feeding
- Grooming
- Locomotion
- Transferring from the bed to the chair

Instrumental Activities of Daily Living (IADL) measure higher-level activities in older adults. These activities also serve as a screening tool to identify possible nutritional problems.

- Shopping
- Cooking
- Handling money
- Using transportation

- Managing medications
- Housekeeping
- Using the telephone

Physical Exam and Anthropometric Data

Weight and weight history are critical parameters for nutrition assessment of older adults. Numerous studies have shown increased morbidity and mortality in patients who are losing weight or who are only 80 to 90 percent of their ideal body weight. Fluid changes in both the hospitalized and nonhospitalized older adult must also be considered. If an older adult suffers from fluid retention (ascites from liver disease or edema from congestive heart failure), a "dry" weight (weight without the excess fluid) should be estimated. The following parameters should be calculated routinely in older adults.

1. Estimation of ideal body weight using the rule-of-thumb method
2. Percent ideal body weight
3. The percent weight change, in the event of a weight loss or gain

Laboratory Tests

A serum albumin level under 3.5g /dL or a total serum cholesterol level under 160 mg/dL, are indicators of protein-malnutrition. Note that albumin levels may appear normal in older patients who are dehydrated because dehydration causes falsely elevated albumin readings. Albumin and cholesterol levels may also be reduced in patients with liver and renal diseases.

Nutritional Requirements of Older Adults

Vitamin and mineral deficiencies are a common problem among older adults. In an attempt to respond to the need for guidelines for this population, in 1989 the Food and Nutrition Board of the National Academy of Sciences established recommended daily allowances (RDAs) for members of the United States population. Requirements for the 51+ age group are listed in Table 5-2. Determining the RDAs proved difficult because of the physiological diversity and heterogeneity of the older adult population and the prevalence of chronic disease in this age group.

Table 5-2 Recommended daily allowances (RDAs) and estimated safe and adequate daily dietary intakes (ESADDIs) for older Americans (51+ years).

NUTRIENT	MEN	WOMEN	NUTRIENT	MEN	WOMEN
Protein (g)	60	46	Folate (mg)	0.2	0.18
Vitamin A (mcg RE)*	1000	800	Vitamin B$_{12}$ (mcg)	2.0	2.0
Vitamin D (mcg)	400	400	Calcium (mg)	1000	1500§
Vitamin E (mcg)	10	8	Phosphorus (mg)	800	800
Vitamin K (mcg)	80	65	Magnesium (mg)	350	280
Vitamin C (mg)	60	60	Iron (elemental) (mg)	10	10
Thiamin (mg)	1.2	1.0	Zinc (mg)	15	12
Riboflavin (mg)	1.4	1.2	Iodine (mcg)	150	150
Niacin (mg NE)†	15	13	Selenium (mcg)	70	55
Vitamin B$_6$ (mg)	2.0	1.6			

*Retinol equivalents.
† IU
NE=niacin equivalents.
§Post-menopausal, not receiving estrogen.

Source: Food and Nurition Board. *Recommended Dietary Allowances.* 10th ed. National Academy of Sciences: Washington DC, 1989.

Nutrient Deficiencies and Related Disorders

Vitamin D Deficiency

Normal Functions of Vitamin D

Vitamin D plays an essential regulatory role in the following bodily functions (see Figure 5-1):

- normal bone mineralization
- intestinal absorption of calcium and phosphorus
- renal reabsorption and homeostasis of amino acids and PO4
- activity of parathyroid hormone (PTH) on bone and kidney

Risk Factors for Vitamin D Deficiency

Factors that have been demonstrated to increase the risk of vitamin D deficiency in older individuals include

- inadequate exposure to the sun attributable to homebound status, living in northern latitudes (40 to 50 percent of institutionalized older adults have vitamin D deficiency)
- avoidance of dietary sources of vitamin D and calcium
- increased use of drugs that interfere with vitamin D status (e.g., anticonvulsants such as phenytoin and phenobarbital, which increase liver catabolism of vitamin D

Figure 5-1   Normal Vitamin D Metabolism

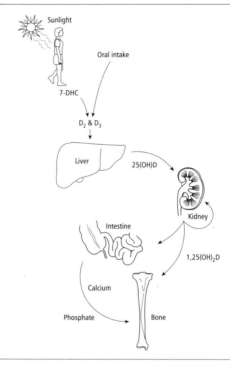

Vitamin D may be ingested as ergocalciferol (D2) or cholecalciferol (D3) or synthesized from 7-dehydrocholesterol (7-DHC) in the skin after exposure to the sun. To become activated, vitamin D must undergo 25-hydroxylation in the liver (calcidiol: 25-(OH)D3) followed by 1-hydroxylation in the kidneys (calcitriol: 1,25-(OH)2D3). Once activated, vitamin D is free to act on bones, kidneys, and intestines to maintain calcium, phosphate, and bone homeostasis.

Source: Adapted from Reichel H, Koeffler HP, Normal AW. *N Engl J Med* 1989;320:980.

- age-related decline in the capacity for cutaneous phototransformation of 7-dehydrocholesterol
- age-related decline in the kidney's ability to form 1,25-(OH)2-D3 even when stimulated by PTH
- malabsorption of fat-soluble vitamins A, D, E, and K in conjunction with certain GI diseases

Symptoms

Vitamin D deficiency should be suspected in patients who present the following symptoms, either individually or in combination:

- deep bone and muscle pain; generalized bone tenderness
- muscle weakness

- appendicular fractures (osteopenia, osteomalacia)
- hyperesthesia (abnormal sensitivity of the skin or an organ to touch)
- osteomalacia

To establish a diagnosis of vitamin D deficiency, obtaining a serum 25-(OH)-D3 to evaluate the body's stores of this nutrient is essential. Normal serum values are as follows:

Summer: 15–80 ng/mL
Winter: 14–42 ng/mL

Osteoporosis

A major affliction among older people, osteoporosis, a reduction in the quantity of bone mass, renders the bones susceptible to fractures as a result of minimal trauma.

Statistics

In the United States, the incidence of osteoporosis has increased in proportion with the aging population. Currently, osteoporosis

- afflicts 20 million Americans, mostly postmenopausal women (one in four of whom develop this disorder)
- leads to 1.5 million fractures every year in the United States, most commonly of the vertebrae, distal radius, and hip
- is the cause of death in 20 percent of afflicted patients within one year of a traumatic event
- leaves half of the survivors unable to walk again
- costs an estimated ten billion dollars annually for treatment of fractures in its victims

Signs and Symptoms

Classic indicators of osteoporosis include
- altered posture caused by deformity of the spine, or postural slumping due to acute pain
- loss of height as a result of vertebral collapse fractures
- changes in physical appearance such as increased thoracic kyphosis (humpback) described as a "widow's hump"
- back pain secondary to compression fracture

The most commonly observed fractures in victims of osteoporosis affect two types of bones:
- spongy trabecular bones of the axial skeleton; vertebrae, ribs, ends of long bones (wrists, humerous, hips)

Contributing Risk Factors

The following genetic, behavioral, iatrogenic, and environmental risk factors are all believed to contribute to the development of osteoporosis.

Development of Osteoporosis

Primary Factors

normal decreases in bone mass with advancing age
family history of osteoporosis
premature menopause
short stature and small bones
sedentary lifestyle
cigarette smoking
alcohol abuse
race (Caucasian and Asian)
diets low in vitamin D and/or calcium throughout life

Secondary Factors

long-term glucocorticoid or anticonvulsant therapy
chronic conditions such as anorexia and malabsorption
chronic obstructive pulmonary disease (COPD)
hyperthyroidism and hyperparathyroidism
renal osteodystrophy

Preventive Measures

Osteoporosis takes a lifetime to develop, and consequently a lifetime to prevent. Proper diet is currently thought to be the most critical and controllable measure individuals can take to avoid osteoporosis. Adequate amounts of calories and sufficient calcium intake to promote optimum bone development are especially important during the first three decades of life. Calcium and vitamin D supplementation (either alone or in a multivitamin) is helpful in patients who have a family history or early signs of osteoporosis or whose dietary calcium intake is known to be poor. Exercise—especially weight-bearing exercise—has been shown to benefit those at risk for osteoporosis by helping to reduce the loss of bone mass that is part of the aging process. Finally, a growing body of evidence supports the positive role of anti-resorptive therapy which includes hormonal therapy (estrogen replacement therapy during menopause), biphosphate therapy, and calcitonin in reducing the incidence of this disorder.

Optimal Calcium Intake

Meeting the calcium requirements throughout life is essential for proper skeletal growth and maturation. Calcium requirements increase as people grow older to compensate for the decreased production of $1,25(OH)_2D$ by the kidney and the accelerated bone mineral losses and to maintain maximal bone mass.

Studies reveal that the usual calcium intake of older adults is between 400 and 500 mg per day (about 1½ cups of milk or yogurt, or 1½ slices of cheese). The NHANES III survey revealed that the average woman consumes less than half of the RDA for calcium.

Because of its pivotal role in the normal development of healthy bone, calcium requirements were a major focus of the NIH Consensus Development Conference on Optimal Calcium Intake held in June 1994. A key outcome of the conference was an increase in the recommended levels of calcium intake compared to the RDA. Clearly the average Americans daily calcium intake falls well below the following recommendations.

NIH Conference Recommendations for Calcium Intake

Men	25–65 years	1000 mg
	Over 65 years	1500 mg
Women	25–50 years	1000 mg
	Over 50 years (postmenopausal)	
	On estrogens	1000 mg
	Not on estrogens	1500 mg
	Over 65 years	1500 mg

Nutrition Questions for the Older Adults History and Physical Exam

Past Medical History

Chronic diseases, including obesity
Medications, including over-the-counter products
Vitamin, mineral, or fiber supplements: use or abuse
Food allergies

Social History

Reliability of the patient
Recent loss of spouse
Alcohol consumption
Tobacco use: frequency and duration
Documentation of dietary habits: 24-hour recall, usual intake, food frequency, or food record
Number of meals eaten daily and percentage actually consumed
Food avoidance or restrictions
Economic situation as it affects the ability to obtain and prepare food
Living situation
Special diet (kosher, vegetarian, medical)

Family History

Diseases such as diabetes, heart disease, osteoporosis, hypertension, and cancer

Functional Status

Activities of daily living and instrumental activities of daily living

Review of Systems

General: Weakness, fatigue, clothes tighter or looser, cold intolerance, weight change (how much and over what period of time?)
Skin: Dryness, roughness, easy bruisability (ecchymosis), itching
Hair: Recent changes in texture, color, pluckability
Eyes: Blurred vision, blindness or blind spots, yellowing of the whites of the eyes
Mouth: Condition of teeth, gums, lips, and tongue, dentures, taste, smell, sores
Cardiac: Palpitations, dyspnea, orthopnea
Nails: Recent changes in texture, shape, brittleness, color
GI/Abdomen: Appetite, food intolerance, swallowing, vomiting, nausea, constipation, diarrhea, stool changes, flatulence
Extremities: Swelling, joint pain, sensitivity to cold
Neurological: Seizures, tingling, headaches, decreased sensation, dizziness
Musculoskeletal: Weakness
Endocrine: Cold or heat intolerance, polyuria, polyphagia, polydipsia

Physical Examination and Anthropometric Data

Vital signs *Temperature, heart rate, respiration, blood pressure*

Anthropometric Data

Current height, weight, usual weight, ideal weight, and weight history
Interpretation of % ideal weight, and % weight change if weight loss has occurred

General: Fever, obesity, edema, cachexia, depression
Skin: Rashes, xerosis, follicular hyperkeratosis, flakiness, dermatitis, pallor, dryness, ecchymosis, pressure ulcers, slow-healing wounds, acanthosis nigricans, petechiae, purpura
Hair: Dyspigmentation, easily pluckability, thinning, alopecia
Head: Temporal muscle wasting
Eyes: Pale, dull conjunctival scleral xerosis, Bitot's spots (thickening of conjunctiva), ophthalmoplegia, arcus cornea, scleral icterus
Mouth: Condition of teeth and gums, state of dentures, dysgeusia

Tongue: Glossitis, edema, atrophic lingual papillae
Lips: Cheilosis, angular stomatitis, fissures, scars
Cardiac: Cardiomyopathy, arrhythmia, tachycardia, bradycardia,
    heart failure
Nails: Brittleness, whiteness, spoon-shaped
Abdomen/GI: Ascites, hepatomegaly, splenomegaly
Extremities: Edema, subcutaneous fat (excess or loss), muscle wasting
    (temporal or subcutaneous)
Neurological: Irritability, weakness, change in deep tendon reflex,
    sensory loss, asterixis, depression, dementia
Musculoskeletal: Muscle wasting, weakness or cramping, growth
    retardation, bone pain and tenderness, fractures, joint tenderness

Laboratory Data

Albumin, prealbumin, transferrin, hematocrit, hemoglobin, glucose,
    cholesterol, BUN, and electrolytes (especially potassium and sodium)

Problem List and Assessment

Primary malnutrition: No pathological process found to explain the
    signs and symptoms of malnutrition. Usually, this form of malnutrition
    is the result of inadequacies, excesses, or imbalances in nutrient intake.
Secondary malnutrition: Nutritional problems of this type occur when a
    pathological process results in
        inadequate food intake
        impaired absorption and utilization of nutrients
        increased losses or excretion of nutrients or increased nutrient
            requirements
        drug-nutrient interactions

Treatment Plan

The following factors have important implications for the treatment of
nutritional disorders in older adults and therefore should be addressed
during the formulation of an appropriate treatment plan.
    Attention to social needs
    Medical and laboratory evaluation, including dental evaluation
    Adjustment of calorie and nutrient intake
    Delivery of nutrition if the patient is disabled
    Bowel regimen adjustment
    Attention to hydration status
    Occupational and physical therapy to improve functional status
    Consultation with a registered dietitian

Case 1

Malnutrition and Depression

Eugenia Siegler and Lisa Hark

Objectives

- To use the history and physical exam to identify factors that affect the nutritional status of older adults.

- To apply nutrition assessment techniques to the older adult.

- To evaluate the appropriateness of an older adult's dietary intake.

- To develop a nutritional care plan for an older adult who became malnourished after a hip fracture.

ML, an 85-year-old woman, visits her geriatrician for a check up after surgery for a hip fracture. The recent death of her husband had caused her to miss her previous scheduled visit. In the office, ML starts to cry and explains how much her life has changed because of her husband's death and the loss of his pension just prior to his death.

History of Present Illness

ML tripped on the steps in her house two months ago, fractured her hip, and underwent surgery to repair the fracture. The surgery went well, and the hip was pinned successfully, but she lost a significant amount of blood during the procedure. ML underwent inpatient rehabilitation for ten days after discharge from the surgical service and has been at home ever since. She ambulates with a cane and can climb stairs with difficulty.

Past Medical History

ML's past medical history is positive for depression. She has no major chronic diseases except for osteoporosis, discovered at the time of her hip fracture two months ago. ML had an appendectomy at age 46. She has no previous history of pneumonia, tuberculosis, hepatitis, or urinary tract infection.

Medications

ML currently takes doxepin (Sinequan) for depression and an iron supplement for anemia (325 mg of FeSO4 three times per day). She has no known food allergies.

Social History

ML lives alone in the four-bedroom, two-story home she has occupied since she married 55 years ago. Her son and daughter both live out of state. Although they call her every few weeks, they have not visited since her husband's death. ML also explains that she used to attend church and visit the local Senior Center regularly with her husband, but has not been to either lately. ML explains that she has no energy to "get up and go" anymore and she falls asleep in front of the television. She also complains of being constipated and that her food does not have much taste. Her reported use of alcohol, tobacco, and caffeine follows.

Alcohol: None

Tobacco: None

Caffeine: One cup of coffee and two cups of tea daily

Dietary Information

At her physician's request, ML provided the following 24-hour dietary re-call, stating that this represents her usual daily intake:

ML's Usual Daily Intake		
Breakfast (home)	Jelly doughnut	1 whole
	White toast	1 slice
	Jelly	2 Tbs.
	Tea	2 cups
Lunch (home)	Butter cookies	2
	Chicken and rice soup	1 cup
	Saltine crackers	6
	Tea	2 cups
Dinner (home)	White bread	1 slice
	Jelly	2 Tbs.
	Peanut butter	2 Tbs.
	Butter cookies	2
	Total calories: 1000 kcal/day	
	Protein: 23 g/day (9% of calories)	
	Fat: 31% of calories	
	Carbohydrate: 60% of calories	

Review of Systems

General: Weakness, fatigue, weight loss, and depression

Mouth: Food lacks taste (hypogeusia)

GI: Poor appetite, constipation

Extremities: Hip pain when climbing stairs, some tenderness at old incision site

Physical Examination

Vital signs

Temperature: 97.0°F

Heart rate: 82 BPM

Respiration: 18 BPM

Blood pressure: 150/80 mm Hg

Anthropometric data

Height: 5'6" (168 cm)

Current weight: 110 lb (50 kg)

Weight 6 months ago: 125 lb (57 kg)

Usual weight: 140 lb (64 kg)

Ideal weight: 130 lb (59 kg)

Percent IBW: 85% (110/130)

Percent weight change: 12% [125–110/125]

General: Thin, elderly woman who appears sad but pleasant. She is well-groomed, but her clothes are loose-fitting.

Skin: Warm to touch

HEENT: Temporal muscle wasting, no enlargement of thyroid

Mouth: Ill-fitting dentures, sore beneath bottom plate

Cardiac: Normal exam

Abdomen: Well-healed appendectomy site scar, no enlargement of liver or spleen, normal bowel sounds

Extremities: Well-healed hip surgery incision with slight surrounding erythema, no edema or sores on feet

Rectal: Hard stool in vault, stool test for occult blood negative

Neurological: Alert, good memory, no evidence of sensory loss

Gait: Slightly wide-based with decreased arm swing, tentative but safe, used cane appropriately

Laboratory Data

Patient's Lab Values	Normal Values
Albumin: 2.5 g/dL	3.5–5.8 g/dL
Hemoglobin: 11.0 g/dL	11.8–15.5 g/dL
Hematocrit: 33.0%	36–46%

Case Questions

1. What information from the case history would cause you concern over ML's functional status? What more would you want to know?

2. Based on that information, what environmental and social factors could lead to nutritional problems in this patient?

3. Do ML's percent of ideal body weight and percent weight change warrant concern?

4. What are ML's calorie and protein requirements for repletion?

5. Using the dietary information obtained during the social history, what general conclusions can you draw regarding ML's diet?

6. Based on ML's typical intake and her complaint of constipation, what specific dietary changes would you recommend?

7. Should a vitamin and/or mineral supplement be prescribed for ML? Why or why not?

8. How can ML's diet be improved to meet her increased requirements and achieve weight gain?

9. What specific recommendations would you offer to improve ML's nutritional status?

Answers begin on the following page.

Answers to Questions: Case 1

Part 1: Assessing Activities of Daily Living

1. **What information from the case history would cause you concern over this woman's functional status? What more would you want to know?**

    In reviewing the parameters of the Activities of Daily Living and the Instrumental Activities of Daily Living, ML's situation reveals the following concerns.

    Activities of Daily Living (ADLs): Although ML can feed herself, she has trouble chewing because of her loose dentures and a sore in her mouth. She has insufficient money for a visit to the dentist. ML also exhibits poor mobility; she walks with a cane, has difficulty with stairs, and fears falling since her hip fracture. Although she is mobile, she reports moving slowly about the house. Finally, ML's dislike of eating alone may have a negative impact on her food intake.

    Instrumental Activities of Daily Living (IADLs): Since her injury, ML fears going outside. Because she does not drive and is unaccustomed to using public transportation, she has difficulty shopping for food and other necessities. ML reports a very limited social life; since her husband's death she has avoided church, community programs, and the Senior Center. Her reported dislike of cooking for one person most likely will have a negative effect on the quality and quantity of her food intake.

2. **Based on that information, what environmental and social factors could lead to nutritional problems in this patient?**

    ML's ill-fitting dentures and hypogeusia may lead to decreased intake. Depression over the loss of her husband may decrease her appetite. Also, ML lives alone in a large house and may be unable to clean and cook for herself because of her poor mobility. Because she is homebound, her exposure to sunlight is limited. Furthermore, she no longer participates in community activities that could provide support, meals, and social interaction. Her children have not visited recently or provided any assistance. Finally, the loss of her husband's pension has significantly reduced her income.

Part 2: Nutrition Assessment

3. **Do ML's percent of ideal body weight and percent weight change warrant concern?**

    Note that in this case the value used for ML's usual weight is 125 pounds, her weight six months earlier. A percent weight change greater than ten percent in a period of six months is a clinically significant indicator of malnutrition.

4. **What are ML's calorie and protein requirements for repletion?**

   An individual's total estimated daily calorie requirements amount to 25 to 30 kcal per kilogram of ideal weight.

   (59 kg) (25 – 30 kcal/kg) = 1480 to 1770 kcal/day

   The estimated total daily protein requirements are 1.5 g/kg of ideal weight.

   (59 kg) (1.5 g/kg) = 89 g/day

   Based on the dietary information ML has provided, her intake falls considerably below the recommended calorie and protein requirements for her current weight.

5. **Using the dietary information obtained during the social history, what general conclusions can you draw regarding ML's diet?**

   ML's usual daily intake provides 1000 kcal and 23 grams of protein. Her diet is low in calories due to her poor selection of foods and decreased appetite. ML's limited consumption of meats and poultry products, resulting in a poor overall protein intake, probably is due to her limited income and poor dentition. Because ML stopped drinking milk many years ago and does not shop for dairy products regularly, her diet is also lower in calcium and vitamin D than her requirements. Fruits, vegetables, and fluids also appear to be below acceptable limits in ML's diet.

Part 3:   Recommendations

6. **Based on ML's typical intake and her complaints of constipation, what specific dietary changes would you recommend?**

   Constipation, very common in older adults, can be corrected by increasing their fiber and fluid intake. Examples of high-fiber foods include fresh fruits, vegetables, bran cereals, and whole-grain products such as whole-wheat bread and brown rice. One bowl of raisin bran cereal or oatmeal every day would most likely be sufficient to achieve bowel regularity. If these measures are not sufficient, fiber supplements can be recommended. Increasing fluid intake will also help alleviate constipation.

7. **Should a vitamin and/or mineral supplement be prescribed for this patient? Why or why not?**

   Based on the analysis of her usual diet, ML is not receiving adequate vitamins and minerals. Her diet is too low in calories and protein to achieve an adequate vitamin and mineral intake. A multivitamin and mineral supplement, with 100 percent of the USRDA for older adults, is therefore appropriate in her situation. In addition, a calcium supplement and increased milk intake should also be recommended. ML's dietary intake of iron also was below the RDA, but her total iron intake is likely to be adequate if she continues to take her iron supplement and consumes additional calories from animal products, as indicated in the previously suggested dietary modifications.

8. **How can ML's diet be improved to meet her increased requirements and achieve weight gain?**

   In light of her weight loss, ML's diet clearly needs to be higher in calories, protein, and calcium to fulfill her current requirements. Specific suggestions for each meal that ML would be able to implement follow.

Revised Diet Plan to Increase ML's Calorie and Protein Intake

Breakfast (home)	Brewed tea	1 cup
	Instant oatmeal	1 single-serving package
	Lactose-free 2% milk	6 oz.
	Orange juice	4 oz.
Lunch (Senior Center)	Chicken drumstick	3 oz.
	Baked potato	1 medium
	Margarine	2 Tbs.
	Green beans	4 Tbs.
Snack (Senior Center)	Lactose-free 2% milk	8 oz.
	Canned peaches	1/2 cup
Dinner (home)	Tuna salad	4 oz.
	Saltine crackers	6
	Tomatoes	3 slices
	Vanilla pudding	5 oz.
Snack (home)	Applesauce	1/2 cup

Total calories: 1718 kcal/day
Protein: 69 g/day (16% of calories)
Fat: 35% of calories
Carbohydrate: 49% of calories

---

9. **What specific recommendations would you offer to improve ML's nutritional status?**

   In addition to the recommended dietary modifications, ML and/or her geriatrician should take the following steps to ensure her continued well-being.

   - Contact her other health care providers regarding recommended changes in medications and make arrangements to have her dentures properly adjusted.
   - Drink high-calorie, high-protein liquid supplements or add nonfat powdered milk to puddings to increase her intake of calories, protein,

vitamins, and minerals.

- Use a microwave oven to prepare convenience foods and decrease cooking time.
- Contact a social worker to help ML get in touch with the area council on aging, Meals on Wheels, and other community resources.
- Consider a home health aid to monitor ML's weekly weight and food intake and assess whether her ambulatory status is improving or whether she is at increased risk of falling again.
- Utilize community volunteers to shop for food or contact a grocery store that delivers.
- Contact her children and other family members for support and to help her arrange to move to an apartment or a smaller, single-story home.
- Undergo further rehabilitation and exercise therapy to increase her diminished mobility.
- Contact a neighbor with whom ML could share meals or travel to the Senior Center daily for a hot lunch.

Case 2

Tube Feeding and Drug-Nutrient Interactions

Lisa D. Unger and Eugenia Siegler

Objectives

- To use the history and physical exam to identify factors that can affect the nutritional status of older adults.
- To apply nutrition assessment techniques to evaluate the adequacy of an older adult's dietary intake.
- To develop a nutritional care plan for an older adult who cannot swallow safely.
- To identify a drug-nutrient interaction commonly seen in older adults.

PJ, a 79-year-old man, was found lying on the floor by his daughter. He was described as conscious but unable to move his right side, and his daughter could not understand what he was saying. She called 911 for an ambulance, which subsequently took him to the closest emergency room. There, the doctors determined that he had had a stroke and admitted him to the hospital.

History of Present Illness

PJ has a history of type II diabetes mellitus and requires two daily doses of insulin (bid). He has had high blood pressure for most of his adult life and takes a diuretic (hydrochlorothiazide) to control it. Four years ago, PJ was in a car accident and hit his head on the windshield. This injury resulted in a seizure disorder that is being treated with phenytoin. He has not had a seizure for the past two years.

Past Medical History

PJ's prior medical history is positive for arthritis. He underwent an appendectomy at age 55. His current regimen of medications includes human NPH insulin, hydrochlorothiazide, phenytoin, and acetaminophen as needed for knee pain due to arthritis. At present he takes no vitamin supplements. He has no known food allergies.

Social History

PJ is divorced and lives with his daughter in a three-story row home. A former construction worker, he retired at age 62. He currently volunteers at the library. His daughter reports the following details concerning his use of alcohol, tobacco, and caffeine:

Alcohol: One beer in the evening.

Tobacco: 50 pack per year smoking history. He quit smoking five years ago when he moved in with his daughter.

Caffeine: Two cups of coffee daily.

Diet: Follows a low-sugar, low-sodium diet.

Review of Systems

The review of systems proved impossible to conduct because PJ's speech is difficult to understand.

Physical Examination

Vital signs

Temperature: 98.6°F

Heart rate: 90 BPM

Respiration: 14 BPM

Blood pressure: 154/72 mm Hg

Anthropometric data

Height: 5'7" (170 cm)

Current weight: 154 lb (70 kg)

General: Robust, elderly man lying quietly in bed, appears comfortable

Skin: Warm

Head/neck: Right facial drooping

Mouth: Saliva pooling in the mouth

Cardiac: Regular rate and rhythm

Abdomen: Well-healed appendectomy scar, no enlargement of liver or spleen, normal bowel sounds

Extremities: No edema or sores on feet, peripheral pulses absent

Rectal: Stool test negative for occult blood

Neurological: Alert, with diminished mobility on his right side; attempts to answer questions, but his speech is slurred, and his voice sounds garbled; has no gag reflex

Gait: Unable to walk

Laboratory Data

Patient's Lab Values	Normal Values
Albumin: 4.5 g/dL	3.5–5.8 g/dL
Hemoglobin: 15.0 g/dL	13.5–17.5 g/dL
Hematocrit: 46.0%	40–52%
Blood urea nitrogen (BUN): 18 mg/dL	10–20 mg/dL
Creatinine: 0.8 mg/dL	0.8–1.3 mg/dL
Glucose: 270 mg/dL	70–110 mg/dL
Potassium: 3.2 mmol/L	3.5–5.3 mmol/L
Phenytoin: 20 mg/L	10–20 mg/L

Progress

PJ received nasoenteric feedings continuously over 24 hours for one week. He progressed to the point where he was able to use his hands, move in bed, and attend physical therapy. His overall strength increased, his voice grew firmer, and he pleaded that his feeding tube be removed, stating that he wanted to eat real food. Reportedly, his family had given him ice chips, which he chewed and swallowed without difficulty. A speech therapist was consulted to evaluate his swallowing function, and a swallowing study using video fluoroscopy was ordered. During the video fluoroscopy, PJ was instructed to swallow foods of different textures, and his swallowing function was assessed radiographically. During this study, PJ aspirated foods of all consistencies and as a result failed the study. Therefore, the speech therapist recommended maintaining PJ's NPO (no food or liquid by mouth) status and using a feeding tube to meet his nutritional requirements and prevent dehydration. If PJ's swallowing improves to the extent that he is no longer at risk for aspiration, the feeding tube can be removed.

PJ tolerated tube feeding well for the first week. Subsequently his feeding schedule was limited to the 12 hours when he was asleep to enable him to attend physical therapy and participate in other rehabilitation activities in the daytime. After one day of receiving tube feeding over 24 hours, PJ had a seizure at 11 A.M. A review of PJ's medication profile showed that he had been receiving regular human insulin twice a day: at 7 P.M., immediately before his evening tube feeding, and at 7 A.M., at the conclusion of his morning tube feeding. PJ also had been receiving 300 mg/day of phenytoin elixir via his feeding tube at the conclusion of the 7 A.M. feedings.

Case Questions

1. What are PJ's risk factors for a stroke?

2. What abnormalities exist with regard to PJ's fluid and electrolyte status? How can they be corrected?

3. What risks are associated with feeding PJ regular food?

4. Assuming that PJ has a nasoenteric tube for postpyloric feedings, how can his nutrient needs be estimated?

5. What are PJ's long-term feeding tube placement options? What types of permanent feeding tubes are available, and which are the most appropriate for PJ?

6. What factors may have caused PJ's seizure?

7. Why did PJ develop hypoglycemia, and what can be done to prevent its recurrence in the future?

8. What drug-nutrient interaction accounts for PJ's low phenytoin level?

Answers begin on the following page.

Answers to Questions: Case 2

1. What are PJ's risk factors for a stroke?

    PJ's risk factors for a stroke are: diabetes mellitus, a history of smoking, and high blood pressure.

2. What abnormalities exist with regard to PJ's fluid and electrolyte status? How can they be corrected?

    PJ is intravascularly depleted (dehydrated), as evidenced by an elevated BUN/creatinine ratio. Therefore, the emergency room physician placed an IV for hydration with 5-percent dextrose and 1/2 normal saline (NS) solution at an infusion rate of 80 ml per hour. The physician also discontinued PJ's diuretic. In addition, PJ's potassium level is low, so he also received 40 mEq IV potassium. To control his elevated glucose level, PJ received 4 units of regular human insulin subcutaneously.

3. What risks are associated with feeding PJ regular food?

    PJ's stroke left him unable to move his right side. He also has a right facial droop, difficulty speaking and swallowing his saliva, and no gag reflex. Given his difficulty swallowing and absence of a gag reflex, he is at risk for aspiration, with subsequent pneumonia, if he is allowed to eat a regular diet. Aspiration pneumonia is a lung infection due to inhalation of foreign material, such as food. Because of this risk, PJ should not be placed on an oral diet at this time. His feeding options include tube feeding (enteral nutrition) or intravenous feeding (parenteral nutrition). Since his gastrointestinal tract is functional, enteral feeding should be instituted. To minimize his risk for aspiration, a nasoenteric feeding tube should be placed in a postpyloric position.

4. Assuming that PJ has a nasoenteric tube inserted for postpyloric feedings, how can his nutrient needs be estimated?

    To estimate PJ's nutrient needs correctly, his protein and calorie requirements should be considered separately. As for protein, PJ should receive 1.5 g/kg/day to account for his increased needs. Because PJ weighs 70 kg, his protein requirements are 105 g/day.

    To estimate his nonprotein calorie needs, use the Harris-Benedict equations or the 25 kcal/kg rule-of-thumb method with appropriate adjustments for an individual confined to bed. Compare the results of the following two calculations. Using the Harris-Benedict equation,

    66 + {13.7 (70 kg) + 5 (170 cm)} – 6.8 (79 years) = 1338 kcal/day

    1338 kcal/day x 1.3 (confined to bed) = 1739 kcal/day

    Using the 25 kcal/kg rule-of-thumb approach,

    (25 kcal/kg) (70 kg) = 1750 kcal/day

    Having determined PJ's nutrient needs, choose the enteral formula that best meets them. Each of the variety of enteral formulas available provides different concentrations of calories and protein to meet patients' requirements. Once an appropriate formula has been selected, determine the quantity of formula that should be administered to PJ on a daily basis.

5. **What are PJ's long-term feeding tube placement options? What types of permanent feeding tubes are available, and which is the most appropriate for PJ?**

   A percutaneous endoscopic gastrostomy (PEG) tube is placed endoscopically into the stomach under local anesthesia. Inability to feed intragastrically due to an obstruction is the chief contraindication to PEG placement. Patients who are at increased risk for aspiration should not receive a PEG tube because aspiration pneumonia can develop if gastric contents are refluxed. A surgical gastrostomy is a tube placed in the stomach via an incision under general anesthesia. This device is appropriate for patients on whom an endoscopy cannot be performed because of obstruction and who therefore are not candidates for PEGs. A jejunostomy is a tube placed in the jejunum, also under general anesthesia. This alternative is used primarily in patients who require a feeding tube but are at increased risk for aspiration, because its postpyloric positioning minimizes that risk. Because PJ is at increased risk for aspiration, a jejunostomy tube was selected, and within 48 hours of its placement, tube feeding was initiated.

6. **What factors may have caused PJ's seizure?**

   PJ's seizure may have been due to hypoglycemia or to a subtherapeutic phenytoin level. A finger stick blood glucose determined that PJ's glucose level was under 80 mg/dL. Subsequent electrolyte and phenytoin levels revealed a blood glucose of 30 mg/dL (normal = 70–110 mg/dL) and a phenytoin level of 5 mg/L (normal = 10–20 mg/L).

7. **Why did PJ develop hypoglycemia, and what can be done to prevent its recurrence in the future?**

   When PJ was tube-fed initially, his feedings were administered continuously over 24 hours, and he required insulin twice a day. When PJ's tube feeding schedule was changed to a 12-hour nocturnal cycle, he no longer received feedings between 7 A.M. and 7 P.M. However, his insulin regimen was not adjusted accordingly, and he still received insulin in the morning. PJ's development of hypoglycemia at 11 A.M. as a consequence of his earlier dose of insulin probably precipitated his seizure. To prevent future recurrences, finger stick blood sugars should be obtained every 6 hours, and PJ's morning insulin dose should be either decreased or discontinued.

8. **What drug-nutrient interaction accounts for PJ's low phenytoin level?**

   Coadministration of phenytoin and tube feeding is likely to result in decreased absorption of phenytoin. The exact mechanism of the interaction is unknown, but it is believed to be due to the protein or the magnesium and calcium content of tube feeding formulas. Administration of phenytoin and scheduled tube feedings should therefore occur two hours apart. The tube feeding may be given either two hours before or two hours after a scheduled phenytoin dose. Monitoring phenytoin levels closely on initiation or discontinuation of tube feeding is very important. Adjustments in the dosage of phenytoin and the timing of its administration should be made as needed. Thus, administering PJ's phenytoin sometime between 9 A.M. and 5 P.M., instead of at the conclusion of his tube feedings, should minimize future recurrences of this drug-nutrient interaction.

See Chapter Review Questions, pages A9–A11.

REFERENCES

Aloia JF, Vaswani A, Yeh JK, et al. Calcium supplementation with and without hormone therapy to prevent postmenopausal bone loss. *Ann Intern Med* 1994;120:97–103.

Anonymous. NIH consensus development panel on optimal calcium intake. *JAMA* 1994;93(1):137–145.

Applegate WB. Hypertension in elderly patients. *Ann Intern Med* 1989;110: 901–915.

Corti MC, Guralnik JM, Salive JD. Serum albumin level and physical disability as predictors of mortality in older persons. *JAMA* 1994;272:1036–1042.

Drickamer MA, Cooney LM. A geriatrician's guide to enteral feeding. *J Am Geriatr Soc* 1993;41:672–679.

Dwyer JT. *Screening Older Americans' Nutritional health: Current Practices and Future Possibilities*. Washington, DC: Nutrition Screening Initiative, 1991.

Dwyer JT, Gallo JJ, Reichel W. Assessing nutritional status in elderly patients. *Am Family Phys* 1993;47,3:613–620.

Food and Nutrition Board. *Recommended Dietary Allowances*. 10th ed. Washington, DC: National Academy of Sciences, 1989.

Ham RJ. Indicators of poor nutritional status in older Americans. *Am Family Phys* 1992;45,1:219–228.

Healthy People 2000: National Health Promotion and Disease Prevention Objectives. Washington, DC: US Department of Health and Human Services, 1990.

Heaney RP. Consensus Development Conference on Osteoporosis: bone mass, nutrition, and other lifestyle factors. *Am J Med* 1993;95(5A):29S–33S.

Johnson RM, Kaiser FE, Kerstetter JE, et al. Maintaining good nutrition in the elderly. *Patient Care* (November 15) 1995:46–67

Lipschitz DA, Ham RJ, White JV. An approach to nutrition screening for older Americans. *Am Family Phys* 1992;45,2:601–608.

Miller PD. A guide to the management of osteoporosis and prevention of hip fractures in women. *Mod Med* 1992;60:46–52.

Morley JE, Glick X, Rubenstein LZ. *Geriatric Nutrition. A Comprehensive Review.* New York: Raven, 1991.

National Center for Health Statistics. *Health statistics on older persons.* United States, 1986.

Nutrition Screening Initiative. *Nutrition screening manual for professionals caring for older Americans.* Washington, DC: Nutrition Screening Initiative, 1991.

Reichel H, Koeffler HP, Normal AW. The role of vitamin D endocrine system in health and disease. *N Engl J Med* 1989;320:980–991.

Reife CM. Involuntary weight loss. *Med Clin North Amer* 1995;79:299–313.

Report of Nutrition Screening I: Toward a common view. Washington, DC: Nutrition Screening Initiative, 1992.

Reuben DB, Greendale GA, Harrison GG. Nutrition screening in the older person. *J Am Geriatr Soc* 1995;43:415–425.

White JV. Risk factors for poor nutritional status. *Prim Care* (March)1994;21: 19–31.

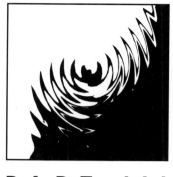

PART III

Nutrition and Pathophysiology

6

Cardiovascular Disease

Daniel J. Rader, Lisa Hark, and Frances Burke

Objectives

- To understand the nutritional manifestations and therapy of hyperlipidemia, hypertension, and congestive heart failure.
- To understand the nutritional and lifestyle factors related to hyperlipidemia, hypertension, and congestive heart failure.
- To identify the causes of cardiac cachexia in patients with congestive heart failure.
- To understand the National Cholesterol Education Program (NCEP) nutritional recommendations for adults with hyperlipidemia.
- To incorporate nutrition into the history, review of systems, and physical examinations for patients with cardiovascular diseases.

Hyperlipidemia

According to the National Center for Health Statistics and the American Heart Association, cardiovascular disease ranks as the number one killer in the United States (see Figure 6-1). Of the more than 2 million Americans who die each year, 43 percent die of heart disease. Epidemiological evidence now suggests that dietary fat, specifically saturated fat, increases serum cholesterol levels, and as a consequence, the risk for coronary heart disease (CHD). According to the NHANES III survey, 34 percent of the calories in the average American diet consists of fat.

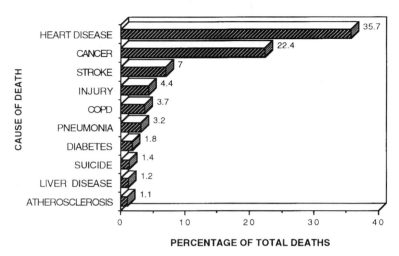

Figure 6-1   The ten leading causes of death in the United States (1987).

National Cholesterol Education Program Guidelines

The National Cholesterol Education Program (NCEP) issued reports in 1987 and 1993 on the detection, evaluation, and treatment of elevated serum cholesterol levels in adults. In both reports, dietary management is considered to be the cornerstone of treatment for patients with high levels of low-density lipoprotein (LDL) cholesterol. The major dietary contributors to elevated LDL cholesterol levels are high intakes of fat, particularly saturated fat, and an imbalance between caloric intake and energy expenditure, leading to obesity. Therefore, physicians, nurses, and registered dietitians should be prepared to counsel their patients on low-fat diets to help them reduce their LDL cholesterol levels and hence their risk of CHD. Helping patients to change their diets and lower LDL cholesterol can be accomplished by a combination of supportive attitudes and the understanding that long-term changes require lifestyle adjustment and take time. Equally important is knowing when to initiate cholesterol lowering dietary therapy. In 1993, the NCEP issued the following guidelines.

NCEP Guidelines for Initiating Dietary Therapy to Reduce Cholesterol

- If the patient is without heart disease and has one or no risk factors, initiate dietary recommendations if the LDL level is greater than 160 mg/dL.
- If the patient is without heart disease and has two or more risk factors, initiate dietary recommendations if the LDL level is greater than 130 mg/dL.
- If the patient has heart disease, initiate dietary recommendations if the LDL level is greater than 100 mg/dL.

Source: National Heart, Lung and Blood Institute.

Assessing Risk Factors for Coronary Heart Disease

When the NCEP revised its guidelines in 1993 for treating patients with elevated serum cholesterol, it placed increased emphasis on CHD risk status to guide cholesterol lowering therapy. By assessing a patient's risk, the appropriate intensity of medical and nutritional treatment can be better determined. In addition to an LDL cholesterol level greater than 130 mg/dL, risk factors for CHD include the following.

Risk Factors for Coronary Heart Disease

- Age
- Men over 45
- Women over 55 (or those who have undergone premature menopause and are not on estrogen therapy)
- Family history of premature cardiovascular disease
- Current cigarette smoking
- Hypertension (>140/90 mm Hg, or individuals taking antihypertensive medications)
- Diabetes mellitus
- Decreased high-density lipoprotein (HDL) level (<35 mg/dL)*

*An HDL level greater than 65 mg/dL has been identified as a negative risk factor.

Source: National Heart, Lung and Blood Institute.

Definition of Terms

Fats and Lipids

Dietary fats are composed chiefly of three fatty acids attached to a glycerol molecule. All fats are a combination of both saturated and unsaturated fatty acids. Fat is the most calorically dense nutrient, supplying nine calories per gram. Therefore, a diet high in fat is generally high in calories. Reducing total fat intake and adhering to an exercise program can help an individual achieve weight loss.

Saturated Fats

Saturated fats are fatty acids with no double bonds. With the exception of palm, palm kernel, and coconut oils, saturated fats are solid at room temperature and come primarily from animal sources. Examples of foods high in saturated fat are butter, lard, beef and chicken fat, hot dogs, sausage, bacon, most cheeses, and milk. In the typical American diet, approximately 13 percent of the calories come from saturated fat. These fats contribute to atherogenesis by raising serum LDL cholesterol levels in animals and humans alike.

Unsaturated Fats

Unsaturated fats are classified as either polyunsaturated or monounsaturated. Fatty acids with one double bond are monounsaturated fats. Fatty acids with two or more double bonds are polyunsaturated fats. Both of these types of fats, found in fish and plant food sources, are generally liquid at room temperature.

Polyunsaturated Fats The two major categories of polyunsaturated fats are omega-3 and omega-6 fatty acids. Vegetable oils such as corn, sunflower, safflower, and soybean contain omega-6 fatty acids. Polyunsaturated fats from these sources provide the essential omega-6 fatty acid, linoleic acid, which is essential because it cannot be synthesized by the body and therefore must be consumed in the diet. It is required by the body to synthesize arachidonic acid, the precursor of prostaglandins. Essential fatty acid deficiency can result in dry, scaly dermatitis, increased susceptibility to infection, and impaired wound healing. Approximately 5 grams of linoleic acid per day (2 to 3 percent of total calories) are required to prevent essential fatty acid deficiency. Substituting foods rich in polyunsaturated fat for those high in saturated fat has been shown to decrease LDL cholesterol levels. Low-fat diets may also lower HDL levels in some individuals.

Fish oils contain omega-3 fatty acids and have been shown to decrease blood pressure and triglyceride levels and increase clotting times. Recent research has also shown that individuals who consumed at least one meal per week of fatty fish rich in omega-3 fatty acids had a lower incidence of heart attacks compared to those who ate fatty fish less often. Because omega-3 fatty acids are concentrated in fish and shellfish, current recommendations advise including these foods in the diet at least once a week. Fresh or canned tuna, salmon, sardines, and herring are good sources of omega-3 fatty acids. Patients with very high triglyceride levels may be prescribed fish oil supplements to produce a more rapid effect.

Monounsaturated Fats Recently, monounsaturated fats have received attention because they do not raise LDL cholesterol levels. Canola and olive oils contain the highest percentage of monounsaturated fat. Oleic acid is the major fatty acid found in these oils. Epidemiological data suggest that people who live in certain Mediterranean countries, such as Italy and Greece where olive oil is the basic cooking oil, have a lower incidence of heart disease. However the typical Mediterranean diet consists of considerably more fruits and vegetables and less meat than the typical American diet. Highly monounsaturated oils are especially good for cooking because they develop fewer free radicals when overheated than polyunsaturated oils.

Trans Fatty Acids

Hydrogenation, the addition of hydrogen atoms to an unsaturated fat, changes the fat's structure, forming a trans fatty acid. This process is often used by food manufacturers to give foods such as crackers, cookies, potato chips, and puddings a longer shelf life by making them less likely to turn rancid. Recent evidence suggests that trans fatty acids may raise LDL cholesterol levels nearly as much as saturated fatty acids. However, the data are controversial because it is unlikely that people actually consume trans fatty acids in amounts significant enough to raise LDL cholesterol levels. Presently there is no way to determine the amount of trans fatty acids Americans consume. However, food manufacturers, pressured into reducing their use of saturated tropical oils (palm and coconut), have switched to using partially hydrogenated oils instead. Although the newly revised food labels do not specify the amounts of trans fatty acids in a product, the following current recommendations may be helpful to individuals who wish to decrease their intake of these substances.

1. Check ingredient labels on foods and limit intake of processed foods containing hydrogenated oils.

2. Limit intake of all fat. Use tub or squeeze margarines; the less solid the vegetable oil, the less hydrogenated fat it contains. Diet margarines are a better choice than regular margarine because they contain more water, half the fat, and half the calories.

3. Whenever possible, use a liquid oil or a nonfat cooking spray on a nonstick pan for cooking.

4. Try olive oil or jelly as a spread on bread instead of butter or margarine.

Nutrition Therapy

The goals of nutrition therapy for a patient with hyperlipidemia are to reduce serum cholesterol levels while providing a nutritionally balanced diet. These goals can be achieved by

-   reducing intake of total fat, saturated fat, and cholesterol
-   maintaining a reasonable body weight
-   increasing intake of complex carbohydrates
-   increasing intake of high-fiber foods

The NCEP has developed nutritional recommendations similar to those of the American Heart Association, the Surgeon General, and most other health organizations in the United States. Adapting these recommendations to each individual and to his or her particular lifestyle is the key to successful dietary counseling. However, long-term adherence to an appropriate diet demands an investment of time and support from family members.

The NCEP guidelines recommend using all fats sparingly and reducing total fat intake to less than 30 percent of the daily intake of calories. The Step I and Step II diets have been designed by the NCEP panel to reduce the intake of saturated fat and cholesterol gradually and to promote weight reduction in overweight patients. In the Step I diet less than 10 percent of calories should come from saturated fat, whereas in the Step II diet less than 7 percent should come from saturated fat. Polyunsaturated fat should not exceed 10 percent of the total calories consumed, and monounsaturated fat can contribute up to 15 percent of total calories. These percentages translate into 2 to 3 tablespoons per day of either polyunsaturated or monounsaturated oils such as those found in margarine, salad dressings, mayonnaise, sour cream, and cream cheese. Products labeled "light" or "fat free" are generally acceptable in terms of fat content and allow patients to reduce their fat intake even further. Table 6-1 summarizes the nutritional recommendations in the NCEP report and the components of the Step I and Step II diets for reducing high serum cholesterol levels. The first step in eating right is buying right. Table 6-2 provides a guide to choosing low-saturated fat and low-cholesterol foods.

Following a low-saturated fat, low-cholesterol diet is a balancing act: getting the variety of foods necessary to supply the nutrients you need without too much saturated fat and cholesterol or excess calories (see Table 6-2). One way to assure variety—and with it, a well-balanced diet—is to select foods each day from each of the following food groups. Select different foods from within groups, too, especially foods low in saturated fat (the left column). How many portions and the size of each portion should be adjusted to reach and maintain your desirable weight. As a guide, the recommended daily number of portions is listed for each food group.

Table 6-1   Characteristics of the Step I and Step II diets for lowering high serum cholesterol (NCEP Report).

RECOMMENDED INTAKE

Nutrient	Step I Diet	Step II Diet
Total fat	<30% of total calories	<30% of total calories
Saturated	8–10% of total calories	<7% of total calories
Polyunsaturated	Up to 10% of total calories	Up to 10% of total calories
Monounsaturated	Up to 15% of total calories	Up to 15% of total calories
Cholesterol	<300 mg/day	<200 mg/day
Carbohydrates	55% of total calories	55% of total calories
Protein	15% of total calories	15% of total calories
Calories	Number required to achieve and maintain desired weight	

Source: National Heart, Lung and Blood Institute.

Table 6-2 The first step in eating right is buying right. A guide to choosing low-saturated fat, low-cholesterol foods.

	CHOOSE	GO EASY	DECREASE

Meat, Poultry, Fish, and Shellfish (up to 6 ounces a day)	Lean cuts of meat with fat trimmed, like:
	• beef
	   round sirloin, chuck loin
	• lamb
	   leg, arm, loin, rib
	• pork
	   tenderloin, leg (fresh), shoulder (arm or picnic)
	• veal—all trimmed cuts except ground
	poultry without skin
	fish
	shellfish
			"Prime" grade
			Fatty cuts of meat, like:
			• beef
			   corned beef brisket, regular ground, short ribs
			• pork
			   spareibs, blade roll, fresh
			goose, domestic duck
			organ meats
			sausage meats
			regular luncheon meats
			frankfurters
			caviar, roe

Dairy Products (2 servings a day, 3 servings for women who are pregnant or breastfeeding)	skim milk, 1% milk, low fat buttermilk, low fat evaporated or non-fat milk low-fat yogurt low-fat cheeses, like cottage, farmer, pot cheeses labeled no more than 2 to 6 grams of fat per ounce sour cream	2% milk yogurt part-skim ricotta part-skim or imitation cheeses, like part-skim mozzarella "light" cream cheese "light" sour cream	whole milk, regular, evaporated, or condensed cream, half and half, most non-dairy creamers, imitation milk products, whipped cream custard style yogurt whole-milk ricotta
Eggs (no more that 3 egg yolks in a week)	egg whites cholesterol-free egg substitutes		egg yolks
Fats and oils (up to 6 to 8 teaspoons a day)	unsaturated vegetable oils: olive, peanut, rapeseed (canola oil), safflower, sesame, soybean margarine; or shortening made from unsaturated fats listed above: liquid, tub, stick, diet	nuts and seeds avocados and olives	butter, coconut oil, palm oil, palm kernel oil, lard, bacon fat margarine or shortening made from saturated fats listed above
Breads, Cereals, Pasta, Rice, Dried Peas, and Beans (6 to 11 servings a day)	breads, like white, whole wheat, pumpernickel, and rye pita; bagel; English muffin; sandwich buns; dinner rolls; rice cakes low-fat crackers, like matzo bread sticks, rye crisps saltines, zwieback hot cereals, most cold dry cereals pasta like plain noodles, spaghetti, macaroni any grain rice	store-bought pancakes waffles, biscuits, muffins, cornbread	croissant, butter rolls, sweet rolls, danish pastry, doughnuts most snack crackers, like cheese crackers butter crackers, those made with saturated oils granola-type cereals made with saturated oils pasta and rice prepared with cream, butter or cheese sauces; egg noodles

Table 6-2 continued

	CHOOSE	GO EASY	DECREASE
Breads (cont.)	dried peas and beans, like split peas, black-eyed peas, chick peas, kidney beans, navy beans, lentils, soy bean curd (tofu), soybeans		
Fruits and Vegetables (2 to 4 servings of fruit and 3–5 servings of vegetables a day)	fresh, frozen, canned or dried fruits and vegetables		vegetables prepared in butter, cream or sauce
Sweets and Snacks	low-fat frozen desserts, like sherbet, sorbet, Italian ice frozen yogurt, popsicles low-fat cakes, like angel food cake low-fat cookies, like fig bars, gingersnaps low-fat candy, like jelly beans hard candy low-fat snacks like plain popcorn, pretzels nonfat beverages like carbonated drinks, juices, tea, coffee	frozen desserts, homemade cakes, cookies, and pies using unsaturated oils sparingly fruit crisps and cobblers	high-fat frozen desserts, like ice cream, frozen tofu high-fat cakes, like most store-bought, pound, and frosted cakes store-bought pies store-bought cookies most candy, like chocolate bars high-fat snacks, like chips, buttered popcorn high-fat beverages, like frappes, milkshakes, floats, and eggnogs
Label Ingredients	Go easy on products that list any fat or oil first or that list many fat and oil ingredients. The following lists clue you in to names of saturated fat ingredients (decrease) and unsaturated ingredients (go easy on).	carob, cocoa oils, like corn, cottonseed, olive, safflower, sesame, soybean or sunflower oil	cocoa butter animal fat, like bacon, beef, chicken, ham, lamb, meat, pork or turkey fats, butter, lard coconut, coconut oil, palm or palm kernel oil cream egg and egg-yolk solids hardened fat or oil hydrogenated vegetable oil milk chocolate shortening or vegetable shortening vegetable oil (could be coconut, palm kernel or palm oil)

Source: National Heart, Lung and Blood Institute.

Incorporating Nutrition into the Medical History and Nursing Assessment

The diet history should focus on the patient's intake of saturated fat and cholesterol. Because animal fats provide two-thirds of the saturated fat and cholesterol in the average person's diet, specific questions to ask during the history include the following:

Specific Foods

Red Meat How many times per week does the patient eat red meat (beef, lamb, veal, pork, or duck), and what is the usual portion size? A general rule of thumb is that a patient who consumes red meat more than four times per week most likely is not following a low-fat diet. The NCEP advises that eliminating red meat altogether from the diet is not necessary because of the value of its high iron, zinc, and vitamin B12 content. Rather, suggest leaner red meat substitutions that are lower in saturated fat, such as round and sirloin steak, and limit intake to less than 6 ounces per day. Because all animal protein sources contain saturated fat and cholesterol, the NCEP recommends limiting protein intake to 10 to 20 percent of total calories. Processed meats such as bacon, sausage, luncheon meats (bologna or salami), and hot dogs also are high in saturated fat and should be eaten only in limited amounts when following the Step I or Step II diets. Patients should be advised to check labels for fat content. Generally, if the food contains more than 3 grams of fat per 100 calories, it contains more than the recommended 30 percent of calories from fat (see Figure 6-2).

Poultry How many times per week does the patient eat poutry and what is the usual portion size? Because white meat turkey and chicken have decreased amounts of total fat and saturated fat compared to red meat, they should be included in the diet as an alternative. White meat turkey, with only 8 percent fat, is leaner than white meat chicken, which contains approximately 24 percent total fat. However, the fat content of both turkey and chicken increases significantly when the skin or the dark meat is eaten. Also, most turkey or chicken hot dogs contain approximately 70 percent fat, little less than a regular beef hot dog containing 80 percent total fat (see Figure 6-3).

Fish and Shellfish How many times per week does the patient east fish and shellfish and what is the usual portion size? Fish and shellfish are good alternatives to meat and poultry because of their low fat and saturated fat content (see Figure 6-4). The cholesterol content in shellfish varies widely, but all shellfish is very low in total fat and saturated fat. As stated above, fish and shellfish are also rich sources of omega-3 fatty acids. Therefore, encourage patients to increase their intake of fish, preparing it with lemon and herbs on the grill or in the broiler rather than frying it.

Dairy Products How often does the patient eat dairy products, and what types of dairy products does he or she consume? Certain dairy products such as regular cheese and whole milk contain a significant amount of saturated fat. Therefore, determining the amounts and types of dairy products consumed daily is important. Because dairy products are an excellent source of calcium, completely eliminating them from the diet is not advised, especially for women. Some brands of low-fat mozzarella, ricotta, cottage, and farmer's cheese are now made from part-skim milk rather than whole milk and can be substituted in moderation. Low- or nonfat yogurt or nonfat sour cream alternatives can be used in dips and salad dressings. Nondairy coffee creamers, whipped toppings,

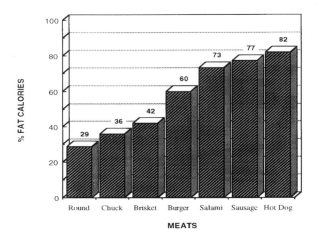

Figure 6-2 Percent of calories from fat in various meats.

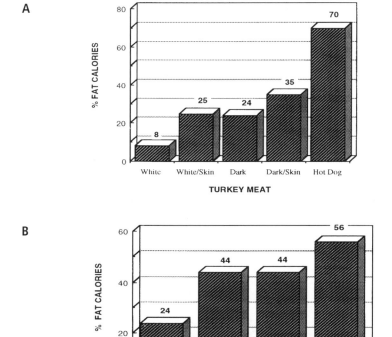

Figure 6-3 A. Percent of calories from fat in turkey meats. B. Percent of calories from fat in chicken meats

A

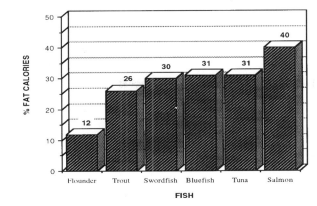

FISH

B

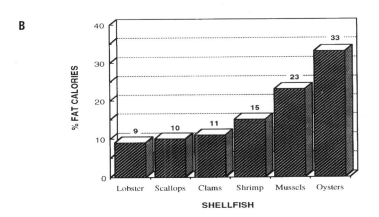

SHELLFISH

Figure 6-4   A. Percent of calories from fat in various fish. B. Percent of calories from fat in shellfish.

and half and half are laden with saturated fats and should be avoided. Evaporated skim milk is an acceptable substitute for whipped cream and coffee creamers and in recipes that call for heavy cream.

Sweets and Desserts   How often does the patient eat desserts and sweets? Most commercial baked products are made with saturated fats such as butter and eggs. Fresh fruit, angel food cake, fat-free frozen yogurt, and sherbet are good alternatives. Although fat-free desserts are readily available in supermarkets, many contain such high amounts of simple sugar in place of fat that their calorie content may well surpass that of the desserts they are intended to replace.

Eating Out

How often does the patient eat away from home? Generally, patients consume more fat from hidden sources when eating out. Most of the time sauces and salad dressings can be ordered on the side. Casserole dishes may have a high saturated fat content because they often contain cheese and eggs, so advise patients to select grilled, poached, baked, or broiled entrees. Most fast food restaurants now offer low-fat alternatives such as grilled chicken breast served on a bun without added sauce, salad with low-fat dressing, and baked potato.

Maintaining a Reasonable Body Weight

Weight reduction in overweight patients has been shown to reduce both LDL cholesterol and triglyceride levels, increase HDL cholesterol, reduce blood pressure, and improve blood sugar levels in patients with diabetes. Successful weight control programs recommend reducing total fat and calorie intake and increasing physical activity.

Assessing Dietary Adherence

Dietary adherence in patients on the Step I diet should be assessed initially after 6 weeks and again after 3 months. For patients with established CHD or another atherosclerotic disease such as peripheral arterial or carotid artery disease, the Step II diet should be prescribed, and the importance of adhering to it should be explained. Referral to a registered dietitian is recommended for patients who need to follow the Step II diet and for those on the Step I diet who do not successfully reduce their LDL cholesterol levels. If the patient has achieved the desired reduction in LDL cholesterol, long-term monitoring can begin. Drug therapy can be considered if the LDL cholesterol level is substantially above the desired goal despite dietary adherence. However, even when drug therapy is initiated, diet therapy should not be suspended, because both are beneficial for lowering cholesterol levels in most patients.

Cardioprotective Effects of Alcohol

Does the patient drink alcohol? How often and what type? Should an individual begin drinking to prevent heart disease or improve lipid levels? Probably not. Because of the known side effects of excessive alcohol consumption—liver damage, cirrhosis, cardiomyopathy, adverse psychological consequences, motor vehicle accidents, and an increased risk of hypertension—the NCEP does not advocate alcohol consumption to reduce the risk of heart disease. Furthermore, excessive alcohol consumption is contraindicated for patients with significantly elevated triglyceride levels. However, moderate alcohol use has been epidemiologically associated with decreased incidence of heart disease, leading to the conclusion that alcohol in any form may be cardioprotective. Moderate alcohol intake is defined as no more than 2 drinks per day for men and 1 drink per day for women. A drink is defined as five ounces of wine, one and a half ounces of 80-proof liquor, or twelve ounces of beer. One mechanism of its protective effect is that alcohol use increases HDL cholesterol levels. It is important, however, to emphasize that the best ways to reduce the risk of heart disease are to avoid smoking, eat a low-fat diet, exercise regularly, and control blood pressure and diabetes.

Hypertension

Hypertension is a major risk factor for the development of cardiovascular disease. Understanding the relationship between diet and blood pressure has important implications for the prevention and treatment of hypertension. Dietary modifications may obviate the need for drug therapy, particularly in patients with mild hypertension. This approach should be pursued whenever possible to avoid potential iatrogenic side effects of medications intended to control hypertension.

Nutritional Factors Associated with Essential Hypertension

Nutritional factors that may contribute to the development of essential hypertension include obesity, high sodium intake, low potassium and calcium intake, and excessive alcohol consumption.

Obesity

Epidemiologic evidence suggests that in industrialized societies obesity is a major risk factor in the development of hypertension. The exact cause-and-effect relationship between obesity and hypertension is not clearly understood, but increased cardiac output and sodium retention related to elevated insulin levels may play a role. The beneficial effects of weight reduction in hypertensive individuals have been clearly documented. Controlled dietary intervention trials have estimated that a mean reduction in body weight of 9.2 kg is associated with a 6.3 mm Hg reduction in systolic blood pressure and a 3.1 mm Hg reduction in diastolic blood pressure.

Dietary Sodium Intake

Research clearly shows that population groups with high-sodium diets have an increased occurrence of hypertension. Although certain patients exhibit a small reduction in blood pressure in response to moderate sodium restriction (2 to 3 grams per day), some may not. Based on results of sodium depletion and sodium loading studies, approximately 30 to 50 percent of hypertensives (and an even smaller number of normotensives) are salt-sensitive. Thus not all individuals with hypertension respond to reduced dietary sodium intake intended to lower their blood pressure. Currently no clear method exists for identifying those hypertensive patients most likely to benefit from sodium restriction. Therefore, initially a low-sodium diet is prescribed for most hypertensive patients.

Dietary Potassium Intake

An inverse correlation appears to exist between potassium intake and blood pressure, especially in individuals consuming a high-sodium diet. Although the exact mechanism remains unclear, potassium supplementation can induce sodium and water excretion, thereby reducing blood pressure. Exactly why low potassium intake leads to elevated blood pressure in some individuals is still uncertain.

Dietary Calcium Intake

Individuals with hypertension tend to have a lower intake of calcium than do nonhypertensive individuals. Furthermore, calcium supplementation has been shown to reduce blood pressure in some populations. Most clinical trials evaluating the effect of high-calcium diets on blood pressure have involved supplementing individuals' diets with 1000 to 1500 mg per day. However, reductions in blood pressure achieved by increased calcium intake have been modest and inconsistent.

Alcohol Intake

Alcohol consumption in amounts over two drinks per day is estimated to account for 5 to 7 percent of the diagnosed cases of hypertension. In controlled studies, reducing alcohol consumption has been associated with a modest reduction in blood pressure. However, the mechanism by which alcohol may affect blood pressure has not been established.

Nutrition Therapy for Hypertension

The goals of nutrition therapy for patients with hypertension are to
  * promote weight reduction in the overweight and obese
  * reduce sodium intake
  * increase potassium intake
  * reduce alcohol consumption
  * encourage healthy eating habits and a balanced intake
  * encourage increased physical activity level

Weight Reduction

Because obesity may contribute to the development of hypertension and weight reduction often improves blood pressure, weight loss should be the primary goal for the overweight hypertensive patient. In addition to its positive effect on blood pressure, weight loss can also improve lipid levels, further reducing cardiovascular risk. A reduction of 500 kcal per day will achieve a weekly weight loss of one pound per week. Increasing physical activity and adhering to a low-fat, low-calorie diet have been shown to be effective means of weight and blood pressure control.

Sodium Intake

On average, a typical American diet contains approximately 4 to 8 grams of sodium per day. Reducing the sodium intake of hypertensive individuals to approximately 2 to 3 grams per day is recommended. Table salt and foods high in sodium, such as salted, smoked, canned, and highly processed foods, should be limited.

Potassium Intake

Because a high-potassium diet may have a beneficial effect on blood pressure and potassium wasting often occurs in patients taking commonly prescribed diuretics such as hydrochlorothiazide or furosemide, these patients' diets should regularly include foods high in potassium. Examples of high-potassium foods are oranges, orange juice, potatoes (especially with the skins), and bananas. Monitoring serum potassium levels is essential when potassium-wasting diuretics are prescribed. If the levels are low, potassium supplements such as Slow K should be prescribed.

Alcohol Intake

Alcohol consumption should be limited to 2 drinks a day. One drink is equivalent to 1.5 ounces of 80-proof distilled liquor, 4 ounces of table wine, or 12 ounces of beer.

Congestive Heart Failure

Congestive heart failure (CHF), which affects an estimated 1 to 2 million adults in the United States, is characterized by decreased cardiac output, venous blood stasis, sodium and fluid retention, multiple organ system failure (kidney, liver, heart, brain), and malnutrition. Appropriate nutritional therapy should be instituted as part of the overall medical care for the patient in congestive heart failure.

Causes of Malnutrition in CHF

Cardiac cachexia is the term used to describe the malnutrition seen in patients with CHF. As myocardial function progressively deteriorates, many patients with a long history of CHF present with loss of adipose tissue and lean body mass secondary to poor nutritional intake and decreased activity. Upper-body and temporal wasting and lower-extremity edema are common clinical features of malnutrition associated with CHF. The mechanisms that have been suggested to explain the malnutrition include

- impaired cellular oxygen supply
- increased nutrient losses
- increased nutritional requirements
- decreased nutritional intake

Impaired Cellular Oxygen Supply

Decreased cardiac output causes a diminished supply of oxygen and other nutrients to cells. Lack of cellular oxygen may lead to inefficient substrate oxidation and inadequate synthesis of high-energy intermediary metabolites.

Increased Nutrient Losses

Lack of oxygen and increased venous pressure may cause bowel edema and subsequent fat and protein malabsorption. Decreased synthesis of hepatic bile salts and pancreatic enzymes caused by oxygen deprivation to the spleen, liver, and pancreas may further contribute to malabsorption. Proteinuria is also exhibited in patients with CHF secondary to the greatly reduced renal blood flow characteristic of this disorder.

Increased Nutritional Requirements

Patients with CHF are hypermetabolic and therefore have increased nutritional requirements. This hypermetabolic state is caused by the increased work required for breathing, the mechanical work of the heart, and oxygen consumption related to alterations in neuroendocrine activity. If additional calories are not ingested to meet these increased demands, the patient loses weight.

Decreased Nutritional Intake

Factors that may result in an inadequate food intake in patients with CHF include

- reduced functional gastric volume secondary to hepatomegaly and ascites, which can lead to early satiety, limiting dietary intake
- dyspnea associated with eating and weakness, which can interfere with the ability of the patient to ingest adequate calories
- prescribed low-sodium diets may be unpalatable, resulting in anorexia
- side effects from medications such as digitalis, which can cause nausea, vomiting, and diarrhea, potentially limiting intake

Nutrition Therapy for CHF

The goals of nutrition therapy for patients with CHF are

- to restore and maintain body weight
- to provide adequate energy, protein, vitamins, and minerals for the increased requirements in CHF
- to control sodium and fluid retention
- to restore protein stores in the patient who has lost lean body mass

Calories

For the cachectic patient with CHF, daily caloric intake should be adequate to promote weight gain. Therefore, to support anabolism, current recommendations advise estimating dietary calories at 1.5 times the basal energy expenditure for these patients. High-protein, high-calorie supplements are often necessary to achieve this calorie requirement, especially when the patient is anorectic. Liquid supplements and special puddings are available that provide a high concentration of calories and nutrients in a relatively small volume of fluid. Note that the sodium and fluid content of these supplements should be considered in the total daily sodium and fluid allowance. Small, frequent meals also may help these patients achieve an adequate dietary intake.

Patients who cannot meet their caloric and protein requirements orally may require enteral tube feeding. Enteral nutritional support is accomplished with one of a variety of tubes designed for the varying needs of individual patients. Some feeding tubes are placed through the nose and empty into either the stomach (nasogastric) or intestine (nasoduodenal or nasojejunal). Alternatively, the tube may be placed percutaneously, or surgically, directly into either the stomach or intestine. When tube feeding a CHF patient, care must be taken to avoid overfeeding. Overfeeding may lead to volume overload and increased metabolic rate, resulting in increased cardiac output and myocardium size, which will worsen the patient's CHF.

Protein

In the malnourished patient with CHF, the amount of protein necessary to promote anabolism and achieve positive nitrogen balance is thought to be 1.5 to 2 grams per day. Again, liquid supplements and special puddings are advisable because they provide a high concentration of calories and protein in a relatively small volume of fluid.

Sodium

Because patients with CHF retain sodium and fluid, dietary sodium restriction is necessary as an adjunct to diuretic therapy. The level of sodium restriction should be individualized according to the severity of the CHF to avoid exacerbating its symptoms. Moderately restricting sodium to approximately 4 to 5 grams per day is often adequate. However, a more drastic sodium restriction to an intake of 2 grams per day may be necessary in severe cases. Keep in mind that the dietary sodium level should be as liberal as possible to maximize nutritional intake, especially in the malnourished patient with CHF. Salt substitutes are available to flavor foods, but many of them substitute potassium for sodium. Patients with renal failure or those taking potassium-sparing diuretics should avoid these products. Careful attention must be paid to sodium, potassium, zinc, and magnesium levels in CHF patients because diuretic therapy may lower them dangerously.

Fluid

Severe CHF associated with dilutional hyponatremia may require restricting fluid intake to 1000 to 1500 ml per day. Some suggest limiting daily fluid intake to an amount equal to the 24-hour urine output volume plus 500 ml. Because of edema and liver impairment, nutrition assessment parameters such as actual body weight or weight change may not accurately reflect nutritional status in patients with CHF. For example, cardiac cachexia may go undetected if body weight is normal or elevated because of sodium and water retention and enlargement of the extracellular fluid compartment. Levels of serum visceral proteins such as albumin also may be decreased secondary to malnutrition or fluid overload.

Case 1

Adult Hyperlipidemia

Gregg J. Fromell and Frances Burke

Objectives

- To review the current National Cholesterol Education Program guidelines for screening, evaluation, and treatment of hyperlipidemia.
- To understand the nutritional recommendations for patients with hyperlipidemia.
- To develop a nutritional care plan for a patient with hyperlipidemia.

DG, a healthy 25-year-old computer operator, consults his family physician for a routine physical examination. He is interested in modifying his diet to reduce his risk of heart disease because his father recently had a heart attack. He wonders if he is eating right.

Past Medical History

DG has no prior history of hospitalizations or chronic illnesses. He is not taking any medications or vitamins and he has no known food allergies.

Family History

DG's family history is positive for heart disease. His father had a heart attack at age 53, and his father's brother had a heart attack at age 50. There is no history of hypertension, diabetes, or obesity.

Social History

DG reports occasional alcohol consumption and daily coffee intake. He has smoked half a package of cigarettes per day for the past five years (a 2.5 pack year history). He is not following a special diet and eats three meals per day. DG works long hours and feels he is under pressure on the job. He states that he does not have time to exercise.

Dietary Intake History

Using the 24-hour recall method, DG's physician obtained the following information about DG's intake from the previous day.

DG's 24-Hour Recall		
Breakfast (Office)	Granola cereal	1/2 cup
	Whole milk	1 cup
	English muffin	1 whole
	Butter	1 Tbs.
Lunch (Restaurant)	Pizza with cheese	3 pieces
	Soda (cola)	10 oz.
Evening (Home)	Sirloin steak	6 oz.
	Macaroni and cheese	1 cup
	Caesar salad	2 cups
	Caesar dressing	3 Tbs.
	Vanilla ice cream	1/2 cup
	Total calories: 2800 kcal/day	
	Protein: 20% of calories	
	Fat: 41% of calories	
	Carbohydrate: 40% of calories	
	Cholesterol: 513 mg/day	

Review of Systems

DG appears generally in good health and voices no complaints.

Physical Examination

Results of the physical exam were normal and unremarkable.

Vital signs

Blood pressure: 120/80 mm Hg

Anthropometric data

Height: 5'10" (178 cm)

Current weight: 175 lb (80 kg)

Ideal body weight (IBW): 166 lb (105% IBW)

Case Questions

1. Based on DG's family history of heart disease, what screening tests should be performed?

2. The results of DG's laboratory tests were
     Total cholesterol = 260 mg/dL (desirable <200 mg/dL)
     HDL = 35 mg/dL (desirable >35 mg/dL)
   What other tests, if any, should be done?

3. A fasting lipid panel produced the following laboratory values.
     Total cholesterol: 260 mg/dL (desirable <200 mg/dL)
     HDL = 35 mg/dL (desirable >35 mg/dL)
     LDL = 200 mg/dL (desirable <130 mg/dL)
     Triglycerides = 100 mg/dL (desirable <200 mg/dL)
   What type of lipid disorder does DG most likely exhibit?

4. What methods could be utilized to assess DG's present intake?

5. Is DG's current diet within the recommended guidelines of the Step I Diet?

6. How can DG translate the Step I dietary guidelines into food selections?

7. Should DG receive a lipid-lowering medication at this time?

Answers begin on the following page.

Answers to Questions: Case 1

Part 1:   Screening and Risk Factors

1.   Based on DG's family history of heart disease, what screening tests should be performed?

The current National Cholesterol Education Program (NCEP) guidelines recommend that all adults over 20 years of age have their cholesterol and HDL cholesterol levels tested at least every five years. Patients can be nonfasting for the initial lipid screening because total cholesterol and HDL are not substantially affected by a recent meal. In addition to cholesterol screening, the general health maintenance screening for a man of this age includes a thorough history and physical examination.

Particularly helpful in the history are questions related to cardiac risk factors because these guide decision making for possible lipid-lowering therapy. Dietary intake and exercise habits are also important areas to explore. Past medical history should reveal any diseases that are either cardiac risk factors or possible secondary causes of hypercholesterolemia (see Table 6-3).

In addition to general health screening, patients suspected to have hypercholesterolemia should undergo an examination of pulses (palpation of all pulses, and auscultation for bruits in the carotids and femoral arteries), thyroid palpation (hypothyroidism is a possible secondary cause of hypercholesterolemia), an eye exam for arcus cornea, and a tendon and skin exam for xanthomas. Often the physical exam is unremarkable, but if abnormalities related to hypercholesterolemia are found, they can be followed up once therapy is begun.

Table 6-3   Causes of secondary hyperlipidemia.

ENDOCRINE/METABOLIC	DRUGS
Diabetes mellitus	Alcohol
Obesity	Sex hormones
Hypothyroidism	Androgens
Hypogonadism	Estrogens
Hypercortisolism	Progestins
Acromegaly	Vitamin A analogs
Renal disease	Antihypertensive agents
Nephrotic syndrome	Beta blockers (without ISA)
Chronic renal failure	Thiazide diuretics
Liver disease	Antiseizure agents
Anorexia nervosa	Phenytoin
Macroglobulinemia and myeloma	Barbiturates
Acute intermittent porphyria	Immunosuppressive agents
Glycogen storage disease	Cyclosporine

2. **The results of DG's laboratory tests were**

> Total cholesterol: 260 mg/dL (desirable <200 mg/dL)
>
> HDL: 35 mg/dL (desirable >35 mg/dL)

What other tests, if any, should be done?

The indications for obtaining a fasting lipid profile are based on the patient's cholesterol level and number of risk factors. Fasting lipid profiles should be obtained if the total cholesterol level is between 200 and 240 mg/dL and the patient has two or more risk factors for heart disease.

Because DG's cholesterol level is greater than 240 mg/dL, a fasting lipid panel should be obtained. This includes the triglycerides, total cholesterol, low-density lipoprotein cholesterol (LDL), and high-density lipoprotein cholesterol (HDL). High LDL levels are associated with an increased risk of cardiovascular disease, whereas high HDL levels are associated with a decreased risk of cardiovascular disease. LDL cholesterol is usually calculated using the following equation, but techniques for measuring LDL cholesterol directly also are available.

> Total cholesterol = HDL + LDL + VLDL or
>
> LDL = Total cholesterol − (HDL + VLDL)
>
> VLDL ≈ $\dfrac{\text{Triglyceride level}}{5}$

Therefore the revised equation becomes

> LDL = Total cholesterol − HDL − Triglyceride/5

In the nonfasting state, chylomicrons formed from dietary fat contribute to the triglyceride level and render the preceding equation inaccurate. In hyperlipidemic states, a triglyceride level greater than 400 mg/dL also invalidates the results of this equation. Even though the patient history and physical examination are unremarkable for secondary causes of hypercholesterolemia, a subclinical disease process that could affect cholesterol levels may be present. A fasting glucose to rule out glucose intolerance or diabetes mellitus and a TSH to rule out hypothyroidism should also be obtained. If lipid-lowering drug therapy is required, baseline liver transaminases (ALT and AST) and uric acid levels may be helpful in choosing the appropriate type of drug therapy.

3. **A fasting lipid panel produced the following laboratory values.**

> Total cholesterol = 260 mg/dL (desirable <200 mg/dL)
>
> HDL = 35 mg/dL (desirable >35 mg/dL)
>
> LDL = 200 mg/dL (desirable <130 mg/dL)
>
> Triglycerides = 100 mg/dL (desirable <200 mg/dL)

What type of lipid disorder does DG most likely exhibit?

The most likely diagnosis is polygenic hypercholesterolemia (PHC), the most common primary etiology of hypercholesterolemia in the hypercholesterolemic patient population of the United States (95 percent of known cases). Unfortunately, PHC is not well understood. Experts believe that certain genetic factors affecting lipid metabolism are enhanced by other factors such as aging, hepatic conversion of cholesterol to bile acids, diet, exercise, tobacco, and other unknown environmental conditions. The fact that lipid values often are normal in childhood and early adulthood supports the theory that these other environmental factors are responsible for the disorder's expression. Furthermore, this finding underscores the importance of follow-up lipid testing at least every five years in persons with normal cholesterol levels.

DG's Risk Factors

Heart disease: No known history of heart disease

Age: Not a risk (DG is 25 years old)

Family history: Mother healthy; father had a heart attack at 53; no history of diabetes

Smoking history: Positive; current smoker

Blood pressure: Normal (120/80 mm Hg)

Medical history: No evidence of diabetes, stroke or peripheral vascular disease

Laboratory Findings

Blood cholesterol level: 260 mg/dL

HDL cholesterol level: 35 mg/dL

LDL cholesterol level: 200 mg/dL

Part 2:   Nutrition Assessment and Therapy

4.   **What methods could be utilized to assess DG's present intake?**

A nutrient intake analysis performed by a registered dietitian is one way of assessing DG's intake. In this approach, the patient completes a 24-hour recall or a food diary (up to three days) for intake evaluation. The dietitian then evaluates the caloric content and the percentages of calories from fat, carbohydrate, and protein using reference tables or a computer program.

Another method that can be used during a routine visit involves simply questioning DG during the medical history about his usual intake. Alternatively, the same questions may be presented on a questionnaire for the patient to complete while he or she is in the waiting room. Because DG has a positive family history of heart disease, emphasis should be placed on the fat content of his diet. Probing questions to ascertain whether DG is consuming foods that are high in fat on a regular basis are:

How often do you eat fried foods?

How often do you eat out?

Where do you eat out and what do your order?

How often do you eat luncheon meats such as bologna or salami?

What types of fats and oils do you use in cooking or at the table?

How often do you use dairy products?

How often do you eat red meat? What type? How much? Has the fat been trimmed?

How often do you eat fish or shellfish?

How many egg yolks do you eat in a week?

What types of sweets, desserts, and snacks do you eat?

How many times a day do you eat fruit and vegetables?

How many times a day do you eat bread, pasta, rice, or cereal?

Part 3: Treatment

5. Is DG's current diet within the recommended guidelines of the Step I Diet?

According to the nutritional analysis of his current intake, DG's fat intake is 41 percent of his total caloric intake, higher than the desired 30 percent. Carbohydrate intake is 40 percent of total calories, lower than the desired 55 percent. Suggestions and substitutions that DG can easily implement over time to reduce his risk of heart disease are summarized in the box on p. 200. Not all of these changes need to be incorporated simultaneously.

These dietary changes decrease DG's fat intake to 25 percent of his total calories and his cholesterol intake to only 86 mg per day, and increase his carbohydrate intake to 62 percent of his calories, all within Step I Diet recommendations. Compared to his previous diet, this modified intake enables DG to eat in greater quantity because the substituted foods are lower in fat and thus in calories.

In addition, DG's dietitian developed a sample revised menu for guidance. (See the box on p. 201)

6. How can DG translate the Step I dietary guidelines into food selections?

To consume a diet low in fat, saturated fat, and cholesterol, DG should eat plenty of vegetables, fruits, and grain products; choose lean meats, fish, white meat poultry without skin, and low-fat dairy products; and use fats and oils sparingly. DG can increase fiber intake by eating a variety of high-fiber foods such as fresh vegetables, dried beans, fresh fruits, and whole grains. He should be advised to consume foods and beverages containing sugar, sodium, and alcohol in moderation.

Dietary Suggestions and Substitutions for DG

Breakfast   Select a high-fiber breakfast cereal.

Use skim or nonfat milk.

Switch to tub margarine, which contains less saturated fat than butter.

Lunch   Select low-fat sandwich meats such as turkey, ham, and lean roast beef.

Complete the meal with low-fat, high-carbohydrate foods such as soup, pasta salads, pretzels, and fresh fruit.

Dinner   Prepare entrees without added fat and avoid frying foods. Select low-fat side dishes such as steamed rather than fried or creamed vegetables, and high-carbohydrate foods such as potatoes, rice, and pasta.

Eat smaller portions of meat, fish, and poultry.

Add whole-grain bread and limit use of butter or margarine.

Use less salad dressing or try low-calorie or fat-free brands at home.

Switch to a low-fat ice cream or frozen yogurt.

Snack   Limit snacking and select low-calorie snacks such as fresh fruit or pretzels.

Revised Low-Fat Menu for DG

Breakfast (Office)	Cheerios	2 cups
	Skim milk	1 cup
	Orange juice	4 oz.
Lunch (Restaurant)	Turkey breast	4 oz.
	Whole-wheat bread	2 slices
	Mustard	2 tsp.
	Pretzels	2 oz.
	Soda (cola)	10 oz.
Snack (office)	Orange (fresh)	1 whole
Evening (Home)	Pasta	2 cups cooked
	Tomato sauce	1 cup
	Pumpernickel bread	1 slice
	Margarine	2 Tbs.
	Lettuce	1 cup
	Caesar dressing	1 Tbs.
	Croutons	2 Tbs.
	Vanilla frozen yogurt	1 cup
Snack (home)	Apple juice	1 cup
	Oatmeal raisin cookies	3 medium

Total calories: 2400 kcal/day
Cholesterol: 86 mg/day
Protein: 13% of calories
Fat: 25% of calories
Carbohydrate: 62% of calories

Part 4: Lipid-Lowering Drug Therapy

7. **Should DG receive a lipid-lowering medication at this time?**

It is too early to answer this question definitively. DG may require drug therapy at some point in the future, but only after an adequate trial of lipid-lowering therapy without drugs has been undertaken. Elimination of treatable risk factors is of prime importance. DG has three risk factors: HDL equal to or less than 35 mg/dL, cigarette smoking, and a family history of heart disease. He also eats a high-fat diet and does not exercise. Therefore, implementing a number of lifestyle and behavioral changes on his own may reduce his cholesterol to a more acceptable level.

DG should be encouraged to stop smoking either with the help of a smoking cessation program or the nicotine patch. DG should return in three months for follow-up and retesting of his cholesterol and LDL levels. Cigarette smoking can have a marked effect on lipids, particularly on HDL, which it may decrease as much as 2 to 9 mg/dL. Cigarette smoking also raises total cholesterol, presumably by raising LDL. This patient needs a careful review of the health risks of cigarette smoking and appropriate treatment suggestions or referral for smoking cessation.

Increasing his level of aerobic exercise is another measure DG should be encouraged to adopt. Exercise can raise HDL (usually only modestly) and lower LDL levels and is therefore an important component in treating hypercholesterolemia without drugs. Regardless of age, patients should begin any exercise program gradually and include 5 to 10 minutes of warming up at the beginning of exercise and warming down at the end. The ultimate goal is to increase the total workout to 20 to 30 minutes per day, at least three days per week.

In summary, the cornerstone of nondrug lipid-lowering therapy is a low-saturated fat, low-cholesterol diet. At the very least, all persons should follow the Step I Diet guidelines for general health maintenance, and many may already be following this diet at the time of presentation to a physician. Although diet therapy should always be individualized, this particular group may be able to progress more readily to a Step II Diet. Diet instruction may require several follow-up visits for adequate training by a registered dietitian. Early initial follow-up (every 4 to 6 weeks) is important because it affords opportunities to verify adherence to and provide support for diet, exercise, and smoking cessation programs. Later, the patient can be followed at intervals deemed appropriate to reinforce the nondrug treatment plan and to monitor cholesterol levels. In a patient such as DG, diet and lifestyle changes should be attempted for at least six months before considering drug therapy, because they may bring about a significant enough decrease in LDL and increase in HDL to maintain an acceptable lipid profile. At that point it is possible to determine whether DG's blood cholesterol is diet-responsive.

See Chapter Review Questions, pages A11–A12.

REFERENCES

Blonk MC, Bilo HJ, Nauta JJ. Dose-response effects of fish oil supplements in healthy volunteers. *Am J Clin Nutr* 1990;52:120–127.

Cook NR, Cohen J, Herbert PR. Implications of small reductions in diastolic blood pressure for primary prevention. *Arch Int Med* 1995;155(7):701–709.

Dobrin-Seckler BE, Deckelbaum RJ. Safety of the American Heart Association Step I Diet in childhood. *Ann NY Acad Sci* 1991;623:263–268.

Dwyer J. Overview: Dietary approaches for reducing cardiovascular disease risks. *J Nutr* 1995;125(3 Suppl):656S–665S.

Freeman LM, Roubenoff R. The nutritional implications of cardiac cachexia. *Nutr Rev* 1994;52(10):340–347.

Gurr MI. Dietary lipids and coronary heart disease: old evidence, new perspective. *Prog Lipid Res* 1992;31(3):195–243.

Kesaniemi YA, Lilja M. Hypertension, plasma lipids and antihypertensive drugs. *Ann Med* 1991;23(3):347–351.

Klatsky AL. Can "a drink a day" keep a heart attack away? *Patient Care* 1995;7: 39–56.

Klatsky AL. Cardiovascular effects of alcohol. *Sci Am* 1995;2:28–37.

Kotchen TA, Kotchen JM. Nutrition, Diet, and Hypertension. In Shils ME, Olson JA, Shike M, eds. *Modern Nutrition in Health and Disease*. 8th ed. Philadelphia: Lea and Febiger, 1994.

National Cholesterol Education Program. Second Report of the Expert Panel on Detection, Evaluation, and Treatment of High Blood Cholesterol in Adults. *NHLBI Publication No. 93-3095*. Washington, DC: National Institute of Health, National Heart, Lung and Blood Institute, 1993.

Nettleton JA. Omega-3 fatty acids: comparison of plant and seafood sources in human nutrition. *J Am Diet Assoc* 1991;91(3):331–337.

Rimm EB, Ascherio A, Giovainnucci E, et al. Vegetable, fruit, and cereal fiber intake and risk of coronary heart disease among men. *JAMA* 1996;275:447–451.

Schaefer EJ, Lichtenstein AH, Lamon-Fava S. Lipoproteins, nutrition, aging, and atherosclerosis. *Am J Clin Nutr* 1995;61(3 Suppl):726S–740S.

Schocken DD, Arrieta MI, Leaverton PE. Prevalence and mortality rate of congestive heart failure in the United States. *J Am Col Cardiol* 1992;20(2):301–306.

Siscovick DS, Raghunathan TE, King I, et al. Dietary intake and cell membrane levels of long-chain polyunsaturated fatty acids and the risk of primary cardiac arrest. *JAMA* 1995;274:1363–1367.

Stender S, Dyerberg J, Holmer G, et al. The influence of trans fatty acids on health: a report from the Danish Nutrition Council. *Clin Sci* 1995;88(4):375–392.

Summary of the second report of the National Cholesterol Education Program (NCEP) expert panel on detection, evaluation, and treatment of high blood cholesterol in adults (Adult Treatment Panel II). *JAMA* 1993;269:3015–3023.

Tyroler HA. Nutrition and coronary heart disease epidemiology. *Adv Exper Med and Biol* 1995;369:7–19.

7

Gastrointestinal Disease

Gary R. Lichtenstein and Frances Burke

Objectives

- To incorporate nutrition into the medical history, review of systems, and physical examination of patients with gastrointestinal diseases.
- To understand the causes of malnutrition in inflammatory bowel disease, liver diseases, and malabsorption syndrome.
- To understand why sodium and fluid restriction may be necessary for patients with liver disease.
- To understand the association between diet and lower esophageal sphincter pressure in patients with gastroesophageal reflux disease.

Peptic Ulcer Disease

The goals of nutritional intervention in the treatment of peptic ulcer disease (PUD) are to reduce and neutralize the secretion of stomach acid and to maintain the resistance of the gastrointestinal epithelial tissue to the acid. Traditionally, patients were prescribed special bland diets that restricted the intake of foods and beverages thought to irritate the gastric mucosa or produce excessive acid secretion. In the past, dietary therapy for PUD included small, frequent feedings with mechanically soft foods such as milk and eggs. Frequent feedings were thought to provide constant buffering, and small feedings were thought to limit the amount of gastric distention and thus acid secretion. However, this dietary treatment has not been sufficiently supported by scientific evidence.

Randomized, controlled clinical trials have shown no differences between unrestricted and therapeutic diets with regard to healing of the ulcer or remission of symptoms. In addition, foods with high protein content, such as milk, were found to be the most powerful stimuli of acid secretion, an outcome contrary to the goals of diet therapy in these patients. Therefore, current nutritional therapy is based on the individual's tolerance of foods and beverages that may cause discomfort. Nutritional advice is offered as an adjunct to conventional medical and pharmacological therapy in order to reduce gastric acid secretion.

Nutrition Therapy for Peptic Ulcer Disease

The acid-secreting parietal cells lie mostly in the fundus of the stomach. The sight or smell of food and distention of the stomach trigger neurally mediated reflexes that stimulate acid secretion from the parietal cells. Caffeine and other alkaloids in coffee, polypeptides and amino acids (products of protein digestion), and alcohol stimulate the release of the hormone gastrin, thereby triggering gastric acid secretion. Although alcohol and caffeine consumption have not been directly implicated in the development of PUD, excessive intake of these substances may cause discomfort. In addition, individuals who abuse alcohol appear to have an increased risk of developing PUD.

According to current recommendations, patients with PUD should be advised to

- limit caffeine intake by reducing consumption of coffee, tea, cola, chocolate, and other foods and beverages that contain caffeine
- limit alcohol intake and avoid drinking on an empty stomach
- avoid cigarette smoking, which may increase gastric acid secretion and delay the healing process and is also associated with an increased frequency of duodenal ulcers
- eat three meals daily, avoid skipping meals, and limit intake of spicy, fatty, or otherwise bothersome foods
- avoid bedtime snacks to prevent acid secretion if symptoms often occur in the middle of the night

Gastroesophageal Reflux Disease

Gastroesophageal reflux (GER) is the regurgitation of gastric contents into the esophagus through the lower esophageal sphincter (LES) due to transient, increased abdominal pressure or relaxation of the LES. When the gastric acid, bile, and pepsin in the stomach are in frequent and prolonged contact with the esophagus, gastroesophageal reflux disease (GERD) may develop, and the patient becomes symptomatic.

Heartburn, described as a burning epigastric or substernal pain, is a major symptom of GERD. Findings associated with GERD include a delayed esophageal clearing rate, weak or incompetent LES, delayed gastric emptying, and irritation of the esophageal mucosa. The role of LES tone in preventing GERD is known to be important. If the pressure of the LES is not greater than the pressure in the stomach, the contents of the stomach back up into the esophagus.

The goals of nutrition therapy for patients with GERD include

- avoiding decreases in LES pressure
- decreasing the frequency and volume of reflux
- reducing irritation of sensitive or inflamed esophageal tissue
- improving esophageal clearing time

Because the severity of symptoms varies greatly among individuals with GERD, nutrition therapy is based on the individual's tolerance of foods and beverages that may cause discomfort.

Nutrition Therapy for GERD

Maintaining Lower Esophageal Sphincter Pressure

A major goal in the treatment of GERD is to avoid decreasing lower esophageal sphincter pressure. From a nutritional standpoint, the following measures have proven to be helpful in patients with this disorder.

- *Limiting dietary fat intake:* High-fat meals tend to decrease LES pressure and delay gastric emptying time. As a consequence, the time that the esophagus is exposed to irritants increases, as does the gastric volume available for reflux.
- *Losing weight:* Obesity affects GERD by increasing abdominal pressure and thus the likelihood of reflux.
- *Limiting alcohol, chocolate, and coffee:* These substances decrease LES pressure. Alcohol is also a powerful stimulus of gastric acid secretion.

Decreasing Reflux Frequency and Volume

The following steps have proven useful to decrease the frequency and volume of gastroesophageal reflux:

- eating small meals and eating more frequently if necessary
- losing weight if overweight
- drinking most fluids between meals rather than with them
- consuming adequate fiber to avoid constipation because straining increases intraabdominal pressure

Decreasing Esophageal Irritation

To decrease irritation in the esophagus, patients with GERD should be counseled to monitor their dietary intake in the following ways.

- Limit intake of citrus fruits (oranges, grapefruits, and lemons), tomato products, spicy foods, and carbonated beverages. Although most of these foods do not irritate the esophagus, they can cause heartburn and other GER symptoms in individuals with a sensitive esophagus.
- Avoid any other foods that regularly cause heartburn.

Improving Esophageal Clearing Time

To improve clearing of food from the esophagus, patients should take the following precautions.

- Do not recline after eating. Sit upright or take a walk.
- Avoid eating within two to three hours before bedtime.
- Elevate the head of the bed.

Malabsorption

Malabsorption involves defective digestion and absorption of carbohydrates, proteins, fats, vitamins, and minerals, either jointly or independently. From a clinical standpoint malabsorption should be differentiated from maldigestion. A thorough history and a careful physical examination are essential to detecting the signs and symptoms of malabsorption. Successful management of malabsorption hinges on identifying the underlying defect and implementing specific therapy to correct it. Malabsorption can be treated, and the treatment invariably improves the patient's quality of life.

Defects Associated with Malabsorption

Four categories of defects have been identified as the major causes of malabsorption.

1. *Impairment of mechanical digestion:* Common underlying problems in this category include:

    poor dentition or lack of dentures

    gastrectomy in individuals with PUD or cancer

    gastroparesis due to autonomic nerve dysfunction associated with diabetes mellitus

    vagotomy for PUD

2. *Impairment of chemical digestion:* Common causes are:

    inadequate secretion of lipase, amylase, and other pancreatic enzymes due to pancreatic insufficiency, often seen in cystic fibrosis

    low bicarbonate secretion also due to pancreatic insufficiency

3. *Impairment of solubilization:* The most frequently encountered underlying factors are:

inadequate amounts of bile salts

interruption of enterohepatic circulation

increased deconjugation of bile salts

impaired secretion of bile salts

4. *Pathological impairment of absorption:* Absorption defects due to specific disorders include:

decreased absorptive surface area in short bowel syndrome, celiac disease, and enteric fistulas

impaired fatty acid esterification in celiac disease, pancreatic insufficiency, starvation, and intestinal bypass

impaired chylomicron synthesis and removal

Malabsorption of Specific Nutrients

Carbohydrate Malabsorption

Malabsorption of carbohydrates causes osmotic diarrhea. The most commonly seen carbohydrate malabsorption is lactose intolerance. Lactose is a disaccharide found in milk and dairy products. Normally, lactose is hydrolyzed to glucose and galactose by an enzyme called lactase. About 15 percent of Caucasians and more than 90 percent of African and Asian Americans are lactase-deficient. The development of clinical symptoms of lactose intolerance—bloating, abdominal cramps, and diarrhea—depends on whether the level of lactase activity is adequate to hydrolyze fully the lactose load delivered to the intestine.

Nutrition therapy for lactose intolerance or lactose deficiency involves the following measures, individually or in combination, according to the severity of the patient's intolerance:

• reducing or avoiding lactose intake (milk and dairy products)

• pretreating milk with lactase derived from bacteria

• ingesting only lactose-treated dairy products such as Lactaid or Dairy Ease

Individuals who avoid all products containing lactose will not meet their daily calcium requirement. Calcium supplementation of 800 to 1200 mg/day is therefore necessary for these patients. Pregnant and lactating women and the elderly require higher levels, depending on their intake of nondairy calcium sources.

Fat Malabsorption

Among the lipids is a group of compounds with drastically different chemical and physical properties: triglycerides, diglycerides, monoglycerides, fatty acids, phospholipids, cholesterol, cholesterol esters, and bile acids. Lipids (primarily triglycerides), a major source of calories, require the most complicated sequence of digestive and absorptive processes. A typical Western diet contains at least 70 grams of fat per day, accounting for approximately 34 percent of total dietary calories. The absorption coefficient of triglycerides in normal individuals is greater than 99 percent. Due to the complexity of the digestive and absorptive processes involved in the body's utilization of fats, a number of problems can arise in individuals whose intake of these substances exceeds their capacity to break them down.

Clinical Manifestations of Fat Malabsorption   Malabsorption of fat can present with a unique clinical manifestation of excessive fat loss in the stool called steatorrhea, the result of impairment of either the digestive or the absorptive process. Clinical manifestations of fat malabsorption include the following general signs and symptoms.

- Weight loss, muscle wasting
- Failure to thrive, growth retardation, fatigue, especially in infants, children, and adolescents
- Tetany, osteomalacia, bone pain, compression fracture of vertebra body due to hypocalcemia secondary to calcium malabsorption
- Infertility, dysmenorrhea, amenorrhea

In addition, malabsorption of fats is often responsible for a number of fat-soluble vitamin deficiencies. Clinical signs vary as follows, according to the vitamin deficiency involved.

Vitamin A: night blindness, hyperkeratosis, skin changes

Vitamin D: hypocalcemia, osteomalacia, rickets, hypophosphatemia

Vitamin K: prolongation of prothrombin time, easy bruisability

Vitamin E: neuropathy, hemolytic anemia

Renal Manifestation of Fat Malabsorption   Oxalate stones, the primary renal manifestation of fat malabsorption, are generally caused by bile salt malabsorption resulting from a pathological disease process in the luminal digestive tract. Most dietary oxalic acid is normally precipitated in the lumen as calcium oxalate and excreted in the feces without being absorbed. However, in the presence of certain pathological processes, such as extensive ileal Crohn's disease, the damaged portion of the intestine is unable to absorb bile salts completely. The resulting excess bile salt loss in the stool eventually leads to bile salt pool depletion, despite the liver's attempts to compensate by increasing the amount of bile salts it produces.

In individuals with extensive ileal disease, an excess of fatty acids in the lumen depletes calcium by binding with it to form calcium soap. Consequently, dietary oxalic acid in these patients bonds with sodium to form sodium oxalate, which is more soluble than the calcium salt. Oxalic acid thus becomes available for absorption, which occurs primarily in the colon. In the presence of bile acid malabsorption, bile acids alter colonic permeability, and as a result the colon absorbs the sodium oxalate produced in the lumen. The kidney excretes this oxalate, which contributes secondary to the formation of oxalate stores. In addition, these patients tend to be volume depleted secondary to diarrhea, with low urine output, another factor contributing to increased oxalate stone formation. To avoid the formation of stones, patients with bile salt malabsorption should avoid foods high in oxalate such as spinach, rhubarb, cocoa, chocolate, tea, green beans, collards, kale, peanut butter, and beer. Oxalate kidney stones are discussed in detail in Chapter 10.

Liver Disease

The liver is involved in many of the body's metabolic processes, including regulation of protein, fat and carbohydrate metabolism, vitamin storage and activation, and detoxification and excretion of waste products. Thus impaired liver function can lead to nutrient deficiencies, and eventually, protein-energy malnutrition. Conversely, malnutrition can further impair liver function by affecting the liver's structural integrity.

Most liver disease in the United States is related to alcohol abuse. Of all active cases of cirrhosis, the end stage of liver disease, in the United States, ninety percent are secondary to alcohol-related liver damage. Regardless of the cause, however, patients with cirrhosis usually present some degree of muscle wasting and malnutrition.

Causes of Malnutrition

The major causes of malnutrition in patients with liver disease are

- poor dietary intake
- maldigestion and malabsorption
- abnormalities in the metabolism and storage of macro- and micronutrients

Protein-energy malnutrition is a common finding in both alcohol- and non-alcohol-related liver disease. The goals of nutritional management in patients with liver disease are to correct preexisting malnutrition and supply adequate calories as well as protein to encourage hepatic regeneration without precipitating hepatic encephalopathy.

Poor Dietary Intake

Alcohol provides 7 kcal/g that can be fully utilized and metabolized, but no vitamins or minerals. Individuals who substitute alcohol for other sources of carbohydrate and fat calories find that their appetite decreases proportionally to the amount of alcohol they ingest, largely because their need for calories is satisfied. To evaluate the risk of alcohol-related liver disease, dietary assessment should therefore include an evaluation of the pattern, quantity, and duration of alcohol intake, usual dietary intake, and various socioeconomic factors affecting eating habits.

Patients with chronic liver disease frequently present with a poor dietary intake resulting from nausea, vomiting, diarrhea, abdominal pain, and early satiety. Ascites, resulting in distention of the abdominal cavity due to the accumulation of fluid, may also contribute to early satiety. Because patients with ascites secondary to cirrhosis are prescribed a low-sodium diet to decrease fluid retention, their dislike of unseasoned food may further decrease their intake. Changes in mental status secondary to hepatic encephalopathy may also contribute to poor dietary intake in patients with advanced liver disease.

Maldigestion and Malabsorption

Individuals with chronic liver disease frequently present with both maldigestion and malabsorption of fat. High concentrations of alcohol can disrupt the gastric and duodenal mucosa, causing diarrhea and malabsorption of thiamin, folate, and vitamin B_{12}. Steatorrhea, the most common manifestation of malabsorption, occurs in approximately 50 percent of patients with cirrhosis. Cholestasis is associated with decreased bile salt secretion due to pancreatic insufficiency, both of which may contribute to fat malabsorption. These patients may have deficiencies of the fat-soluble vitamins A, D, E, and K. Clinical manifestations include night blindness caused by vitamin A deficiency, osteomalacia caused by vitamin D deficiency, neuropathy caused by vitamin E deficiency, and easy bruisability or hemorrhaging caused by vitamin K deficiency.

Abnormal Metabolism and Storage of Nutrients

Liver disease causes many metabolic problems and also affects the assessment parameters commonly used to evaluate nutritional status. Therefore the patient's stage of liver disease and the amount of fluid on board should always be considered when assessing the degree of malnutrition present.

Protein Reduced hepatic synthesis of transport proteins often results in low serum albumin and transferrin values in these patients. Likewise, reduced synthesis of serum proteins, which can decrease serum oncotic pressure, is the most probable cause of ascites and edema. Hepatic synthesis of clotting factors is also reduced, interfering with blood coagulation, as evidenced by an abnormal Prothrombin Time (PT and PTT). Therefore, albumin and transferrin levels are not an accurate indicator of visceral protein status in patients with advanced liver disease.

BUN levels are reduced, and plasma ammonium levels may be increased in liver disease because of decreased hepatic urea synthesis. The failure to detoxify ammonia and the abnormal amino acid profile (increased aromatic amino acids and decreased branched chain amino acids) seen in patients with cirrhosis may raise their risk of hepatic encephalopathy. Therefore, in patients with acute encephalopathic conditions, decreased dietary protein intake for a few days may be helpful.

Carbohydrate Liver disease can also lead to disturbances in glucose metabolism, resulting in hypoglycemia or hyperglycemia. The hypoglycemia sometimes seen in acute liver disease may be due to impaired glycogenesis, glycogenolysis, and gluconeogenesis. Hyperglycemia, often observed in cirrhosis and chronic hepatitis, may be associated with increased glucagon levels and insulin resistance.

Fat Disturbances in fat metabolism can lead to decreased lipid clearance and increased serum triglyceride and cholesterol levels. Excessive alcohol consumption is associated with increased accumulation of triglycerides in the liver and the development of fatty liver. Poor utilization of fat increases dependence on gluconeogenesis as an energy source.

Vitamins and Minerals Poor absorption and reduced storage of vitamins and minerals occurs commonly in patients with liver disease. Chronic liver disease also contributes to their frequent deficiencies in thiamin, folate, pyridoxine, and vitamin D by decreasing the conversion of these vitamins to their active forms.

Nutrition Therapy for Liver Disease

The goals of nutrition therapy for patients with liver disease are to provide adequate protein and calories to maintain nitrogen balance and support liver regeneration, while preventing such complications as encephalopathy. Abstinence from alcohol is an essential part of managing alcohol-related liver disease.

Calories

An unrestricted diet is indicated for most patients with liver disease. Studies show no significant increase in energy requirements in patients with liver disease and estimate them at 25 to 30 kcal/kg of ideal body weight. In patients with ascites, calorie and protein requirements must be based on estimated "dry" weight, or total weight minus the weight of the ascites fluid. One liter of fluid is said to be equivalent to approximately 1 kg of body weight. When fluid is seen only in the abdominal cavity, the amount is estimated at 5 liters, or 5 kg of body weight. If fluid is present in both the abdominal cavity and the extremities, the amount is estimated at 10 liters, or 10 kg of body weight. Additional adjustments must be made for infection, trauma, surgery, or loss of nutrients due to disorders such as steatorrhea, because additional calories are needed to minimize endogenous protein catabolism.

Fat

Fat intake amounting to 20 to 40 percent of daily caloric requirements should be encouraged as tolerated in the absence of steatorrhea, because fat contributes to the nonprotein calories and increased palatability of the diet. Providing fat calories in the form of oil composed solely of medium-chain triglycerides (MCTs), may be necessary in the presence of fat malabsorption. MCTs are more efficiently absorbed than long-chain triglycerides (LCTs) because they are absorbed directly into the portal vein and subsequently are transported to the liver.

Protein

Positive nitrogen balance in patients with cirrhosis can be attained with daily amounts of dietary protein similar to those required by healthy individuals: 0.8 to 1.0 g/kg of ideal body weight, or approximately 4 to 6 ounces of meat, fish, or chicken per day. At the onset of hepatic encephalopathy, precipitating factors such as infection, electrolyte imbalance, and GI bleeding should be identified and treated, but dietary intervention should be initiated only if hepatic encephalopathy persists. Dietary protein may be restricted to lower plasma ammonium levels because ammonia, a by-product of protein metabolism, contributes to the development of hepatic encephalopathy. However, drastic, long-term protein restriction is not indicated because these patients are depleted already when they present for treatment. Additional protein deprivation may promote catabolism of lean body tissue and contribute to malnutrition, reducing host defenses to infection. Protein restriction should be individualized and based on tolerance. Forty grams of protein per day (2 to 3 ounces per day of meat, fish, or chicken) is the initial recommendation. With improvement in mental status, protein intake can be increased by increments of 10 to 15 grams to attain the maintenance levels of 0.8 to 1.0 g/kg daily.

Studies have been conducted to determine if vegetable protein, versus meat protein, improves the clinical status of cirrhotic patients with encephalopathy. Possible mechanisms for greater tolerance of vegetable proteins include their lower levels of aromatic amino acids, alterations in the patient's absorption and intestinal bacteria flora, and fiber content. Most results show only marginal improvement in encephalopathic symptoms and often reflect poor tolerance of pure vegetable protein diets. Use of branched-chain amino acids has been extensively investigated, but remains controversial, especially in light of their cost. Most of the literature indicates no benefit to incorporating branched-chain amino acids over standard amino acids in the majority of patients.

Sodium

In the severely sodium-retentive patient who has liver disease with ascites, sodium and fluid restrictions are necessary. How restricted dietary sodium needs to be is controversial. Some support the view that moderate sodium restriction (2 to 3 g/day) coupled with effective diuretics can make the diet more palatable and nutritious, while minimizing biochemical complications such as hyponatremia, hypokalemia associated with potassium-wasting diuretics, or hyperkalemia and uremia resulting from the treatment of ascites. However, cirrhotic patients have limited ability to excrete sodium, and those who are severely sodium-retentive should be restricted initially to not more than 500 mg of sodium per day. Once the patient shows rapid diuresis, the diet can be liberalized.

Fluid

By consensus, patients with hyponatremia (serum sodium under 130 mEq/L) require a fluid restriction of 1000 to 1500 cc/day. Fluid imbalances in patients with liver disease generally make body weight, skinfold measurements, and serum albumin levels unreliable indicators of nutritional status. Serum albumin levels may be falsely elevated if the patient is dehydrated or falsely decreased if the patient is in fluid overload. Massive fluid shifts result from edema, ascites, and diuretic therapy in these patients. Malnutrition is associated with a fluid shift from the intravascular space to the extravascular space and a concurrent decrease in lean body mass. Body weight can increase by as much as 10 kg in cirrhotic patients with both ascites and peripheral edema.

Vitamins and Minerals

Patients with chronic liver disease are at risk for vitamin and mineral deficiencies secondary to poor intake, malabsorption, impaired metabolism, and decreased storage. The physical examination therefore should include evaluation of the physical signs and symptoms of vitamin and mineral deficiency. A combined multivitamin and mineral preparation should be routinely provided for patients with chronic liver disease. If the patient is still consuming alcohol, thiamin and folate supplements must be prescribed to prevent Wernicke's encephalopathy and macrocytic anemia, respectively. Patients with advanced chronic liver disease may have problems with vitamin storage, metabolism, and transport, and thus may require subcutaneous injections of vitamins. Serum potassium, magnesium, and zinc levels should be monitored closely when diuretics are prescribed for these patients (see Case 1).

Inflammatory Bowel Disease

Inflammatory bowel disease (IBD) refers to idiopathic, chronic, inflammatory conditions affecting the gastrointestinal tract, primarily Crohn's disease and ulcerative colitis. Because of the chronic involvement of the GI tract, most patients with IBD have some form of nutritional deficiency. Therefore, careful attention to the diet can prevent nutritional deficiencies and help in the medical and surgical management of these diseases.

Protein-energy malnutrition is prevalent among patients with IBD. Nutrition assessment is essential because of the consequences of malnutrition which include the following: growth retardation in children, impaired healing of the inflamed and damaged bowel, and enhanced susceptibility to infection in children and adults. In addition, a malnourished patient with IBD may present with defects in GI function that further limit the absorption and utilization of nutrients.

Causes of Malnutrition

Malnutrition occurs in patients suffering from IBD as a consequence of

- decreased dietary intake
- increased nutrient losses
- increased nutrient requirements

Decreased Dietary Intake

The most important factor contributing to the poor nutritional status seen in patients with IBD is inadequate dietary intake. Gastrointestinal symptoms such as nausea, diarrhea, and recurrent abdominal pain at mealtimes often decrease appetite and food intake. Also, eating certain foods can increase the likelihood of particular complications of IBD. For example, in Crohn's disease, where the lumen of the small bowel is narrower, impaction of bulky food in an inflamed area may precipitate an obstruction.

Increased Nutrient Losses

In Crohn's disease, small and large bowel inflammation, bacterial overgrowth, and multiple bowel resections can decrease the absorptive surface area of both the small and large intestine and cause malabsorption of essential nutrients. Resections of the ileum can cause bile salt deficiency, resulting in steatorrhea or fat malabsorption and subsequent deficiency of the fat-soluble vitamins, A, D, E, and K. Vitamin B_{12} is coupled with intrinsic factor secreted by the parietal cells of the stomach. Because the vitamin B_{12}–intrinsic factor complex is absorbed in the ileum, complete ileal resection produces a vitamin B_{12} deficiency that requires treatment with intramuscular injections of this vitamin.

IBD also results in protein-losing enteropathy, or excessive intestinal secretion of protein-rich fluids through the inflamed bowel wall. Severe diarrhea causes depletion of electrolytes, minerals, and trace elements such as zinc. Gastrointestinal bleeding can contribute to iron deficiency anemia.

Increased Nutrient Requirements

The inflammatory process of IBD may increase resting energy expenditure, thereby contributing to weight loss and depleted fat stores if patients are not consuming adequate calories and protein. Patients with fever or sepsis and those undergoing surgery also have greater requirements for protein, calories, and other nutrients than do patients who are less severely ill. Increased intestinal cell turnover can also raise nutrient requirements in patients with IBD.

Nutrition Therapy for IBD

The goals of nutrition therapy for patients with IBD are to prevent symptoms associated with malabsorption such as diarrhea; to correct and prevent nutritional deficiencies; to promote healing of the intestinal mucosa; to minimize stress on the inflamed and often narrowed segments of the bowel (Crohn's disease); and in children, to promote normal growth and development. Oral nutritional repletion may be difficult to achieve during symptomatic, active IBD, since most patients' symptoms worsen both during and following meals. Therefore to decrease both the symptoms associated with eating and bowel activity during the healing process, patients hospitalized for IBD are sometimes placed on bowel rest. However, prolonged bowel rest without enteral or parenteral nutritional support can lead to nutritional depletion.

An oral diet may be tolerated when active IBD is less severe. To control diarrhea and malabsorption, a low-fat, low-fiber, low-lactose diet is often prescribed. Small, frequent feedings may help to limit gastrointestinal secretions as well as reduce the volume of food that the damaged bowel must handle at any one time. The diet should be individualized according to the patient's clinical condition and food tolerances.

Calories

In adults, calories should be provided in amounts sufficient to maintain or restore body weight. In children, the amount of calories should be adequate to support growth and development, generally measured on the pediatric growth charts. Complications such as sepsis and fistulas may increase caloric requirements to as high as 35 to 45 kcal/kg per day, or approximately 1.5 to 1.7 times the basal energy expenditure according to the Harris-Benedict equation. Supplemental calories can be given in the form of glucose polymers or MCT oil, which are undetectable when added to foods or beverages.

Protein

Protein needs may be as high as 1.5 to 2.5 g/kg per day, compared to the RDA of 0.8 g/kg per day. The exact value depends on the degree of catabolism and protein losses in individual patients.

Vitamins and Minerals

Because patients with IBD are at higher risk for vitamin, mineral, and trace element deficiencies, their diets should be supplemented with a multivitamin and mineral preparation 1 to 5 times the normal recommended dietary allowance. High doses of specific nutrients are indicated if clinical or laboratory evidence shows a deficiency due to possible poor absorption or increased requirements due to complications such as anemia, peripheral neuropathy, or night blindness. Patients with Crohn's disease who have extensive damage and/or have undergone resection of the terminal ileum are likely to suffer from defective vitamin

B12 absorption and thus require supplementation with intramuscular injections of this vitamin. IBD patients with persistent, watery diarrhea may have trouble maintaining adequate zinc and magnesium levels and require supplementation of these minerals.

Chronic blood loss and altered iron absorption, frequently observed in IBD, can cause iron deficiency anemia. However, iron supplements in full therapeutic doses may exacerbate symptoms. In particular, oral iron irritates the gastric mucosa, causing nausea, diarrhea, and abdominal cramping. Slower iron supplementation along with ascorbic acid may be more effective, because ascorbic acid enhances the absorption of iron by converting the ferric ions to the ferrous form, which is absorbed primarily in the duodenum.

Long-term treatment with corticosteroids requires calcium and vitamin D supplementation because steroids decrease calcium absorption and increase calcium excretion. Patients treated with sulfasalazine (Azulfidine) should receive folate supplements because this medication inhibits folate conjugation in the jejunum.

Fiber

A low-fiber diet is often prescribed for patients with narrowed sections of bowel to decrease the possibility of intestinal obstruction, minimize physical irritation to the inflamed bowel, reduce stool weight and frequency, and slow the rate of intestinal transit. The diet consists of white bread and refined cereals and avoidance of high-fiber fresh fruits and vegetables, nuts, skins, and seeds. Some controversy exists over the benefits of a low-fiber diet for these patients because its efficacy in managing symptoms or affecting the course of IBD remains unclear.

Lactose

Patients with IBD may malabsorb lactose because of decreased brush border epithelial cell lactase activity and rapid intestinal transit. The incidence of lactose intolerance among those suffering from IBD is similar to that of the general population. Symptoms of lactose intolerance include bloating, cramps, and diarrhea. Total elimination of dietary lactose is not always required to control symptoms. When necessary, patients may be advised to resort to lactose-treated milk and lactose pills, available in most supermarkets. The major dietary sources of lactose—milk and milk products—are also significant sources of protein, calcium, vitamin D, and calories. Consequently, they should not be removed routinely from the diet. In the event that they are eliminated from the diet, calcium supplementation is usually necessary to meet their requirements.

Fat

Decreased fat intake may help control the symptoms of steatorrhea, especially in patients with Crohn's disease involving the small bowel. Currently under way are experiments in using omega-3 fatty acids to treat patients suffering from ulcerative colitis who are unresponsive to other treatment modalities.

Oxalate

Calcium oxalate kidney stones following ileal resection are a common complication in patients with Crohn's disease. Limiting fat intake and foods with a high oxalate content is recommended to help reduce the formation of these stones.

Nutrition Support

Enteral or parenteral nutrition support is indicated in severe cases of IBD whenever bowel rest is considered necessary to decrease bowel activity during healing, when the patient is unable to consume an adequate diet, or when short bowel syndrome occurs as a complication of the primary disease. The liquid formula used to provide enteral or parenteral nutrition support in patients with IBD should be low in fat and residue and lactose-free. Elemental formulas for enteral tube feeding that contain protein in the form of free amino acids have been used successfully in this population. Because these formulas are completely absorbed in the upper small intestine and seem to be effective in reducing residue in the bowel, they are particularly appropriate for patients with Crohn's disease. Elemental formulas are also well tolerated because of their low-fat content. (See Chapter 11.)

Alcohol and Vitamin Deficiencies

Patricia Charlton, Gail Morrison, and Lisa D. Unger

Objectives

- To learn how excessive alcohol consumption contributes to nutritional deficiencies.
- To understand the biochemical and pathophysiological abnormalities that occur with excessive alcohol intake.
- To develop nutritional recommendations for patients who consume alcohol.

CT, a 52-year-old car salesman, presents to his family physician for his yearly physical complaining of fatigue, numbness in his hands and feet, loss of balance, decreased memory, and heartburn. He also has noticed a recent weight gain around the waist and decreased endurance when exercising. He denies blurred vision, headaches, night sweats, or hearing loss.

Past Medical History

CT has no prior history of heart disease, stroke, or peripheral vascular disease. He has been told in the past that his liver is damaged, but he has never received treatment. He is not taking any medications and has no known drug or food allergies.

Social History

CT states that he consumes three meals every day and his diet is healthful, but his appetite has been poor for the past week. He has smoked one pack of cigarettes per day for 30 years (30 pack year history).

Family History

CT's family history is negative for heart disease, stroke, cholesterol and lipid disorders, and neurological diseases.

Review of Systems

General: Lethargic, decreased appetite, recent bloating; patient reports that his pants are tighter in the waist than usual.

GI/Abdomen: No vomiting or diarrhea.

Neurological: No history of seizures; no tinnitus or syncope; reported short-term memory loss for recent events.

Physical Examination

Vital signs

Temperature: 98.2°F

Heart rate: 104 BPM

Respiratory rate: 16 BPM

Blood pressure: 120/90 mm Hg

Anthropometric data

Height: 5'8" (173 cm)

Current weight: 160 lb (73 kg)

Usual weight (1 month ago): 150 lb (68 kg)

Ideal body weight (IBW): 154 lb (70 kg)

General: Well-dressed male who appears to be in mild distress

Eyes: Pale conjunctiva, sclera anicteric; no ophthalmoplegia or nystagmus

Skin: Jaundiced; spider angiomas on the upper chest (central artery feeding small, dilated vessels, characteristic of chronic liver disease)

Cardiac: Resting tachycardia

GI/Abdomen:

Protuberant abdomen

Presence of an abdominal fluid wave and shifting dullness, consistent with ascites (physical finding of fluid accumulation in the peritoneal cavity associated with severe liver disease)

Enlarged liver (14 cm span) with a firm, nontender edge

No splenomegaly

Pulmonary: Lungs clear bilaterally

Neurological:

Decreased vibratory sensation in the lower legs

Bilaterally decreased knee reflexes

No asterixis

Normal sensation and position sense in upper and lower extremities

Cranial nerves II through XII grossly intact

Laboratory Data

Patient's Values	Normal Values
Red blood cells: 3.8 million/mm^3	4.3–5.8 million/mm^3
Hemoglobin: 10 mg/dL	Males: 13.5–17.5 mg/dL
Hematocrit: 35%	Males: 40–52%
Mean corpuscular volume (MCV): 104 fl	80–100 fl
Mean corpuscular hemoglobin (MCH): 34 fmol/cell	27–33 fmol/cell
Albumin: 3.0 g/dL	3.5–5.8 g/dL
Prothrombin time: 15 seconds	0–15 seconds
Total bilirubin: 5 mg/dL	0–1.2 mg/dL
AST: 140 U/L	0–40 U/L
ALT: 80 U/L	0–36 U/L
Sodium: 135 mg/dL	133–143 mg/dL

Case Questions

1. What additional information is important to obtain from a patient who presents with these complaints?

2. What are the biochemical consequences of excessive alcohol consumption?

3. What are the nutritional consequences of excessive alcohol consumption?

4. What evidence from CT's physical exam and the following laboratory data suggests complications of alcoholism and nutritional deficiencies?

5. What does CT's serum albumin level indicate? (Take into account his prothrombin time of 15 seconds and the finding of ascites during his physical exam.)

6. What additional laboratory tests would you request before giving CT a folate supplement?

7. What additional nutritional recommendations would you give CT?

Answers begin on the following page.

Answers to Questions: Case 1

Part 1:   Diagnosis

1. **What additional information is important to obtain from a patient who presents with these complaints?**

    Alcohol intake should always be included in the social history because the majority of persons who actively drink alcohol may not voluntarily admit to having a drinking problem. In addition, particular attention must be paid to those signs, symptoms, and lab tests that are likely to be abnormal in the alcoholic patient. Neurological signs, combined with fatigue, ascites, enlarged liver, and possible gastroesophageal reflux, all alert the clinician to probe for chronic alcohol ingestion. Once the patient admits to drinking, specific information regarding quantity, type, frequency, and duration of consumption should be ascertained. CT has been drinking heavily for ten years. His daily routine consists of two cocktails with hard liquor before dinner, a few glasses of wine with dinner, and two drinks of hard liquor after dinner, totaling six drinks per day.

    Considering that CT is a heavy drinker, as evidenced by his consumption of 42 drinks per week, he is a candidate for the CAGE test. The CAGE test was developed as a diagnostic tool for alcoholism. CT is asked the following questions, which are assigned a value of one point when answered "yes."

    Have you ever felt you should **C**ut down on your drinking?   ___(Yes)
    Have people **A**nnoyed you by criticizing your drinking?   ___(No)
    Have you ever felt bad or **G**uilty about your drinking?   ___(Yes)
    Have you ever had a drink the first thing in the morning (**E**ye
    opener) to steady your nerves or to get rid of a hangover? ___(No)

    When interpreting the CAGE test, take into account the patient's answers to the preliminary questions about alcohol use. A key question is "When was the last time you had a drink?". Because CT reports drinking within the past 30 days and scored two on the CAGE test, he is very likely to have a current alcohol problem. A detailed dietary history to assess CT's calorie and protein intake also is important, especially because he reports a decreased appetite over the past week.

2. **What are the biochemical consequences of excessive alcohol consumption?**

    Excessive alcohol consumption can cause metabolic acidosis by interfering with the oxidation of acetyl CoA in the TCA cycle. Ethanol is oxidized to acetaldehyde by alcohol dehydrogenase, which also simultaneously reduces NAD^+ to $NADH + H^+$. Acetylaldehyde dehydrogenase also reduces another NAD^+ to $NADH + H^+$ and simultaneously oxidizes acetaldehyde to acetyl CoA. Both enzymes require NAD^+ to accept the hydrogen ions.

    The high ratio of NADH to NAD^+ in the presence of excess alcohol, called an altered redox state, drives pyruvate to lactate instead of to acetyl CoA. High levels of lactate generated from pyruvate suggest an abnormality in the recycling of NADH to NAD^+ caused by excessive alcohol ingestion. In addition, instead of entering the TCA cycle, where more NADH is produced, acetyl CoA is converted to ketone bodies and fatty acids. As a result, a ketoacidotic state develops, and fatty acids are converted to triglycerides. In turn, a significant rise in triglyceride levels can lead to fatty liver (Figure 7-1).

3. What are the nutritional consequences of excessive alcohol consumption?

Alcohol provides 7 kcal/g, which can be fully utilized and metabolized when substituted for calories from food, but provide no vitamins or minerals. Drinking causes a decrease in appetite that generally is proportional to the amount of ingested calories from alcohol and can significantly affect the nutritional adequacy of a patient's diet. High concentrations of alcohol can also disrupt the gastric and duodenal mucosa, affect the digestive and absorptive processes, and as a consequence, reduce significantly the absorption of vitamins and minerals.

One of the most important vitamin supplements routinely given to alcoholics is thiamin (vitamin B_1), since alcohol interferes with thiamin absorption, even in healthy individuals. Thiamin is a cofactor for the enzyme thiamin pyrophosphate (TPP), which converts pyruvate to acetyl CoA. Inadequate thiamin intake forces pyruvate to convert to lactate, further contributing to the development of lactic acidosis (see Figure 7-1). Thiamin deficiency manifests as anorexia, irritability, and weight loss. Later stages present with weakness, peripheral neuropathy, headache, and tachycardia. Therefore, thiamin is routinely prescribed for patients suspected of alcohol abuse.

Alcohol also affects folate levels by decreasing intake, impairing absorption and metabolism, and increasing urinary excretion of this nutrient. Folate is involved in one-carbon-unit transfers and thus takes part in several amino acid conversions, among them, homocysteine to methionine, with methyl tetrahydrofolate (THF) as a coenzyme for methionine synthase. Vitamin B_{12} acts as a cofactor in the methylation of this homocysteine-to-methionine reaction, in which methyl THF is converted to its active form, THF. As a result, in vitamin B_{12} deficiency, the demethylation of methyl THF is prevented, blocking folate metabolism, or trapping folate.

Folate is also required for normal purine synthesis. The methylation of deoxyuridine monophosphate (deoxyuridylate) to thymidine monophosphate for normal thymidylate synthase requires 5,10-methylene THF, which is synthesized from THF. Because thymidine is a component of DNA, folate deficiency alters red blood cell production, resulting in enlarged, oval erythrocytes, manifested as megaloblastic anemia. Megaloblastic anemia is a blockage in the normal erythrogenic pathway at one or more of these early stages.

High concentrations of alcohol also induce vitamin B_{12} deficiency by decreasing production of intrinsic factor, a protein secreted by the gastric parietal cells and required for vitamin B12 absorption in the ileum. As described previously, vitamin B12 acts as a cofactor in the methylation of homocysteine to methionine, the reaction that converts methyl THF to THF. Elevated plasma methyl THF levels are observed commonly in patients with vitamin B12 deficiency because methyl THF cannot be converted to THF, the active form of folate, in the absence of this nutrient. In vitamin B12 deficiency, the demethylation of methyl THF is prevented, and folate metabolism is once again blocked or trapped. Therefore, vitamin B12 deficiency also ultimately causes megaloblastic anemia.

Vitamin B12 is also required for myelin formation of the large nerve fibers in the spinal cord. Symptoms of vitamin B12 deficiency therefore include neuropathy and myelopathy. Axonal degeneration occurs as a consequence of insufficient myelin in a deficiency state. Paresthesias in the feet and hands and loss of vibration and position sense are the earliest clinical signs of this condition. Impaired deep tendon reflexes, ataxia, and mild cerebral manifestations such as depression, irritability, and memory impairment are also common. Not all patients exhibit these abnormalities, and the mechanism that produces these neurological lesions is unclear.

4. **What evidence from CT's physical exam and the following laboratory data suggests complications of alcoholism and nutritional deficiencies?**

Decreased lower-leg reflexes, loss of lower-leg vibratory sensation, cold-

Figure 7-1   Alcohol metabolism and the altered redox state.

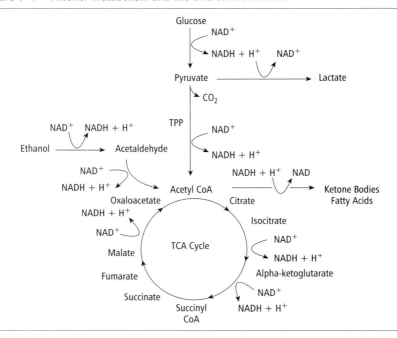

Adapted from: Stryer L. *Biochemistry*, 4th edition. New York: W.H. Freeman, 1995.

ness of extremities, nystagmus, and paresthesias are all neurological symptoms associated with thiamin deficiency due to prolonged alcohol abuse. Because this patient has been drinking heavily for ten years, the diagnosis of thiamin deficiency is highly likely. This condition is considered a medical emergency because, if untreated, it can progress quickly and cause irreversible damage.

This patient's hematology lab data reveal that anemia is present, which may explain his fatigue. Anemia is diagnosed when the red blood cell count (RBC), hemoglobin, and hematocrit are below normal. An elevated mean corpuscular volume (MCV) indicates large red blood cells, characteristic of megaloblastic anemia. Megaloblastic anemia can be caused by either vitamin B_{12} or folate deficiency as previously explained. Folate deficiency alters DNA metabolism and diminishes the production of red blood cells, which normally multiply rapidly, by inhibiting pronormoblast (immature red blood cell) division and maturation rates.

5. **What does CT's serum albumin level indicate? (Take into account his PT of 15 seconds and the finding of ascites during his physical exam.)**

   CT's serum albumin value may reflect moderately depleted visceral protein stores. Depleted albumin, however, may not accurately reflect visceral protein status in patients with severe liver disease because albumin is synthesized in the liver and is also influenced by hydration status (remember CT's ascites). Usually, the liver retains its capacity to produce albumin until end-stage liver disease. The liver also synthesizes the vitamin K-dependent clotting factors, which explains CT's prolonged prothrombin time, since the liver's ability to produce factors II, VII, IX, and X can be affected early in liver disease.

6. **What additional laboratory tests would you request before giving this patient a folate supplement?**

   Serum and red blood cell folate and serum vitamin B_{12} levels should be checked. RBC folate is a good indicator of folate stores over the preceding two weeks. Serum folate levels are more responsive to the patient's recent folate intake and thus are not as reliable. If CT's megaloblastic anemia is due to vitamin B_{12} deficiency, prescribing folate without vitamin B_{12} will improve the anemia but mask the vitamin B_{12} deficiency and its progression. Left unchecked, the GI and neurological lesions caused by vitamin B_{12} deficiency may lead to irreversible, progressive neuropathy, permanent spinal column damage, or even death. Thus it is important to remember that neurological impairments do not respond to folate supplementation alone, whereas hematological abnormalities do respond both to folate and to vitamin B_{12}. CT's results from the recommended tests support the diagnosis of both vitamin B_{12} and folate deficiency.

CT's Values	Normal Values
Serum vitamin B₁₂: 72 pg/mL	>200 pg/mL
Serum folate: 2 ng/mL	>3.7 ng/mL
RBC folate: 120 ng/mL	>150 ng/mL

7. **What additional nutritional recommendations would you give CT?**

The most important recommendation for CT is to reduce or eliminate drinking alcohol. Alcoholics Anonymous, a hospital rehabilitation program, and family counseling to help him achieve this goal are all options that should be discussed.

Considering that CT's physical exam revealed ascites, his weight without fluid, or dry weight, is most likely close to his ideal weight of 154 lb. Because his usual weight is about the same as his ideal weight and his typical diet consists of three meals a day, he is not presently at risk for malnutrition. However, if CT's appetite does not return to normal and his intake decreases as a consequence, he may soon run this risk. Therefore CT should be encouraged to continue eating three meals a day consisting of a wide variety of foods.

Based on his lab data, CT should receive thiamin, folate, vitamin B_{12}, and multivitamin supplements, especially if he continues to drink alcohol. Thiamin, folate, and vitamin B_{12} may be given in pill form because alcoholics can absorb these nutrients if given large doses. Because alcohol decreases intrinsic factor production, vitamin B_{12} injections may also be needed in addition to the pill.

Case 2

Malabsorption

Gary R. Lichtenstein and Donna H. Mueller

Objectives

- To evaluate the clinical, anthropometric, and laboratory data of a patient with malabsorption.
- To explain how dietary factors affect a patient with malabsorption.
- To identify vitamin and mineral deficiencies associated with malabsorption syndrome and develop a nutritional care plan to treat these problems.

JR, a 27-year-old graduate student, sustained a gunshot wound to his abdomen five years ago and subsequently underwent resection of approximately 75 percent of his small intestine. Postoperatively he noted about five liquid bowel movements daily, described as oily and foul-smelling, which persist until the present time. After surgery he did not seek medical follow-up.

Past Medical History

JR's history is significant for a gunshot wound requiring intestinal resection of the ileum and most of the jejunum and anastomosis, or surgical connection, of the proximal jejunum to the cecum. JR takes no medications.

Social History

At the time of his surgery he was instructed to follow a high-calorie diet and to take a daily multivitamin and mineral supplement, but he self-discontinued this vitamin and mineral supplement one year ago. JR does not smoke cigarettes, but he reports drinking two beers per week and three cups of coffee daily. He states that he does not have the energy to exercise.

Diet History

At his physician's request, JR provided the following 24-hour dietary recall, which he states represents his "typical" intake.

JR's 24-Hour Dietary Recall

Breakfast (Diner)	Fried eggs with margarine	2 large
	Bacon	3 slices
	White toast with butter	2 slices (enriched), 2 Tbs.
	Coffee with sugar	2 cups, 4 packets
Snack (Food Truck)	Coffee with sugar	2 cups, 4 packets
	Jelly doughnut	1

Lunch (Fast-Food Restaurant)

	Cheeseburger	1
	French fries	2 small orders
	Soda (cola)	16 oz.
Dinner (Home)	Baked ham	8 oz.
	Baked potato with butter	1 medium, 2 Tbs.
	White bread with butter	2 slices (enriched), 2 Tsp.
	Apple pie	1/6 of 9" pie
	Coffee with sugar	1 cup, 2 packets
Snack (Home)	Corn chips	3 oz. bag
	Beer	12 oz.

Total calories: 4472 kcal/day
Protein: 12% of calories
Fat: 46% of calories
Carbohydrate: 42% of calories

Review of Systems

General: Weight loss, fatigue, and weakness

Skin: Dry and scaly

Eyes: Difficulty driving at night

GI: Five liquid bowel movements daily, described as oily and foul-smelling.

Appetite good, but patient complains that he must eat "twice as much food" as he did prior to his operation and that he still continues to lose weight.

Physical Exam

Vital signs

Temperature: 98.0°F

Heart rate: 80 BPM

Respiration: 16 BPM

Blood pressure: 94/60 mm Hg

Anthropometric data

Height: 5'10" (178 cm)

Current weight: 125 lb (57 kg)

Usual body weight: 165 lb (lost 40 pounds since surgery five years ago)

Ideal body weight: 166 lb (75 kg)

General: 27-year-old male who appears very thin and wears loose-fitting clothes

Skin: Flaky dermatitis, ecchymosis

Head: Temporal muscle wasting

Mouth: Glossitis, cheilosis

GI/Abdomen: Protuberant abdomen

Extremities: Skeletal pain, interosseous muscle wasting, subcutaneous fat wasting, skeletal muscle wasting

Laboratory Data

Patient's Lab Values   Normal Values

Patient's Lab Values	Normal Values
Albumin: 2.5 g/dL	3.5–5.8 g/dL
Calcium: 5.5 mg/dL	8.5–10.5 mg/dL
Vitamin B12: 100 pg/mL	>200 pg/mL
Vitamin A: 13 µg/dL	28–94 µg/dL
Vitamin E	
Alpha tocopherol: 3 mg/L	4.6–14.5 mg/L
Beta gamma tocopherol: 0.6 mg/L	1.4–4.8 mg/L
Prothrombin time: 16.0 seconds	0–15 seconds
Folate: 2.5 ng/mL	>3.7 ng/mL
Zinc: 300 µg/dL	550–1400 µg/dL
Magnesium: 1.2 mg/dL	1.8–2.9 mg/dL

Case Questions

1. Explain why JR continues to lose weight even though he eats so much.

2. What is the cause of JR's steatorrhea?

3. What are the causes and associated clinical signs or symptoms of each laboratory abnormality that JR presents?

4. Using JR's actual body weight, calculate the percentage change from his usual weight.

5. What conclusions can you draw regarding the fat, calorie, vitamin, and mineral content of JR's diet?

6. How does JR's present caloric intake compare to his requirements?

7. JR notes that his symptoms worsen when he eats fried or fatty foods. What should be done to correct these symptoms and his laboratory abnormalities?

8. When should JR be scheduled for a follow-up visit? What should follow-up entail in JR's case, and what information should be obtained during subsequent visits?

Answers begin on the following page.

Answers to Questions: Case 2

Part 1:   Diagnosis

1.   Explain why JR continues to lose weight even though he eats so much.

Profound weight loss may be a result of the fat malabsorption that often accompanies steatorrhea. Moreover, while luminal digestion of starch into oligosaccharidases and proteins into oligopeptides should be unaffected, decreased small bowel surface area interferes with brush border and cytoplasmic digestion, as well as transport across enterocytes. Transit time through the small intestine is decreased in patients who have undergone partial resection. Therefore reduced exposure of nutrients to the intestinal mucosa also interferes with optimal absorption.

2.   What is the cause of JR's steatorrhea?

JR does not have an ileum and thus is unable to absorb bile salts. Bile salts are essential for the absorption of fats and fat-soluble vitamins. Normally, bile salts are reabsorbed through the ileum, transported to the liver via the enterohepatic circulation, and recycled back to the intestinal lumen to meet the need for bile salts. Following ileal resection, bile salt loss through the stool increases because these salts are no longer being absorbed. The liver increases bile salt production in an attempt to compensate for the losses, but often fails to accommodate them. As a result, absorption of fat and fat-soluble vitamins A, D, E, and K decreases as the bile salt pool becomes depleted. Even in the face of greatly increased hepatic synthesis of bile salts, a deficiency of conjugated bile salts may result.

Bile salt deficiency leads to impairment in the body's ability to incorporate ingested dietary lipids into the micellar phase. This inability leads to decreased mucosal absorption of ingested lipids and fat-soluble vitamins and subsequent steatorrhea, a condition called cholerrheic enteropathy.

When dealing with patients who have undergone ileal resection, it is important to remember that although bile salt absorption occurs passively throughout the upper small intestine, active sodium-coupled uptake in the ileum normally is responsible for retrieval of over 95 percent of the intraluminal bile salts.

Part 2:   Laboratory Evaluation

Several laboratory abnormalities were observed in this patient. JR's nutritional problems reflect his decreased small bowel absorptive area, which renders him less able to absorb fat, protein, carbohydrate, vitamins, and minerals.

3. **What are the causes and associated clinical signs or symptoms of each laboratory abnormality that JR presents?**

Albumin   JR's value: 2.5 g/dL   Normal value: 3.5–5.8 g/dL

A serum albumin level of 2.1 to 2.7 g/dL is associated with a moderate degree of visceral protein depletion caused by decreased calorie and protein absorption.

Calcium   JR's value: 5.5 mg/dL   Normal value: 8.5–10.5 mg/dL

Most calcium absorption occurs in the duodenum, but all small intestinal segments absorb calcium. When adjustments are made for transit time and the relative lengths of the different intestinal segments, both the jejunum and ileum therefore contribute substantially to overall calcium absorption. JR's resection has substantially reduced the available absorptive surface area of the small intestine and thus accounts in part for his low calcium value.

A second cause for the low calcium level seen in this patient is the reduction in the size of the bile salt pool with impairment of micellar solubilization. This condition leads to decreased calcium absorption due to intraluminal binding of dietary calcium to unabsorbed fatty acids (soap formation). Third, vitamin D malabsorption and deficiency also lead to calcium malabsorption.

Because calcium is bound to albumin, it is always important to determine the corrected calcium based on the patient's albumin level to account for the ionization of calcium in serum which is determined by an equilibrium between calcium and protein. We use the following equation to determine the corrected calcium.

(Normal albumin – Patient's albumin) (Correction factor) + Patient's calcium

Correction factor = 0.8
Normal albumin = 4.0

Therefore, in JR's case

Corrected calcium = (4 – 2.5) (0.8) + 5.5 = 1.2 + 5.5 = 6.7 mg/dL

This calcium value of 6.7 mg/dL, corrected for JR's albumin level, still is not in the normal range of 8.5 to 10.5 mg/dL, and he also suffers from hypocalcemia, a low serum calcium level. Clinical manifestations of calcium deficiency include skeletal pain, tetany, paresthesia, osteoporosis, and stunted growth in children.

Dietary sources high in calcium and thus often recommended to such patients are milk, cheese, yogurt, and other related dairy products.

Vitamin B$_{12}$ JR's value: 100 pg/mL   Normal value: >200 pg/mL

After vitamin B$_{12}$ complexes with the binding protein intrinsic factor, which is produced in the stomach, it is absorbed in the terminal ileum. Patients who have undergone removal of the terminal ileum thus cannot absorb vitamin B$_{12}$ and require intramuscular injections of this nutrient to prevent long-term deficiency and associated peripheral neuropathy, which generally first becomes apparent after five to ten years.

Clinical manifestations of vitamin B12 deficiency include megaloblastic anemia, peripheral neuropathy, glossitis, and cheilosis.

The only dietary sources of vitamin B12 are foods of animal origin such as meat, chicken, fish, eggs, and dairy products.

Vitamin A   JR's value: 13 μg/dL   Normal value: 28–94 μg/dL

Vitamin A, in the form of dietary retinyl esters, is hydrolyzed to retinol by pancreatic and intestinal brush border esterases prior to uptake from the gut lumen. Absorption occurs in the proximal small intestine and is aided by the presence of bile salts. Another source of retinol is the vitamin precursor ß-carotene. After uptake and transport, vitamin A is stored in the liver.

Clinical manifestations of vitamin A deficiency include xerophthalmia (with clinical findings ranging from night blindness to corneal ulceration and irreversible blindness), poor wound healing, and loss of epithelial integrity (in the skin, GI tract, and urinary and respiratory systems). Dietary sources of vitamin A and ß-carotene among plants include dark green, leafy vegetables and deep yellow fruits. These nutrients also are found in meats, wheat and rice germ, nuts, and legumes.

Vitamin E   JR's alpha tocopherol value: 3.0
Normal value: 4.6–14.5 mg/L

JR's beta gamma tocopherol value: 0.6
Normal value: 1.4–4.8 mg/L

Vitamin E is absorbed passively in the proximal small intestine. Bile salts serve as an important factor in normal vitamin E absorption. Like other fat-soluble vitamins, vitamin E is packaged into chylomicrons and delivered into the mesenteric lymphatics. It is stored primarily in the liver and in the adipose tissue.

Clinical manifestations of vitamin E deficiency include neurological dysfunction in the form of cerebellar ataxia, loss of deep tendon reflexes, and diminished vibratory and position sense. Hemolytic anemia is another significant consequence of vitamin E deficiency.

Dietary sources of vitamin E are whole grains, vegetables, vegetable oils, and meats.

Vitamin K   JR's PT: 16.0 seconds   Normal PT: 0–15 seconds

Vitamin K is obtained from dietary sources and also produced by colonic flora. Absorption of vitamin K occurs primarily in the proximal small bowel and requires bile salts. Following intestinal absorption, vitamin K is taken up largely by the liver and accumulated in the microsomal fraction. In the liver, vitamin K is a required cofactor for the enzymatic gamma-carboxylation of glutamic acid on vitamin K-dependent coagulation proenzymes (factors II (prothrombin), VII, IX, and X) and other proteins involved in coagulation and fibrinolysis (proteins C, S, M, and Z).

Clinical manifestations of vitamin K deficiency include prolonged clotting time resulting in bleeding problems (oral, genitourinary, gastrointestinal, and skin). Patients on long-term antibiotics may eliminate bacterial production of vitamin K and therefore are particularly prone to clinical deficiency if they do not receive exogenous sources of vitamin K. Dietary sources of vitamin K are the green, leafy vegetables (spinach and kale), whole grains, liver, and nuts.

Folate   JR's value: 2.5 ng/mL   Normal value: >3.7 ng/mL

The jejunum absorbs folate for subsequent delivery into the portal circulation. Following intestinal resection, the remaining portions of the small intestine may increase their uptake of folate to compensate for poor absorption. Serum folate levels reflect very recent dietary ingestion rather than total body folate stores. Therefore, a normal serum folate test does not exclude folate deficiency. A better reflection of total body folate stores would be an erythrocyte folate level.

Clinical manifestations of folate deficiency include megaloblastic anemia, glossitis, cheilosis, heartburn, constipation, depression, and confusion.

Dietary sources of folate are dark green, leafy vegetables, oranges, orange juice, potatoes, yeast, red meat, eggs, and whole grains. Folate is easily destroyed in cooking or processing.

Zinc   JR's value: 300 μg/dL   Normal value: 550–1400 μg/dL

Zinc absorption occurs throughout the small intestine, but its rate of absorption is greater in the jejunum than in the ileum or duodenum. In patients who have undergone intestinal resection, transit time and surface area for absorption decrease, especially for zinc absorption. Intestinal reabsorption of zinc is impaired further in these patients because the jejunum and ileum have been removed.

Clinical manifestations of zinc deficiency include anorexia, hypogeusia, alopecia, delayed onset of puberty, dermatitis, and poor wound healing. Oysters, meats, nuts, and legumes all constitute excellent dietary sources of zinc.

Magnesium   JR's value: 1.2 mg/dL   Normal value: 1.8–2.9 mg/dL

Magnesium is absorbed primarily in the jejunum and ileum by a passive mechanism. In patients with steatorrhea, unabsorbed fatty acids inhibit Mg^{2+} absorption by forming insoluble complexes in a reaction called chelation. Magnesium absorption is reduced in patients who have undergone small intestinal resections because of the decreased surface area available for this process.

Clinical manifestations of Mg^{2+} deficiency include neuromuscular weakness, confusion, fatigue, tetany, paresthesias, and hypokalemia.

Dietary sources of magnesium include milk, cheese, yogurt, fruits, legumes, cereals, vegetables, fish, poultry, and meats.

Part 3:   Anthropometric and Clinical Assessment

4. Using JR's current body weight, calculate the percentage change from his usual weight.

$$\% \text{ Weight change} = \frac{\text{Usual weight} - \text{Current weight}}{\text{Usual weight}} \times 100$$

$$= \frac{165 \text{ lb} - 125 \text{ lb}}{165 \text{ lb}} \times 100 = 24\%$$

A value of this magnitude indicates a clinically significant weight loss.

5. What conclusions can you draw regarding the fat, calorie, vitamin, and mineral content of JR's diet?

According to JR's 24-hour dietary recall, his diet is high in fatty and salty foods and sweets. JR's diet lacks foods from three major food groups: fruits, vegetables, and dairy products. The fact that he rarely selects foods from these groups places him at high risk for vitamin and mineral deficiencies, compounded by malabsorption of several vitamins and minerals.

6. How does JR's present caloric intake compare to his caloric requirements?

Using 35 kcal/kg Ideal Body Weight (35 kcal/kg × 75.5 kg I Bw) JR should consume 2650 kcal/day to meet his caloric requirements. However, according to JR's actual intake, he is consuming 4472 kcal. Normally, weight gain can be expected even when excess intake amounts only to a few hundred calories, but JR's significant malabsorption problem has resulted in weight loss instead.

Part 4:   Treatment

7. JR notes that his symptoms worsen when he eats fried or fatty foods. What should be done to correct these symptoms and his laboratory abnormalities?

JR is experiencing malabsorption secondary to his surgery. Prone to fat malabsorption because his ileum was resected, JR cannot reabsorb the bile acids required for fat digestion. Thus his dietary fat intake, at 46 percent of total calories, far exceeds his ability to digest and absorb fat properly. Referral to a registered dietitian for individualized counseling and reinforcement of the following suggestions is highly recommended in JR's case.

Low-fat foods should be substituted for fried and fast foods. However, because JR may find gaining weight difficult if his diet is too low in fat, monitoring his weight carefully is important. Note, too, that not all patients with malabsorption require a low-fat diet.

JR should consume a wide variety of foods, including fruits, vegetables, and enriched or whole grains, to obtain adequate nutrients. Because many patients with malabsorption due to intestinal resection tend to be lactose-intolerant as a consequence of their reduced levels of lactase enzyme, a lactose-free diet may be beneficial.

Consider supplementation with oral, medium-chain triglycerides (MCTs). MCTs are triglycerides with fatty acyl groups of 8 to 12 carbon chain lengths. Their luminal and intracellular metabolism differs in several respects from that of LCTs, and MCT absorption does not require bile salts. MCTs may be more efficiently absorbed than long-chain triglycerides (LCTs) by patients with short bowel syndrome and bile salt depletion. However, in some individuals, MCT oil can cause osmotic diarrhea.

Vitamin and mineral supplementation is indicated, since his surgery has significantly increased his intestinal motility and decreased transit time and the available absorptive area for the vitamins and minerals described previously. In addition, as a result of bile salt depletion, his absorption of fat and fat-soluble vitamins A, D, E, and K also has decreased.

8. **When should JR be scheduled for a follow-up visit? What should follow-up entail in JR's case, and what information should be obtained during subsequent visits?**

Schedule an appointment for JR immediately with a registered dietitian to implement the preceding suggestions. Repeat a 24-hour dietary recall at the follow-up visit to ensure that the dietary goals are being met. Have JR record abdominal symptoms and visually check his stools daily. JR needs to gain weight because currently he is only at 75 percent of his ideal body weight. His weight therefore should be monitored weekly. Retest JR's blood levels of calcium and magnesium after intravenous repletion. Recheck JR's PT after vitamin K supplementation. Also recheck his albumin, vitamin B$_{12}$, and folate in one month.

AIDS with Esophagitis and Diarrhea

Rob Roy MacGregor, Lisa Hark, and Mary Langan

Objectives

- To assess the nutritional status of a patient with late-stage AIDS.
- To understand nutritional consequences of AIDS such as weight loss, anorexia, and odynophagia.
- To determine appropriate nutritional recommendations for patients with esophagitis and diarrhea secondary to AIDS.
- To understand the indications for nutritional support for patients with AIDS.

TF, a 30-year-old man diagnosed with AIDS one year ago was admitted to the hospital complaining of severe odynophagia (pain on swallowing) for the previous eight weeks due to esophagitis secondary to thrush (mucosal candida infection). He also has thrush of the oropharynx. He reports pain and a feeling that food is stuck in his chest when he swallows and mentions that the odynophagia worsens when he eats spicy or rough foods. TF also reports having had a fair appetite and stable weight until eight weeks ago, but states that now he is only able to tolerate gelatin, soup, and juice. He has lost 21 pounds during this eight-week period and complains of feeling lightheaded and weak.

Past Medical History

TF reports having had a previous bout of esophageal candidiasis one year ago. His current medication regime includes fluconazole, rifabutin, AZT, and cotrimoxazole. Presently, he takes no vitamin supplements.

Social History

TF was married 10 years ago, but is now divorced. An avowed homosexual whose main supports are his sister and brother, he formerly worked as a painter until recently, when he became too weak to continue.

Alcohol intake: None

Tobacco: None

IV drug abuse: None

Broth, apple juice, and gelatin: 500 kcal/day

5% dextrose in normal saline IV at 85 mL/hour which provides 350 kcal/day

Total daily caloric intake: 850 kcal/day

Review of Systems

General: Poor appetite, weakness, fatigue, and weight loss (21 lb in 8 weeks)

Mouth: Oral lesions consistent with thrush (candidiasis of the oral mucosa, with formation of raised, whitish spots overlying shallow ulcers)

GI: No diarrhea, nausea, or vomiting

Neurological: No sensory loss

Musculoskeletal: No muscle pain

Physical Examination

Vital signs

Temperature: 98.6 °F

Heart rate: 84 BPM

Respiration: 12 BPM

Blood pressure: 107/70 mm Hg

Anthropometric data

Height: 5'10"

Current weight: 119 lb (54 kg)

Usual weight: 140 lb (64 kg)

Ideal weight: 166 lb (75 kg)

Triceps skinfold (TSF): 6.0 mm (10th percentile)

Mid-arm muscle circumference (MAMC): 250 mm (10th percentile)

General: Cachectic man resting comfortably

Skin: Cold and extremely dry, especially on scalp and feet

Head/Neck: Bitemporal wasting, dry, thinning hair, sclera anicteric

Mouth: All teeth present, good dentition; several raised white oral lesions visible (thrush)

Cardiac: Regular rate and rhythm

Abdomen: Soft, nontender, bowel sounds present, no hepatosplenomegaly

Extremities: Muscle wasting in upper and lower extremities, no edema

Neurological: Cranial nerves II–XII intact, sensorium intact throughout

Laboratory Data

Patient's Lab Values	Normal Values
CD4 count: 50 µL blood	600–1800 µL blood
Albumin: 2.3 g/dL	3.5–5.8 g/dL
Hemoglobin: 10.0 g/dL	13.5–17.5 g/dL
Hematocrit: 31%	39–49%
ALT: 22 IU/L	0–35 IU/L
AST: 22 IU/L	0–35 IU/L
PT: 11 seconds	0–15 seconds
PTT: 30 seconds	25–35 seconds

Follow-up

TF returns to his physician six months later complaining of diarrhea, which has persisted for two weeks. He reports that after treatment of his esophagitis his weight increased from 119 pounds to 125 pounds, in large measure because of liquid nutritional supplements and a high-protein, high-calorie diet. However, over the past two months his appetite has decreased, and his weight has declined again to 117 pounds. During the past two weeks, his weight has decreased even further, to 112 pounds. TF attributes his weight loss to his diarrhea and decreased appetite.

Case Questions

1. Using TF's current weight, calculate his percent ideal body weight (IBW) and his percent weight change. What do these values imply with regard to TF's nutritional status?

2. What factors are contributing to TF's weight loss?

3. Using the evidence from TF's medical history, anthropometric data, and lab data, evaluate his nutritional status.

4. Based on TF's current weight and odynophagia, what would you advise him with regard to an oral diet?

5. Is a vitamin and mineral supplement indicated for TF?

6. What are the causes of diarrhea in patients diagnosed with AIDS?

7. Are large amounts of fluid lost because of diarrhea? How can the amounts be assessed?

8. Considering TF's current weight of 112 lb (51 kg), which is 68 percent of his ideal body weight, is enteral or parenteral nutrition support indicated at this time?

Answers begin on the following page.

Answers to Questions: Case 3

Part I: Nutrition Assessment

1. **Using TF's current weight, calculate his percent ideal body weight (IBW) and his percent weight change. What do these values imply with regard to TF's nutritional status?**

$$\% \text{ IBW} = \frac{\text{Current weight}}{\text{Ideal weight}} \times 100$$

$$= \frac{119 \text{ lb}}{166 \text{ lb}} \times 100 = 72\%$$

This value indicates moderate malnutrition.

$$\% \text{ Weight change} = \frac{\text{Usual weight} - \text{Current weight}}{\text{Usual weight}} \times 100$$

$$= \frac{140 \text{ lb} - 119 \text{ lb}}{140 \text{ lb}} \times 100 = 15\% \text{ weight change}$$

Note in the preceding equation that the value used for the usual weight was 140 lb, the weight TF reported from 8 weeks ago. Thus TF's weight loss during that period represents a 15% change. Any change greater than 7.5 percent over three months is considered a severe weight loss, sufficient to place TF at risk for malnutrition

2. **What factors are contributing to TF's weight loss?**

    TF has significantly reduced his intake because of severe pain when swallowing (odynophagia) due to esophagitis, secondary to esophageal candidiasis. TF's chronic fatigue contributes to decreased ability to perform activities of daily living (ADLs), including shopping for food and preparing meals. This patient also has the poor appetite characteristic of late-stage AIDS. Although the etiology of this anorexia is unclear, it probably is multifactorial, involving high levels of tumor necrosis factor (TNF) and other catabolic mediators of inflammation, medication side effects, and depression. As a result, he has only been able of late to consume 500 kcal/day, significantly less than his requirements, and he is in negative calorie balance. In addition, he may be hypermetabolic due to his HIV status and esophageal candidiasis. Therefore, his caloric requirements may be elevated over the baseline requirements, further contributing to his weight loss.

3. **Using the evidence from TF's medical history, anthropometric data, and lab data, evaluate his nutritional status.**

    In light of his severe weight loss (a 15-percent change in 8 weeks) and the fact that he is only at 72 percent of ideal body weight, TF is considered moderately malnourished in terms of energy and calories. His TSF and MAMC are currently at the 10th percentile, indicating that his fat and muscle stores are severely depleted. TF's albumin reflects moderately depleted visceral protein stores. From these values, TF can be diagnosed with protein-energy malnutrition (PEM). TF's nutritional status is deteriorating quickly, and early intervention should be instituted to help prevent further weight loss and visceral protein depletion.

Part 2:   Recommendations

4. **Based on TF's current weight and odynophagia, what would you advise him with regard to an oral diet?**

TF should be advised to consume a high-protein, high-calorie diet. A registered dietitian can recommend and help calculate the amount of supplementation necessary to meet his estimated nutritional needs. During this period, drinking liquid supplements such as milk shakes, Carnation Instant Breakfast, and nutritional supplements through a straw to bypass any painful oral lesions may help. If milk products increase mucous production in the throat, drinking a glass of water after milk to rinse the throat may prove helpful. Milk, an excellent protein source, can be fortified with powdered skim milk or powdered protein amino acid supplements to maximize nutrient intake. Polycose also can be added to juices or shakes to increase calorie intake. Raw eggs, meats, and unprocessed dairy products should be avoided because opportunistic infections can occur from eating these raw foods.

After TF's esophagitis improves, he can return to soft foods, and eventually solids. Examples of soft, high-protein foods include omelets, yogurt, cottage cheese, ground chicken, ground beef, tuna, and other fish. TF also can try eating baby foods and homemade, mashed, and blended foods, which are all less irritating to the oral mucosa. Using butter, gravies, and sauces will add calories and make food easier to swallow. Acidic and spicy foods may be painful to swallow; bland foods served cold or at room temperature are therefore recommended. Rough, fibrous foods such as raw vegetables, fruits, and hard crackers should be limited, as they may irritate the mucosa and cause pain. Lidocaine, a local anesthetic, can be used prior to eating to reduce pain on swallowing.

5. **Is a vitamin and mineral supplement indicated for TF?**

Assessing a patient's diet history before recommending supplements is essential. TF is not meeting all of his vitamin and mineral needs because his intake is poor, and a vitamin and mineral supplement will help him to do so. A vitamin C supplement may also be required, because TF's esophagitis causes him to avoid citrus fruits and vegetables. Many studies report decreased serum levels of vitamins B_6, B_{12}, A, E, and zinc in patients with AIDS.

Part 3:   Follow-up

6.   **What are the causes of diarrhea in patients diagnosed with AIDS?**

The specific etiology of most cases of HIV-associated diarrhea is unknown. However, especially because of the frequent finding of low CD4 counts, diarrhea may result from a multitude of infections in patients with AIDS. Some of the causes of diarrhea in AIDS patients are:

Protozoal diseases: Cryptosporidiosis, coccidiosis, microsporidiosis, *giardiasis*, amebiasis, leishmaniasis, *Blastocystis hominis* infection

Viral disorders: Cytomegalovirus, herpes simplex virus, adenovirus, and perhaps HIV itself

Intestinal neoplasms: Lymphoma, Kaposi's sarcoma

Bacterial infections: Shigellosis, salmonellosis, campylobacteriosis, *Clostridium difficile* colitis, small bowel bacterial overgrowth

Other infections: Tuberculosis, *Mycobacterium avium* complex infection, histoplasmosis, coccidiomycosis

Pancreatic insufficiency: Secondary to cytomegalovirus, *Mycobacterium avium* complex

After evaluating stool specimens for bacterial enteric pathogens, ova, parasites, and acid-fast bacilli, consider flexible sigmoidoscopy to obtain both a biopsy and a tissue culture for viruses and protozoa. If the results are unremarkable, then consider esophagogastroduodenoscopy, with aspiration of small bowel secretions and biopsy to search for pathogens.

7.   **Are large amounts of fluid lost because of diarrhea? How can the amounts be assessed?**

The amount of diarrhea can be quantified by a 24- to 72-hour stool collection. A normal stool weight is less than 200 grams per day. To assess fluid losses, determine whether axillary sweat is decreased, assess skin turgor, look for dry mucous membranes, verify whether eyeballs are "sunken," and check for orthostasis, decreased urine output, hypernatremia, and elevated BUN to creatinine ratio.

8.   **Considering TF's current weight of 112 lb (51 kg), which is 68 percent of his ideal body weight, is enteral or parenteral nutrition support indicated at this time?**

This is a controversial decision. Most HIV experts do not recommend enteral or parenteral nutrition support in AIDS patients except for brief applications at times of acute weight loss secondary to a specific cause, such as GI surgery, esophagitis, pneumonia, or pancreatitis. Not only is nutrition support expensive, it also can lead to metabolic, infectious, and mechanical complications. Furthermore, the use of enteral or parenteral nutrition support has not been shown to improve the clinical outcome of AIDS patients.

See Tables 7-1 and 7-2 for more information about the nutritional consequences of HIV and its medications.

Table 7-1   Manifestations of HIV infection with nutritional implications.

	BODY SITE AFFECTED	MANIFESTATION
Malignancies		
Kaposi's Sarcoma (KS)	50% of patients with KS lesions of the skin may have involvement of the GI tract, including hard and soft palate	Odynophagia, dysphagia, abdominal pain, obstruction, nausea, vomiting, bleeding, rarely diarrhea
Non-Hodgkins lymphoma and Burkitt's lymphoma	GI tract	Nausea, vomiting, dysphagia, hematemesis, lower GI tract bleeding, obstruction, abdominal pain, diarrhea
Fungi		
Candida albicans	Oral and esophageal involvement with dense plaques of exudate	Dysgeusia, dysphagia, decreased salivation, burning, odynophagia, nausea, and upper GI bleeding
Cryptococcus neoformans	Meningitis	Fever, nausea, vomiting, dementia
Histoplasma capsulatum	Lung, bone marrow, liver, spleen, ulcerated lesions of oropharynx	Fever, weight loss, dysphagia
Viruses		
Herpes simplex virus (HSV)	Lesions of oral cavity, esophagus, anorectal area	Odynophagia, dysphagia, esophagitis, proctitis, local pain, constipation
Cytomegalovirus (CMV)	Identified in 90% of patients with AIDS at autopsy. Ulcerative lesions may appear in entire GI tract especially esophagus, stomach, small intestine, colon, biliary tract	Esophagitis, retrosternal pain, gastritis, enteritis, colitis, proctitis, watery or bloody diarrhea, biliary disease, perforations of afffected organ
Epstein-Barr virus (EBV)	Tongue	Oral hairy leukoplakia
Human immunodeficiency virus (HIV)	Low-grade small bowel atrophy; also found in gastric mucosa	May contribute to diarrhea, malabsorption, gastritis
Protozoa		
Cryptosporidium spp	Entire GI tract, especially microvilli of small intestine and biliary tract	Profuse, watery diarrhea, malabsorption, steatorrhea, lactose intolerance, abdominal pain, cholecystitis, pancreatitis, nausea, vomiting, dehydration, malnutrition, low electrolytes
Isospora belli	Microvilli of small intestine	Often indistingishable from *Cryptosporidium spp.* Symptoms may include diarrhea, steatorrhea, abdominal pain, anorexia, vomiting, fever
Microsporidia	Small intestine	Diarrhea, malabsorption
Giardia lamblia	Small intestine	Nausea, bloating, abdominal cramping, diarrhea, fever, malaise, weight loss, increased flatus
Entamoeba histolytica	Large intestine	Diarrhea, proctocolitis
Pneumocystis carinii pneumonia	Lungs, may be disseminated	Dypsnea, fever, coughing, weight loss
Toxoplasma gondii	Encephalitis	Fever, dementia
Bacteria		
Mycobacterium avium intracellulare (MAI)	Intestine, liver, spleen, lymph nodes, bone marrow	Fever, weight loss, cachexia, malaise, diarrhea, malabsorption, steatorrhea
Salmonellae	Large intestine	Diarrhea, abdominal pain, fever, high propensity for recurrence

Table 7-1 continued

Shigellae	Large intestine	Abdominal pain (cramping), tenesmus, fever, bloody diarrhea, bacteremia, high propensity for recurrence
Campylobacter jejuni	Large and small intestine	Abdominal pain, fever, bloody diarrhea
Oral manifestations		
Periodontal disease, gingivitis	Gingival erythema resulting in spontaneous bleeding, rapid loss of periodontal attachment and bone	Severe mouth pain, tooth loss, halitosis

Source: Nutrition Management of HIV Infection and AIDS in Manual of Clinical Dietetics, 4th edition, American Dietetic. Association 1992.

Table 7-2   Nutrition-related side effects of commonly prescribed medications in HIV infections and AIDS.

MEDICATION	CONDITION TREATED	NUTRITIONAL SIDE EFFECTS
Acyclovir	HSV, herpes zoster virus	Nausea, vomiting, altered taste
Alpha interferon	Kaposi's sarcoma	Nausea, vomiting, anorexia
Amphotericin B	Cryptococcosis, disseminated candidiasis	Hypokalemia, renal failure, severe nausea and vomiting, anemia
Clotrimazole	Candidiasis	Abdominal cramping and pain, nausea, vomiting, diarrhea
Fluconazole	Cryptococcus	Nausea, abdominal pain
Ganciclovir	CMV	Elevated liver enzymes, nausea, anorexia
Ketoconazole	Candidiasis	Hepatitis, nausea, vomiting, diarrhea
Megestrol acetate	Cachexia	Increased appetite; no nutritional side effects
Nystatin	Candidiasis	Hepatitis, nausea, abdominal pain
Octreotide	HIV-related diarrhea	No nutritional side effects noted
Pentamidine	*Pneumocystis carinii* pneumonia	Hypotension, nausea, vomiting, abnormal liver function tests, hypoglycemia and hyperglycemia (pancreatitis)
Phosphonoformate	HIV infection, CMV, acyclovir-resistant HSV	Increased thirst, nausea, anorexia, increased serum creatinine
Pyrimethamine	Toxoplasmosis	Folic acid malabsorption necessitating folinic acid supplement
Sulfadiazine	Toxoplasmosis	Skin rash and itching, dysphagia, anorexia, nausea, vomiting
Trimethoprim and sulfamethoxazole	PCP	Same as sulfadiazine
Zidovudine	HIV infection	Altered taste, nausea, anemia

Source: Nutrition Management of HIV Infection and AIDS in Manual of Clinical Dietetics, 4th edition, American Dietetic Association, 1992.

See Chapter Review Questions, pages A12–A14.

REFERENCES

Estruch R, Nicolas JM, Villegas E, et al. Relationship between ethanol-related diseases and nutritional status in chronically alcoholic men. *Alcohol and Alcoholism,* 1993;28(5):543–550.

French SW. Nutrition in the pathogenesis of alcoholic liver disease. *Alcohol and Alcoholism* 1993;28(1):97–109.

Gallagher LK, Shaffer AT, Aaronson SM (eds.). Nutritional Management in Inflammatory Bowel Disease. In *Thomas Jefferson University Hospital Nutrition Manual.* Gaithersburg, MD: Aspen, 1993.

Klesges RC, Mealer CZ, Klesges LM. Effects of alcohol intake on resting energy expenditure in young women social drinking. *Am J Clin Nutr* 1994;59(4): 805–809.

Leibel RL, Dufour M, Hubbard VS, et al. Alcohol and calories: a matter of balance. *Alcohol* 1993;10(6):427–434.

Lieber CS. Alcohol, liver and nutrition. *J Amer College of Nutrition* 1991;10(6): 602–632.

Lieber CS. Mechanisms of ethanol-drug-nutrition interactions. *J Toxicology-Clinical Toxicology* 1994,32(6):631–681.

Manual of Clinical Dietetics. 4th ed. Chicago: The American Dietetic Association, 1992.

Marsano L, McClain CJ. Nutrition and alcoholic liver disease. *J Parent Ent Nutr* 1991;15:337–344.

Meyer JH. The Stomach and Nutrition. In Shils ME, Olson JA, Shike M (eds.), *Modern Nutrition in Health and Disease.* 8th ed. Philadelphia: Lea and Febiger, 1994:1003–1035.

Rosenberg IH, Mason JB. Inflammatory Bowel Disease. In Shils ME, Olson JA, Shike M (eds.), *Modern Nutrition in Health and Disease.* 8th ed. Philadelphia: Lea and Febiger, 1994:1043–1049.

Zeman FJ. *Clinical Nutrition and Dietetics.* 2nd ed. New York: Macmillan, 1991.

Zeman FJ, Ney DM. Liver Disease and Alcoholism. In *Application of Clinical Nutrition.* Englewood Cliffs, NJ: Prentice Hall, 1988:312–317.

8

Endocrine Disease

Seth Braunstein and Frances Burke

Objectives

- To incorporate nutrition into the history, review of systems, and physical examination of individuals with diabetes mellitus.

- To identify the goals of nutritional management for individuals with diabetes mellitus.

- To differentiate individuals with insulin-dependent diabetes mellitus (IDDM) and non-insulin-dependent diabetes mellitus (NIDDM) when establishing strategies for achieving nutritional goals.

- To understand the advantages of high-carbohydrate diets for individuals with diabetes mellitus.

- To recommend appropriate amounts and types of dietary fat for individuals with diabetes mellitus.

- To identify the effects of alcohol on individuals with diabetes mellitus and provide appropriate recommendations.

Nutrition therapy is an essential component in the management of both insulin-dependent diabetes mellitus (IDDM) and non-insulin-dependent diabetes mellitus (NIDDM). The goals of nutrition therapy are to assist people with diabetes in making lifestyle changes, especially in the areas of diet and exercise, to normalize blood glucose, and to improve lipid levels. Nutritional recommendations are individualized to meet the person's physiological and psychological needs and should be flexible enough to allow a relatively normal lifestyle. Individualizing the meal plan requires conducting a thorough nutrition assessment and obtaining a detailed social history. The information elicited should include food preferences, cooking facilities, alcohol consumption, physical activity, and daily employment or school schedules. Ongoing blood glucose monitoring is necessary to evaluate blood glucose levels.

Insulin-Dependent Diabetes Mellitus (IDDM)

Strategies for Achieving Nutritional Goals

Timing of Meals and Snacks

Individuals with IDDM (type I) must be precise in balancing food intake with exogenous insulin and activity. Ideally, since insulin is injected at approximately the same times each day, meals also should be eaten at regular times for optimal glycemic control. The source, action, and concentration of the prescribed insulin will determine its onset, peak, and duration of action. Animal insulins from the pancreas of cows and pigs are absorbed at different rates than human insulin, which is synthetic (Tables 8-1 and 8-2). The various types of insulins also differ in their actions, which may be short (regular), intermediate (NPH and Lente), and long-acting (Ultralente). Often, different types of insulin are used in combination to achieve the desired glucose-lowering effect. The choice of insulin and the way it is prescribed should be tailored to meet the individual's target glucose goals, eating pattern, and ability to adhere to a particular regimen. Individual instruction on its use should include planning meals and snacks to cover the peak periods of an insulin dose and eating 15 to 30 minutes after insulin administration to allow for the insulin's absorption and prevent hypoglycemia.

Table 8-1 Pharmacology of animal insulin.

TYPE	ONSET (h)	PEAK (h)	USUAL EFFECTIVE DURATION (h)
Regular	0.5–2	3–4	4–6
Intermediate-acting (NPH and Lente)	4–6	8–14	16–20
Long-acting (Ultralente)	8–14	Minimal	24–36

Source: American Diabetes Association. *Maximizing the Role of Nutrition in Diabetes Management*. Alexandria, Va: American Diabetes Association, Inc., 1994.

Table 8-2   Pharmacology of human insulin.

TYPE	ONSET (h)	PEAK (h)	USUAL EFFECTIVE DURATION (h)
Regular	0.5–1	2–3	3–6
Intermediate-acting (NPH and Lente)	2–4	4–12	10–18
Long-acting (Ultralente)	6–10	?	18–20

Source: American Diabetes Association. *Maximizing the Role of Nutrition in Diabetes Management.* Alexandria, Va: American Diabetes Association, Inc., 1994.

Consistency of Diet

Individuals wih IDDM must be consistent with regard to the amounts and nutrient content of the foods they consume. Once an insulin dose that provides optimum blood glucose levels is established, the calorie and carbohydrate content of meals should be consistent from day to day to avoid large fluctuations in blood glucose. Consistency also aids in regulating total caloric intake. Ideally, individuals can be taught to adjust their insulin doses to changes in food intake or blood glucose levels. However, doing so may be difficult and even dangerous for some people.

Monitoring Blood Glucose Levels

Regular self-monitoring of blood glucose levels, periodic evaluation of glycosylated hemoglobin, and determination of fructosamine levels are three methods used to monitor the effectiveness of treatment for diabetes.

Exercise

Most people with IDDM can benefit from regular exercise because it improves overall fitness, flexibility, endurance, and muscle strength while helping to preserve lean body mass. Metabolically, for individuals with type I diabetes whose blood gucose is well controlled, exercise contributes to a reduction in blood glucose levels by decreasing hepatic glucose output and increasing peripheral utilization of glucose (Table 8-3). Although individuals with IDDM respond differently to exercise, certain general guidelines are necessary to ensure their safety. Many factors, including the individual's level of physical fitness, the duration and type of exercise, and the timing of exercise in relation to meals or insulin administration, can affect blood glucose levels. Thus, self-monitoring of blood glucose levels, both before and after exercise, is advisable to determine the need for additional food and/or insulin adjustments to prevent hypoglycemia. In general, to avoid postexercise hypoglycemia, 10 to 15 grams of carbohydrate (1 slice of bread or a fresh orange) must be ingested for every hour of exercise performed.

Table 8-3 Metabolic effects of exercise in type I diabetes mellitus.

INSULIN	HEPATIC GLUCOSE OUTPUT	PERIPHERAL GLUCOSE USE	COUNTER-REGULATORY HORMONES		BLOOD GLUCOSE
Adequate	↓	↑	↓	→	↓
Inadequate	↑	↓	↑	→	↑

Source: American Diabetes Association. *Maximizing the Role of Nutrition in Diabetes Management.* Alexandria, Va: American Diabetes Association, Inc., 1994.

Individuals with poorly controlled IDDM, evidenced by blood glucose levels greater than 250 mg/dL and urinary ketones, can have a negative response to exercise. In the presence of insulin deficiency, hepatic glucose output is increased and peripheral use of glucose is decreased. This results in a further increase in blood glucose levels and ketone bodies.

Preventing Hypoglycemia

Hypoglycemia requires immediate treatment with some form of glucose, preferably Glucotabs, because they provide a consistent amount of readily available glucose. Individuals should check their blood glucose level before consuming any food or beverage because relying on symptoms alone can lead to overtreatment, and over time, excess calories may result in weight gain and increased blood glucose levels.

Non-Insulin-Dependent Diabetes Mellitus (NIDDM)

Strategies for Achieving Nutritional Goals

Weight Loss

Approximately 80 percent of individuals with NIDDM (type II) are overweight. Moderate weight loss (10 to 20 pounds), regardless of starting weight, has been shown to reduce hyperglycemia, hyperlipidemia, and hypertension among this group of individuals. However, if metabolic parameters do not improve with moderate weight loss, these individuals may need oral hypoglycemic agents (OHA) or insulin.

Spacing of Meals

Research suggests that dividing total food intake into smaller meals and snacks spread throughout the day may be the best way to achieve optimal glucose control and avoid variation in blood glucose levels. However, some experts recommend eating only three meals a day at four- to five-hour intervals and avoiding snacks to limit total calorie intake. Long-term comparison studies are needed to determine the ideal spacing of food intake.

Exercise

Regular, aerobic exercise (a minimum of 20 minutes, 3 to 5 times a week) is especially beneficial for individuals with type II diabetes because exercise improves insulin sensitivity which results in the increased peripheral utilization of glucose and helps to control weight (Figure 8-1). Exercise also reduces cardiovascular risk by lowering both blood lipid values and blood pressure in persons with mild to moderate hypertension. Because persons with type II diabetes are not prone to ketosis, having enough insulin "on board" to cover blood glucose reduction attributable to exercise is not as great a concern as it is in individuals with type I diabetes. However, persons with type II diabetes who take an oral hypoglycemic agent should be made aware of the possibility of postexercise hypoglycemia.

Nutrition Therapy for People with Diabetes

Dietary Intake Recommendations

The American Diabetes Association (ADA) recently published its revised nutritional guidelines, "Nutrition Recommendations and Principles for People with Diabetes Mellitus." These ADA guidelines follow the USDA's "Food Guide Pyramid and Dietary Guidelines."

Figure 8-1   Metabolic effects of exercise in type II diabetes mellitus

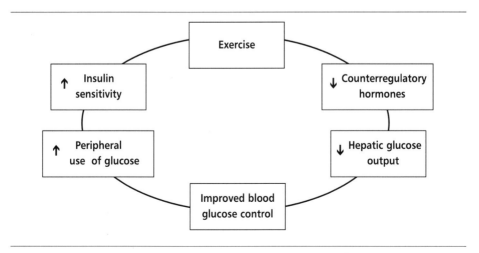

Source: American Diabetes Association. *Maximizing the Role of Nutrition in Diabetes Management.* Alexandria, Va: American Diabetes Association, Inc., 1994.

Calories

Adult calorie requirements vary according to activity level, age, and desired weight change. Calorie levels for children and adolescents must be adequate to support normal growth and development.

Fat

The recommended percentage of calories from fat depends on the individual's blood glucose and lipid levels and weight goals. For people with normal lipid levels and a reasonable body weight, fat intake of 30 percent or less of total calories, with under 10 percent of total calories from saturated fat, is appropriate. When weight loss is of primary concern, a reduction in total dietary fat and a controlled calorie intake will help to achieve this goal.

Reducing saturated fat and cholesterol intake also helps to reduce the strong risk of cardiovascular disease that diabetes poses. Diabetic individuals with lipid abnormalities respond well to nutrition therapy. Those with elevated LDL-cholesterol should be advised to follow the Step II guidelines developed by the National Cholesterol Education Program. For individuals with NIDDM, who commonly present with elevated triglyceride and very-low-density lipoprotein cholesterol levels, increasing intake of monounsaturated fat over other sources of fat may be beneficial. Monounsaturated fats can be increased to 20 percent of total calories, while limiting the intake of saturated and polyunsaturated fats to less than 10 percent each. Reducing total carbohydrate intake is also advised. Sources of monounsaturated fat include olives, peanuts, olive and canola oils, avocados, almonds, pistachio nuts, and pecans. In persons with triglyceride levels greater than 1000 mg/dL, limiting all types of dietary fat is advisable to reduce levels of plasma dietary fat in the form of chylomicrons.

Carbohydrate

Historically, low-carbohydrate, high-fat diets were prescribed for type II diabetics to prevent elevated postprandial blood glucose, poor glycemic control, and increased fasting serum triglycerides. Now, however, total fat intake, especially saturated fat, is limited in the diabetic diet, primarily to reduce the risk of cardiovascular disease. Current recommendations liberalize the carbohydrate content of the diabetic diet to as much as 55 to 60 percent of total calories. The amount of carbohydrate should be individualized however, depending on its impact on blood glucose and lipid levels.

For individuals with normal triglycerides, the advantages of high-carbohydrate diets outweigh the disadvantages. Individuals are more sensitive to insulin when they consume high-carbohydrate rather than high-fat diets, because they have increased numbers of insulin receptors. High-carbohydrate diets also enhance intracellular glucose metabolism and increase the rates of glycogen synthesis and glycolysis in the liver and skeletal muscle.

Carbohydrates in foods have traditionally been labeled as either simple (sugars) or complex (starches). Experts generally have believed that simple sugars are more rapidly absorbed into the blood, causing a greater elevation in blood glucose and an increased need for insulin than their complex counterparts. However, recent studies indicate that sucrose and other simple sugars do not have a more negative effect on blood glucose levels than do starches and that they are absorbed in a similar manner. According to the American Diabetes Association, sucrose can be eaten as part of the total amount of carbohydrate in the meal plan. It is important to keep in mind that the total amounts of food and carbohydrate consumed have a greater effect on blood glucose levels than the source of the carbohydrate.

Protein

Currently, the ideal percentage of total calories that should come from protein is undetermined for individuals with diabetes mellitus. Insufficient evidence exists to recommend a protein intake either higher or lower than the RDA for the general population. Therefore, the guidelines advise a protein intake of 12 to 20 percent of total calories. Limiting dietary protein intake may be effective in slowing the progression of renal disease in individuals with type I diabetes who present with diabetic nephropathy and macroalbuminuria. Therefore, a moderate dietary restriction of 0.6 to 0.8 grams of protein per kilogram of body weight daily is recommended.

Fiber

Although certain types of soluble fiber (guar and oat gums) may delay the absorption of glucose from the small intestine, the effect of dietary fiber on glycemic control probably is not significant. Therefore the recommended fiber intake for individuals with diabetes mellitus is the same as for the general population: daily consumption of 20 to 35 grams of dietary fiber from a wide variety of food sources such as fruits, vegetables, legumes, and grains.

Non-Nutritive Sweeteners

Non-nutritive sweeteners currently approved by the Food and Drug Administration include saccharin, aspartame, and acesulfame K. These sweeteners are considered safe and are used extensively by people with diabetes mellitus to satisfy their taste for sweets without affecting blood sugar control. Often referred to as alternative sweeteners, they are many times sweeter than ordinary table sugar.

Saccharin, 300 times sweeter than table sugar and heat-stable, is not metabolized in the digestive tract, but instead is excreted in the urine. Saccharin was the first non-nutritive sweetener available in the United States. Because it was thought to be a weak carcinogen in rats, potentially causing increased incidence of bladder cancer, saccharin was banned by the FDA in 1977. Due to strong public opposition, Congress passed the Saccharin Study and Labeling Act, which allowed continued use of saccharin until the FDA withdrew its ban in 1991. To date, most evidence obtained from studies involving population groups considered to be heavy saccharin users fails to confirm a link between saccharin and bladder cancer.

Aspartame, commonly known as Nutrasweet, is approximately 200 times sweeter than table sugar. Because it contains 4 kcal/g, aspartame is technically nutritive; however, the amounts necessary to achieve desired level of sweet taste are so small that the numbers of calories ingested by users generally are negligible. When aspartame came on the market, the FDA began to recommend acceptable daily intakes (ADIs), defined as the amount of a food additive that can be consumed safely on a daily basis over an individual's life span. The ADI for aspartame is 50 mg/kg of body weight. One packet of Nutrasweet contains 35 mg of aspartame. Comprehensive studies have failed to confirm that long-term use of aspartame is associated with any adverse effects.

Acesulfame K, marketed as Sweet One and used in candies, baked products, and soft drinks, is heat-stable and 200 times sweeter than table sugar. In summary, both nutritive and non-nutritive sweeteners are safe to consume in moderation, as part of a well-balanced diet for individuals with NIDDM and IDDM.

Alcohol

Moderate amounts of alcohol can be included in the diabetic diet. Blood glucose levels usually are not affected if they are well controlled. Moderation for individuals with diabetes is defined as two equivalents of an alcoholic beverage once or twice a week. Alcohol equivalents are defined as 1.5 ounces of distilled liquor, 4 ounces of wine, and 12 ounces of beer. Drinks that contain mixers, sweet wines, and liqueurs should be avoided. Alcohol does not require insulin for its metabolism. If it is not used as a source of energy, it is converted to fat. Because alcohol impairs gluconeogenesis, and inhibits the release of glucose from glycogen in the liver, hypoglycemia can result when alcohol is consumed without food. Alcoholic beverages provide "empty calories," approximately 7 kcal/g, and have no other nutritional value. Diabetic individuals with elevated triglyceride levels should avoid alcohol consumption because alcohol can lead to hypertriglyceridemia.

The Diabetes Control and Complications Trial

The Diabetes Control and Complications Trial (DCCT) was a 10-year multicenter, randomized clinical trial designed to compare intensive versus conventional diabetes therapy with regard to the development and progression of complications associated with the disease. The intensive therapy regimen sought to bring blood glucose levels as close to the normal range as possible using three or more daily insulin injections, diet therapy and frequent interactions with the health care team. Participants were counseled to adjust their pre-meal insulin dose depending on blood glucose monitoring results, food intake, and whether or not they were exercising. The conventional therapy consisted of one or two daily insulin injections, self-monitoring of urine or blood glucose, quarterly physician visits, and nutrition education as requested by the participant. The study concluded that intensive therapy does significantly delay the onset and slows the progression of long-term complications in individuals with diabetes mellitus. Specifically, there was a 76 percent reduction in retinopathy, a 60 percent reduction in neuropathy, a 54 percent reduction in albuminuria, and a 39 percent reduction in microalbuminuria. The DCCT also demonstrated that even small improvements in blood glucose levels reduced the rate of complications and reaffirmed the role of nutrition in helping individuals with diabetes achieve their target blood glucose goals. The results can also be applied to people with type II diabetes because the pathogenesis by which elevated blood glucose levels cause long-term complications are similar in both type I and type II diabetes mellitus. However, one major adverse effect was the increased incidence of hypoglycemic episodes in the intensive therapy group.

Other Strategies for Controlling Blood Glucose

Meal Planning

Exchange lists for meal planning, developed by the American Diabetes Association and the American Dietetic Association, are used frequently to develop individualized meal plans and to educate persons with diabetes mellitus about nutrition. The exchange lists group foods of similar nutrient composition and includes breads, meats, fruits, milk, vegetables, and fats. All recommended serving sizes or portions on a given exchange list provide similar amounts of energy, carbohydrate, protein, and fat. Exchange-based nutrition plans offer flexibility and choice while maintaining daily consistency in the total caloric, protein, fat, and carbohydrate composition of the diet. Meals consist of servings from each of the six exchange lists or food groups. Combination foods such as pizza, or Chinese and Mexican dishes such as chicken and broccoli or chicken enchiladas also can be planned into the diabetic diet using the exchange approach.

Insulin Delivery and Management

According to the American Diabetes Association, there is no preferred form of therapy for achieving tight control of blood glucose levels. The decision regarding whether to prescribe multiple insulin injections or use an insulin pump that allows for a small, continuous inflow of insulin therefore depends on the patient and the health care team providing the necessary support.

Case 1

Insulin-Dependent
Diabetes Mellitus (IDDM)

Seth Braunstein and Frances Burke

Objectives

- To understand the diagnosis and differentiation between types I and II diabetes mellitus.
- To apply nutrition assessment techniques to persons with insulin-dependent diabetes mellitus.
- To understand why nutrition therapy is a vital component in managing diabetes mellitus.
- To increase awareness of the behavioral and lifestyle factors involved in diabetes management.
- To develop a dietary plan suitable for a person with insulin-dependent diabetes mellitus.

MS, a 24-year-old student, presented to the Student Health Center complaining of fatigue, weight loss, blurred vision, frequent urination, and increased thirst for the past six months. Originally, MS had attributed these symptoms to the stress of his third-year clinical rotations, but during the last two months he lost approximately ten pounds despite his reportedly good appetite.

Past Medical History

MS reports no previous illness or hospitalizations. He is not presently taking any medications or vitamins and has no known food allergies.

Family History

MS's grandmother and father have diabetes. There is no family history of heart disease, hypertension, or obesity.

Social History

MS reports drinking alcohol on weekends, but does not exceed four to six 12-ounce beers per week. He does not smoke cigarettes. His caffeine intake is limited to several cups of coffee daily. MS is not following any special diet. In fact, he reports that his diet is erratic. He skips breakfast, eats late dinners, and snacks throughout the day. MS exercises moderately at the gym several days per week.

MS's Usual Intake (24-Hour Recall)		
Snack (7 A.M.)	Coffee with sugar	1 cup, 2 packets
	Whole milk	3 Tbs.
Breakfast (10 A.M.)	Orange juice	16 oz.
	Bagel	1
	Cream cheese	1 oz. (2 Tbs.)
Lunch (1:30 P.M.)	Beef bologna	4 oz.
	American cheese	2 oz.
	White bread, enriched	4 slices
	Mayonnaise	2 Tbs.
	Corn chips	1 oz.
	Coca-Cola, regular	12 oz.
Snack (5 P.M.)	Frozen yogurt	1 cup
Dinner (8 P.M.)	Pizza	2 slices (1/4 of 15" pie)
	Coca-Cola, regular	12 oz.
Evening Snack (11 P.M.)	Doughnut, jelly	1
	Whole milk	1 cup
	Total calories: 3239 kcal/day	
	Protein: 13% of total calories	
	Fat: 38% of total calories	
	Carbohydrate: 49% of total calories	

Review of Systems

General: Fatigue, weight loss

Eyes: Blurred vision

Endocrine: Increased thirst (polydipsia), frequent urination (polyuria)

Physical Examination

Vital signs

Temperature: 98.4°F

Heart rate: 80 BPM

Respiration: 12 BPM

Blood pressure: 102/70 mm Hg

Anthropometric data

Height: 5'10" (178 cm)

Current weight: 166 lb (75.5 kg)

Usual weight: 176 lb (80 kg)

Ideal body weight: 166 lb (75.5 kg)

General: Thin male resting comfortably

Head/neck: Facial pallor

Cardiac: Regular rate and rhythm, no murmurs or gallops

Abdomen: Soft, nontender, no hepatosplenomegaly

Extremities: Subcutaneous muscle wasting, no edema

Laboratory Data

Patient's Values	Normal Values
Glucose: 300 mg/dL	70–110 mg/dL
Sodium: 133 mg/L	133–143 mg/L
Potassium: 3.3 mg/L	3.5–5.3 mg/L
Chloride: 101 mg/L	97–107 mg/L
Bicarbonate: 22 mg/L	24–32 mg/L
Plasma ketones: 1:8 dilution	None
Urinary ketones: 4+	None

Diagnosis

Based on MS's history and test results, his diagnosis is clearly diabetes mellitus. MS was referred to the diabetes clinic at the outpatient medical center.

Case Questions

1. Differentiate between the two types of diabetes mellitus.

2. Explain why MS experienced the symptoms of fatigue, polydipsia, polyuria, and weight loss despite his good appetite.

3. What criteria are used to confirm the diagnosis of diabetes mellitus?

4. How may the patient's laboratory data be interpreted?

5. What additional information is needed to assess MS's nutritional status?

6. Using the Harris-Benedict equation, calculate MS's caloric requirements.

7. Comment on MS's diet, given his diagnosis of diabetes mellitus. What recommendations would you give to MS?

8. MS's neighbor has type I diabetes mellitus and was taught a diet using an exchange system for meal planning. MS would like to know if this diet would be suitable for him. What is the appropriate response?

9. Why should MS be encouraged to exercise?

10. MS would like to know if he can continue to drink alcohol on the weekends with his classmates. What is the appropriate response?

11. Based on the current nutritional guidelines for individuals with diabetes mellitus, what specific dietary modifications would you recommend for MS?

12. When should a follow-up appointment with the nutritionist be scheduled for MS?

Answers begin on the following page.

Answers to Questions: Case 1

Part 1:   Diagnosis

1. **Differentiate between the two types of diabetes mellitus.**

    Insulin-dependent diabetes mellitus (IDDM), also called type I diabetes, accounts for 10 percent of all cases of diabetes mellitus. Because the pancreas produces little or no insulin, these patients depend on exogenous insulin for their survival. Characteristically, type I diabetes develops before age 20; the peak incidence occurs at 6 to 11 years of age. Patients generally are prone to ketosis (ketoacidosis). Type I diabetes has been linked to specific HLA antigens and is thought to be a weakly inherited trait. Often, type I diabetes develops acutely as the result of an autoimmune insult to the pancreatic beta cells. Patients typically are of normal body weight.

    Non-insulin-dependent diabetes mellitus (NIDDM), or type II diabetes, accounts for 90 percent of all cases. This disorder is characterized by decreased production of insulin and insulin resistance due to decreased tissue sensitivity to this hormone. Exogenous insulin may be required to control persistent hyperglycemia in these patients. No linkage to specific HLA antigens has been observed in type II diabetes. There is, however, a strong association with family history. Eighty percent of patients with type II diabetes are obese, and their glucose tolerance often improves with weight loss.

2. **Explain why MS experienced the symptoms of fatigue, polydipsia, polyuria, and weight loss despite his good appetite.**

    Insulin deficiency reduces glucose uptake and utilization by insulin-sensitive tissues, predominately in the liver and skeletal muscle. As a result, the conversion of glucose to glycogen in the liver is greatly diminished, and gluconeogenesis—the formation of glucose from noncarbohydrate sources such as amino acids—is increased. Together, these effects contribute to an accumulation of glucose in the blood called hyperglycemia.

    When the blood glucose level surpasses the kidney's ability to reabsorb glucose from its ultrafiltrate, an osmotic diuresis ensues, resulting in excessive loss of free water and glycosuria, the elimination of excess glucose in the urine. Polydipsia (increased thirst) and polyuria (increased urinary frequency and volume) therefore are frequently associated with hyperglycemia.

    Lipolysis is greatly increased in the absence of insulin, as fatty acids released from adipose tissue provide an alternative energy source to glucose. When excessive amounts of these fatty acids are released, the liver produces three ketone bodies from acetyl CoA: acetoacetate, D-beta-hydroxybutyrate, and acetone. Because the body has a limited capacity to metabolize ketone bodies as an energy source, excess ketone bodies accumulate in the blood (ketonemia) and are excreted in the urine (ketonuria). The production of increased amounts of ketone bodies, called ketosis, can cause metabolic acidosis.

Although serum glucose levels are elevated, insulin must be present for cellular uptake of glucose to occur. In insulin-dependent diabetes, the cells are in a "starved" state that causes increased appetite, or polyphagia. As serum glucose levels and ketone bodies rise, the renal threshold is overwhelmed, and glucose and ketones are lost in the urine. Thus, individuals with recent onset diabetes experience rapid weight loss.

3. **What criteria are used to confirm the diagnosis of diabetes mellitus?**

According to the American Diabetes Association, a random plasma glucose level of 200 mg/dL or greater, plus classic signs and symptoms such as polydipsia, polyuria, polyphagia, and weight loss, are sufficient cause for diagnosis of diabetes mellitus. Alternatively, a fasting plasma glucose level of 140 mg/dL or greater on at least two occasions is also considered diagnostic in the absence of acute illness or administration of glucocorticoids such as prednisone.

4. **How may the patient's laboratory data be interpreted?**

Biochemical abnormalities accompany sustained hyperglycemia. Serum sodium levels usually are low because the osmotically active glucose draws water from the cells into the intravascular space. This process effectively dilutes the serum sodium level, which therefore should be corrected in hyperglycemia. Serum sodium decreases approximately 1.6 mEq/L for each 100 mg/dL increase in the serum glucose level above the normal value. The resulting osmotic diuresis also causes a loss of free water, potassium, and other electrolytes.

The markedly increased hydrogen ion concentration, reflected in the low bicarbonate level, is caused by the accumulation of ketone bodies. Ketone bodies are relatively weak acids that generate large numbers of hydrogen ions by dissociation, thereby causing metabolic acidosis. As these excess hydrogen ions are buffered by bicarbonate ions and other buffer systems, the serum bicarbonate level decreases.

Part 2: Nutrition Assessment and Therapy

5. **What additional information is needed to assess MS's nutritional status?**

Nutrition intervention is an essential component in the management of both type I and type II diabetes mellitus. Recommendations must be individualized to meet the person's physiological and psychological needs. Furthermore, they must be flexible enough to allow a normal lifestyle. Individualizing the meal plan requires a thorough nutrition assessment that takes into account the patient's nutrition history and pertinent social and economic information. Specific parameters of the assessment include

  alcohol consumption (type, amount, and frequency)

  living situation (e.g., who prepares meals)

cooking facilities

ethnic or religious considerations (i.e., kosher or vegetarian diet)

employment (type of job, hours) and/or school schedule

previous diets and/or any prior diet instructions

meal frequency (approximate timing of meals and snacks)

meals eaten away from home

physical activity level

6. Using the Harris-Benedict equation, calculate MS's caloric requirements.

Recall from Chapter 1 that the Harris-Benedict equation calculates an individual's basal energy expenditure (BEE) based on certain anthropometric data adjusted by an activity factor that reflects individual circumstances. The accepted activity factor for most nonhospitalized patients is 1.5.

For men,

BEE = [66 + 13.7 (Weight in kg) + 5.0 (Height in cm) − 6.8 (Age)] x 1.5

Thus, in MS's case,

BEE = [66 + 13.7 (75.5 kg) + 5.0 (178 cm) − 6.8 (24 years)] x 1.5

= 1827 x 1.5

= 2740 kcal/day

7. Comment on MS's diet, given his diagnosis of diabetes mellitus. What recommendations would you give to MS?

The current nutritional recommendations for individuals with diabetes mellitus call for a diet composed of 55 to 60 percent carbohydrate, 12 to 20 percent protein, and 25 to 30 percent fat. These recommendations are similar to those advocated by the American Heart Association, the National Cancer Institute, and other national health organizations. MS's dietary intake is not optimal given his diagnosis of diabetes mellitus because his calorie and fat intakes exceed the recommended levels. Even though MS is consuming an adequate caloric intake overall, he is losing weight because his tissues are unable to utilize the nutrients.

In the past, individuals with diabetes mellitus were taught to limit carbohydrates for optimal glucose control, but the resulting diets were high in fat and therefore potentially atherogenic. Because diabetes is a major risk factor for coronary artery disease, the American Diabetes Association now recommends a low-fat diet and emphasizes increasing the complex carbohydrate intake in the diet and fiber in the form of breads, cereals, grains, vegetables, beans, and pastas. Other health organizations also recommend increasing fiber intake because of its many benefits, notably: decreased fasting and postprandial triglyceride levels, decreased serum cholesterol, and increased insulin sensitivity. MS's total fiber intake (soluble and insoluble) is approximately 11 grams. A fiber intake of 20 to 35 grams per day appears to be beneficial. Sources of soluble fiber include oat bran, beans, citrus fruits, and pectin, which is found in apples and most fruits. Wheat bran, whole-wheat bread, bran cereals, brown rice, and some green vegetables are good sources of insoluble fiber.

Recent studies have concluded that simple sugars (concentrated sweets) consumed with meals do not cause as rapid a rise in postprandial blood glucose levels as was once thought, but intake of these substances should still be limited. Sources of simple sugars in MS's diet include table sugar, sodas, jelly doughnuts, and frozen yogurt.

Total fat should be limited to less than 30 percent of total calories. Of this amount, saturated fat and polyunsaturated fat should each constitute less than 10 percent of total calories, whereas up to 15 percent can come from monounsaturated fat. Sources of fat in MS's diet include cream cheese, bologna, cheese, mayonnaise, corn chips, cheese pizza, doughnuts, and whole milk, most of which contain saturated fats.

8. **MS's neighbor has type I diabetes mellitus and was taught a diet using an exchange system for meal planning. MS would like to know if this diet would be suitable for him. What is the appropriate response?**

A traditional meal planning approach developed by the American Diabetes Association in conjunction with the American Dietetic Association uses an exchange system. Foods are grouped according to their nutrient and calorie content, and patients can substitute foods within the same group. The six food groups are: dairy products, meat (low-fat, medium-fat, and high-fat), starches and breads, fruits and fruit juices, vegetables, and fats. Grouping foods in this manner allows for greater flexibility in meal planning without sacrificing the consistency that the person with type I diabetes needs to maintain good glycemic control. This is one meal planning approach that would be suitable for MS.

9. **Why should MS be encouraged to exercise?**

Exercise is an important management tool for people with either type I or type II diabetes mellitus because it improves insulin sensitivity and lipoprotein profiles (increasing HDL), helps maintain desirable body weight, and lowers blood pressure. These considerations are all important in preventing complications associated with diabetes mellitus.

Exercise usually requires food and/or insulin adjustments. Because exercise affects individuals differently, adjustments must be based on self-monitoring of blood glucose levels and previous experiences of the individual. Education about exercise and its effects is critical in avoiding the risks of immediate and delayed hypoglycemia and increased hyperglycemia and ketosis.

10. **MS would like to know if he can continue to drink alcohol on the weekends with his classmates. What is the appropriate response?**

The same precautions regarding the use of alcohol that apply to the general public apply to people with diabetes mellitus. However, moderation is essential for individuals with type I diabetes, who should limit their intake to two equivalents of an alcoholic beverage once or twice a week because of the risk of hypoglycemia. Alcohol metabolism impairs gluconeogenesis and inhibits the release of glucose from glycogen in the liver. As a result, the person on evening NPH insulin who drinks excessively at night (more than 2 drinks per evening) may experience very low blood sugars in the middle of the night or early in the morning when their long-acting insulin is peaking. Eating while drinking an alcoholic beverage and avoiding sweet drinks and sugar-containing mixes are recommendations that may help MS and others avoid these unpleasant potential consequences of alcohol intake.

11. **Based on the current nutritional guidelines for individuals with diabetes mellitus, what specific dietary modifications would you recommend for MS?**

    With the assistance of the Diabetes Center's registered dietitian, MS developed the following revised sample meal plan. The total daily caloric intake of 2830 kcal consists of 28 percent fat, 20 percent protein, and 51 percent carbohydrate.

The Diabetes Center's Revised Meal Plan for MS

Breakfast	Bagel, plain	1
(7–7:30 A.M.)	Margarine	2 Tbs.
	Fresh orange	1 medium
	Coffee	1 cup
	1% low-fat milk	2 Tbs.
Lunch (12–12:30 P.M.)	Turkey sandwich	2
	Light mayonnaise	2 Tbs.
	Nonfat yogurt with Nutrasweet	4 oz.
	Pretzels	2 oz.
	Diet cola	12 oz.
Dinner (5:30–6 P.M.)	Pasta/tomato sauce	2 cups/1/2 cup
	Lettuce and tomato	1 cup
	Olive oil/vinegar dressing	2 Tbs.
	Apple	1 medium
	Diet cola	12 oz.
Evening Snack	1% low-fat milk	6 oz.
(9:30–10 P.M.)	Tuna salad	2 oz.
	Whole-wheat bread	1 slice
	Low-fat mayonnaise	1 Tbs.
	Total calories: 2830 kcal/day	
	Protein: 20% of total calories	
	Fat: 28% of total calories	
	Carbohydrate: 51% of total calories	

12. When should a follow-up appointment with the nutritionist be scheduled for MS?

A follow-up appointment should be scheduled approximately one to two weeks after the initial counseling session and on a monthly basis thereafter. This frequency allows for monitoring blood glucose control, weight maintenance, and progress in working with dietary recommendations. Because the amount of new information that a person with newly diagnosed diabetes mellitus receives can be overwhelming, monthly follow-up with the registered dietitian should be encouraged.

Non-Insulin-Dependent Diabetes Mellitus (NIDDM)

Seth Braunstein and Frances Burke

Objectives

- To apply nutritional assessment techniques to persons with non-insulin-dependent diabetes mellitus.
- To understand the current nutritional recommendations for people with non-insulin-dependent diabetes mellitus.
- To understand why maintaining a reasonable body weight and increasing physical activity are important treatment modalities for people with non-insulin-dependent diabetes mellitus.

DR, a 45-year-old male who has had NIDDM for 5 years, visits his family physician because he has not been feeling well. He suspects that his blood sugar is elevated and complains of polyuria and fatigue. Presently, he is not taking medication and does not test his blood sugar at home.

Past Medical History

DR has no history of previous hospitalizations or other illnesses.

Family History

DR's family history is positive for diabetes. His grandmother developed non-insulin-dependent diabetes mellitus at age 60. There is no family history of hypertension, heart disease, or obesity.

Social History

DR, an architect, is single, lives alone, and does not follow a special diet. He reports drinking 2 beers every day when he comes home from work. He has no history of smoking. DR does not exercise or take vitamin supplements. He has no known allergies to foods or drugs. At his physician's request, DR prepared the following 24-hour diet recall.

DR's Diet History (24-Hour Recall)		
Breakfast	Raisin bran cereal	2 cups
	Banana	1 large
	Whole milk	1 cup
	Orange juice	8 oz.
Lunch	Corned beef	4 oz.
	Swiss cheese	1 oz.
	Rye bread	2 slices
	Coleslaw	1/2 cup
	Russian dressing	2 Tbs.
	Potato chips	1 small bag
	Cranberry juice cocktail	12 oz. bottle
Dinner	Fried rice (Chinese)	1 cup
	Hunan chicken (fried)	4 oz.
	Shrimp and cashews	4 oz.
	Beer	2 bottles
	Orange	1 large

Total calories: 3411 kcal/day

Protein: 14% of total calories

Fat: 40% of total calories

Carbohydrate: 46% of total calories

Review of Systems

General: Fatigue, weakness

Endocrine: Increased thirst (polydipsia) and frequent urination (polyuria)

Physical Examination

The physical exam revealed no noteworthy findings other than obesity.

Vital signs

Temperature: 98.8°F

Heart rate: 72 BPM

Respiration: 14 BPM

Blood pressure: 120/80 mm Hg

Anthropometric data

Height: 5'9" (175 cm)

Current weight: 215 lb (98 kg)

Laboratory Data

DR's laboratory tests, conducted one hour after lunch, resulted in the following values.

Serum glucose: 285 mg/dL

Urinary glucose: 2+

Case Questions

1. What are the normal postprandial and fasting glucose levels used to diagnose individuals with diabetes mellitus?

2. What is DR's ideal body weight? What percent of DR's ideal body weight does his current body weight represent? Is this result clinically significant?

3. What is a reasonable weight goal for DR? What information may be useful in making this determination?

4. How many calories does DR require for weight maintenance, assuming that he leads a sedentary lifestyle?

5. What are the current nutritional goals for individuals with NIDDM?

6. Is DR's diet appropriate for a person with type II diabetes? What recommendations are indicated for DR based on his current diet?

7. How can DR's compliance be evaluated when he returns to the doctor's office one month later?

8. What additional treatment modalities are indicated for DR at this time?

9. DR often snacks on cookies containing unsweetened fruit juice and sugar-free candy. He asks the doctor whether he can eat these foods on   a regular basis. What is the appropriate response?

Answers begin on the following page.

Answers to Questions: Case 2

Part 1:   Diagnosis and Assessment

1. **What are the normal postprandial and fasting glucose levels used to diagnose individuals with diabetes mellitus?**

   According to the National Diabetes Data Group and the American Diabetes Association, glucose levels may be interpreted as follows.

   - Fasting blood sugar levels should be under 140 mg/dL.

   - Postprandial levels one hour after eating should be under 200 mg/dL.

   - Postprandial levels two hours after eating should be under 165 mg/dL.

2. **What is DR's ideal body weight? What percent of DR's ideal body weight does his current body weight represent? Is this result clinically significant?**

   DR is a 5'9" man whose ideal body weight may be calculated using the rule-of-thumb estimate.

   106 lb + (9 in. x 6 lb) = 160 lb

   $$\text{Percent ideal body weight (IBW)} = \frac{215}{160 \text{ lb}} = 134\%$$

   DR's current weight, at 134 percent of his IBW, is clinically significant because it represents mild obesity. Eighty percent of individuals with NIDDM are obese, and they tend to be insulin-resistant. Even a moderate weight loss of ten pounds can help these individuals improve their blood sugar levels.

3. **What is a reasonable weight goal for DR? What information may be useful in making this determination?**

   To determine reasonable weight, defined as a weight that an individual can achieve and maintain, ask the following questions.

   1. What weight do you feel is an achievable weight?

   2. How long have you been overweight?

   3. How much time do you expect losing weight to take?

   A reasonable weight goal for DR is 175 lb.

4. **How many calories does DR require for weight maintenance, assuming that he leads a sedentary lifestyle?**

   The first step is to determine DR's adjusted body weight, based on his status as an obese person.

Adjusted weight = 0.25 (Current weight − Ideal weight) + Ideal body weight

= 0.25 (215 − 160) + 160

= 13.75 + 160 = 174 lb (79 kg)

Next, using the 25 kcal/kg rule of thumb, we can estimate the number of calories DR requires for weight maintenance.

25 kcal x 79 kg = 1975 kcal/day

Because DR's glycemic control will improve with weight loss, he can be advised to reduce his intake by at least 500 kcal/day. This will result in a weight loss of one pound per week.

Part 2: Nutrition Therapy

5. **What are the current nutritional goals for individuals with NIDDM?**

The current nutritional goals for a patient with NIDDM are:

- maintaining blood glucose levels as close to normal as possible
- achieving optimal serum lipid and blood pressure levels
- providing adequate calories for maintaining a reasonable body weight

Nutrition therapy is a key component of medical therapy for persons with NIDDM. The nutritional plan should be individualized to accommodate the person's lifestyle, ensure adherence to the diet, and help them achieve his or her personal goals. Specific dietary recommendations include the following.

Fat: Fat intake generally should account for less than 30 percent of total calories, and less than 10 percent of total calories should come from saturated fat. However, this allowance also depends on the individual's eating habits, desired weight, glucose levels, and lipid goals. If weight loss is the priority, reducing total fat intake will help reduce calories, because fat is the most calorically dense nutrient.

Carbohydrate: Carbohydrate intake may account for up to 55 to 60 percent of total calories. This amount varies depending on the persons eating habits, glucose and lipid level goals. Formerly, it was widely believed that the diet's carbohydrate content should consist mostly of starches, such as breads, pasta, rice, potatoes, and beans. However, scientific evidence has shown that sucrose-containing foods, as part of the total allowable carbohydrate content and within the context of a mixed meal, do not impair blood glucose control in persons with IDDM or NIDDM.

Protein: At present little scientific evidence supports recommending a different dietary protein allowance for diabetics without renal disease from that recommended for the general population. Therefore, current recommendations advise that 12 to 20 percent of total dietary calories should come from protein-containing foods. However, high-protein foods usually contain fat, so individuals should be advised to select leaner red meats, fish, and white-meat chicken and turkey as protein sources.

Fiber: Recommendations regarding fiber are the same for diabetics as for the general population: 20 to 35 grams per day from a variety of sources. Although some forms of soluble fiber may delay the absorption of glucose from the small intestine, fiber's overall effect on improving glycemic control is probably insignificant.

Alcohol: Alcohol intake should amount to no more than one to two alcoholic drinks less than two times per week. Because alcohol may increase a person's risk of hypoglycemia, especially if he or she is taking insulin or an oral hypoglycemic agent, experts advise against ingesting alcohol without food.

Vitamins and minerals: Most people with diabetes mellitus do not need to take a vitamin and mineral supplement if they are consuming a balanced diet. However, for individuals on low-calorie diets (i.e., 1000 calories or less) for weight reduction, a supplement is recommended.

6. **Is DR's diet appropriate for a person with type II diabetes? What recommendations are indicated for DR based on his current diet?**

Because diabetes is a risk factor for cardiovascular disease, individuals with NIDDM should be counseled to follow a low-fat diet and reduce their intake of concentrated sweets. According to a nutritional analysis of his current diet, DR's caloric intake is 3411 kcal/day, far higher than the approximately 2000 kcals he requires for weight maintenance. His total fat intake was 40 percent, again higher than the desired 30 percent of total calories. DR's consumption of fried foods, potato chips, whole milk, and large portions of meat and poultry contribute to his high fat and calorie intake. By limiting these foods and substituting foods lower in fat, DR will reduce his calorie intake, improve his blood sugar levels, and most likely lose weight. Suggested substitutions that DR can implement over time are as follows:

Dietary Alternatives to Reduce Fats

Use skim or low-fat milk (1%).

Select turkey breast, water-packed tuna, lean imported ham, or roast beef for sandwiches.

Use mustard instead of high fat salad dressings or mayonnaise.

Choose pretzels, not chips.

Substitute steamed white rice for fried rice.

Skip the nuts and seeds in Chinese dishes.

Try steamed or stir-fried rather than fried chicken and vegetables.

Dietary Alternatives to Reduce Sugars and Concentrated Sweets

Use low-sugar cereals such as Corn Flakes, Rice Krispies, or Rice Chex.

Reduce portion sizes of banana and orange juice.

Substitute diet soda, seltzer, or water for fruit juice and soda.

7. **How can DR's compliance be evaluated when he returns to the doctor's office one month later?**

    DR's physician should take the following measures when DR returns for follow-up.

    1. Evaluate symptoms of polyuria and fatigue.

    2. Monitor weight change.

    3. Monitor fasting and postprandial blood sugars.

    When DR returns to the office for long-term monitoring in six months, his fructosamine or hemoglobin A_1C levels may be drawn to evaluate his compliance. Fructosamine measures the percentage of sugars glycosylated to albumin. Because it has a 21-day half-life, fructosamine testing is a short-term laboratory assessment tool. Hemoglobin A_1C measures the percentage of sugars glycosylated to hemoglobin and has a 120-day half-life. It represents the average glucose level for the preceding two to three months. This test can therefore assess long-term compliance and is more widely used. Glycosylated hemoglobin normally ranges between 4 and 7 percent of total hemoglobin (see Table 8-4).

8. **What additional treatment modalities are indicated for DR at this time?**

    Increased physical activity would help DR to lose weight and control his blood sugars. Exercise increases the number and binding capacity of insulin receptors, lowers blood glucose levels in NIDDM, reduces insulin requirements in persons who use insulin to control persistent hyperglycemia, and improves lipid levels, thereby reducing risk of CHD. Also, education regarding self-monitoring of blood glucose would improve DR's understanding of his diabetes and promote appropriate self-regulation.

Table 8-4   Indices of glycemic controls.*

BIOCHEMICAL INDEX	NORMAL	GOAL	ACTION SUGGESTED**
Preprandial fasting glucose (mg/dL)	< 115	80–120	<80 >140
Bedtime glucose (mg/dL)	<120	100–140	<100 >160
Hemoglobin A_1C*** (%)	<6	<7	>8

*For nonpregnant individuals.

**Depending on individual patient circumstances.

***Referenced to hemoglobin A_1C nondiabetic range (4%–6%).

Source: American Diabetes Association. *Maximizing the Role of Nutrition in Diabetes Management.* Alexandria, Va: American Diabetes Association, Inc., 1994.

9. DR often snacks on cookies containing unsweetened fruit juice and sugar-free candy. He asks the doctor whether he can eat these foods on a regular basis. What is the appropriate response?

    The principal dietary sugars are fructose, sucrose, lactose, and glucose. Sugars provide only energy to the diet; they have no nutritional value. Both unsweetened fruit juice and fresh fruit contain the monosaccharide fructose, a naturally occurring simple sugar. Fructose is also added as a sweetener to soft drinks, jam, cookies, and other baked products. Compared to sucrose (ordinary table sugar), fructose may raise serum glucose levels less in patients with well-controlled NIDDM and IDDM. Initially, fructose metabolism does not require insulin, but after its conversion to glucose in the liver, it requires insulin just as does glucose derived directly from dietary sources. In addition, fructose contains 4 kcal/g, which must be considered when planning a calorie-controlled diet. Finally, eating large amounts (greater than 50 g) of fructose has been shown to cause osmotic diarrhea.

    For most people with diabetes mellitus, foods containing simple sugars do not necessarily influence blood glucose control differently than do starches. Rather, it is the combination of these two forms of carbohydrate that must be planned in the diabetic diet to produce the optimal blood glucose control depending on the goals of the individual.

    Sugar-free candy generally is sweetened with sorbitol, a sugar alcohol, or polyol, that tends to be half as sweet as table sugar. Other examples are xylitol and mannitol. Sugar alcohols also are used as fillers and food bulking agents and are a major ingredient in hard candy, sugarless chewing gum, jams, and jellies. They are absorbed slowly in the jejunum and converted rapidly to fructose in the liver. Because sugar alcohols can cause abdominal gas and osmotic diarrhea, eating them in large amounts is not recommended. Like fructose, polyols contribute 4 kcal/g to the diet. Therefore the best response to DR is to use these products in moderation because "sugar-free" does not necessarily mean "calorie-free" or "fat-free."

See Chapter Review Questions, pages A14–A15.

REFERENCES

American Association of Diabetes Educators. Nutrition. In Peragallo-Dittko V. (ed.). *A Core Curriculum for Diabetes Education.* 2nd ed. Chicago: , 1993: 131–177.

American Diabetes Association. Standards of medical care for patients with diabetes mellitus. *Diabetes Care* 1994;17:616–623.

American Diabetes Association. Detection and management of lipid disorders in diabetes. *Diabetes Care* 1993;16(Suppl 2):106–112.

American Dietetic Association. Position of the American Dietetic Association: use of nutritive and nonnutritive sweeteners. *J Am Diet Assoc* 1993;7:816–821.

Anderson JW, Geil PB. Nutritional Management of Diabetes Mellitus. In Shils ME, Olson JA, Shike M (eds.). *Modern Nutrition in Health and Disease.* 8th ed. Philadelphia: Lea and Febiger, 1994:1259–1284.

Atkinson MA, Maclaren NK. The pathogenesis of insulin-dependent diabetes mellitus. *N Engl J Med* 1994;331(21):1428–1436.

Beebe CA, Pastors JG, Powers MA, et al. Nutrition management for individuals with non-insulin-dependent diabetes in the 1990s: a review by the Diabetes Care and Education Dietetic Practice Group. *J Am Diet Assoc* 1991;91(2):196–207.

Bernard RI, Jung T, Inkeles SB. Diet and exercise in the treatment of NIDDM. *Diabetes Care* 1994;17(12):1469–1471.

Brodsky IG, Robbins DC, Hiser E, et al. Effects of low protein diets on protein metabolism in insulin-dependent diabetes mellitus patients with early nephropathy. *J Clin Endocrinol Metab* 1992;75:351–357.

Cryer PE, Fisher JN, Shamoon H. Hypoglycemia. *Diabetes Care* 1994;17: 734–755.

Delahanty L. Nutritional recommendations for cardiovascular complications of diabetes. *Diabetes Educator* 1992;18(6):543–544.

Franz MJ. Avoiding sugar: Does research support traditional beliefs? The *Diabetes Educator* 1993;19(2):144–150.

Franz MJ. Alcohol and diabetes, part I. *Diabetes Spectrum* 1990;3(3):136–140, 144.

Franz MJ, Horton ES, Bantle J, et al. Nutrition principles for the management of diabetes and related complications. *Diabetes Care* 1994;17:490–519.

Henry RR. Protein content of the diabetic diet. *Diabetes Care* 1994;17: 1502–1514.

Horton ES. Prescription for exercise. *Diabetes Spectrum* 1991;4(5):250–257.

Nuttall FQ. Dietary fiber in the management of diabetes. *Diabetes* 1993;42: 503–508.

Patterson CM, Levin S. Diabetes mellitus: Helping NIDDM patients achieve control through diet and weight loss. *Consultant* 1994;9:1319–1335.

Schneider SH, Ruderman NB. Exercise and NIDDM. *Diabetes Care* 1990;13: 785–789.

The Diabetes Control and Complications Research Group. The effect of intensive treatment of diabetes on the development and progression of long-term complications in insulin-dependent diabetes mellitus. *N Engl J Med* 1993;329(14): 977–996.

Vessby B. Dietary carbohydrates in diabetes. *Am J Clin Nutr* 1994;59(Suppl 3): 742S–746S.

Wasserman DH, Zinman B. Exercise in individuals with IDDM. *Diabetes Care* 1994;17:924–937.

Wilson JP. New diabetes nutrition guidelines: do you know the score? *Nursing.* 1995;25(7):65–66.

9

Pulmonary Disease

Scott Manaker and Frances Burke

Objectives

- To understand nutritional deficits, requirements, and therapy in patients with chronic obstructive pulmonary disease and cystic fibrosis.
- To examine available feeding options and their indications for mechanically ventilated patients and the risks associated with nutritional support.
- To understand appropriate preoperative and postoperative nutritional therapy for patients undergoing lung transplantation.
- To appreciate the association between obstructive sleep apnea syndrome and obesity.
- To incorporate nutrition into the history, review of systems, and physical examinations of patients with pulmonary diseases.

Chronic Obstructive Pulmonary Disease

Between 25 and 50 percent of patients with chronic obstructive pulmonary disease (COPD) have some degree of nutritional depletion. Weight loss is exceedingly common among patients with COPD, as are reductions in fat reserves and muscle mass. Patients who experience progressive weight loss to the extent that their current weight is less than 90 percent of their ideal body weight are considered malnourished. The more severe the COPD, the greater the associated malnutrition and weight loss. The greater the weight loss, the smaller the weight of the respiratory muscles and diaphragm.

Patients with COPD require nutritional assessment because the consequences of malnutrition include adverse effects on respiratory muscle mass and function that result in decreased respiratory muscle strength. Furthermore, because malnutrition also is associated with decreased cell-mediated immunity, altered immunoglobulin production, and impaired cellular resistance of the tracheobronchial mucosa to bacterial infection, malnourished patients are at increased risk for respiratory infections, especially pneumonia and bronchitis.

Causes of Weight Loss

Hypermetabolism

Two major causes of hypermetabolism result in increased energy requirements in patients with COPD.

Increased work of breathing: In patients with normal lung function, breathing expends 36 to 72 calories per day. Patients with COPD may have up to a tenfold increase in their daily energy expenditure from breathing. Both the increased resistive load and the reduced respiratory muscle efficiency experienced by these patients contribute to this increased daily energy expenditure from breathing. This increased work of breathing results in an increased daily energy requirement. If patients do not ingest additional calories to meet these increased needs, they lose weight.

Frequent, recurrent respiratory infections: Respiratory infections may increase metabolic rate, depending on the severity of the illness, further contributing to weight loss.

Poor Nutritional Intake

Factors that may result in inadequate intake in patients with COPD include

- chronic sputum production and frequent coughing, which may alter desire for and taste of food
- shortness of breath and fatigue, which can interfere with the ability to prepare and ingest adequate meals
- depression from the illness, a possible cause of anorexia
- flattening of the diaphragm and pressure on the abdominal cavity during eating, resulting in early satiety
- oxyhemoglobin desaturation during eating, resulting in increased dyspnea, which further limits dietary intake
- side effects of medications such as nausea, vomiting, diarrhea, dysgeusia, dry mouth, and gastric irritation, which may limit dietary intake

Nutrition Therapy

Because patients with COPD have increased energy requirements combined with poor nutritional intake, they have difficulty meeting their caloric requirements and frequently lose weight. It is safe to assume that patients who are not ingesting their caloric requirements and present with weight loss also suffer from vitamin and mineral deficiencies. Certain electrolytes (calcium, magnesium, potassium, and phosphorus) are especially important in malnourished COPD patients because depletion of these electrolytes may contribute to the impairment of respiratory muscle function. When severely malnourished COPD patients are rapidly refed with glucose infusions, careful attention must be paid to these electrolytes because the need for them increases during anabolism. Inadequate electrolyte repletion in this setting can produce refeeding syndrome with severe metabolic consequences.

Therefore, the goals of nutrition therapy for COPD patients are to

- supply adequate calories, protein, vitamins, and minerals
- provide small, frequent meals with nutrient-dense foods such as peanut butter and jelly sandwiches, and soft-textured, easily consumed foods such as omelettes, yogurt, cottage cheese, and casseroles
- add high-calorie, high-protein, liquid nutritional supplements or milk shakes to the diet
- recommend foods that require little preparation, such as frozen dinners heated in a microwave oven
- recommend timing the main meal to correspond to the time when the patient's energy level is the highest
- encourage patients to rest before mealtime
- prescribe a daily multivitamin and mineral supplement

Mechanical Ventilation

Rationale for Nutrition Support

Patients with respiratory failure requiring mechanical ventilation cannot ingest food through the mouth because of the endotracheal tube, unless a tracheostomy (breathing tube transcutaneously inserted into the trachea) has been placed. Because many patients require mechanical ventilation for prolonged periods, nutrition support is necessary to prevent malnutrition.

Malnutrition associated with critical illness impairs cell-mediated immunity, alters immunoglobulin production, and impairs cellular resistance to infection. Therefore patients who are not fed for more than 7 to 10 days are at increased risk of infection and may take longer to be weaned from the ventilator. Conversely, ventilated patients with preexisting malnutrition who are fed have improved respiratory muscle strength and function, which may hasten weaning from the ventilator.

Feeding Options

The two methods available for feeding mechanically ventilated patients who cannot be fed through the mouth are tube feeding directly into the gut (enteral feeding) or through peripheral or central veins (parenteral feeding). Patients on mechanical ventilation are at risk for aspiration with enteral nutritional support. Those who have an altered mental status are at even greater risk of aspiration because they have incompetent swallowing and gag reflexes. In general, patients given postpyloric feedings into the duodenum or jejunum have a lower risk of aspiration compared with gastric feedings, in which the tube empties into the stomach.

Parenteral nutrition is indicated for patients who are malnourished and do not have a functioning gut (e.g., patients with bowel obstruction or ileus). The decision to begin parenteral nutritional support is made if the patient is not a candidate for enteral feedings and will be unable to eat for more than 7 to 10 days. (See Chapter 11 for fundamentals of nutrition support.)

Minimizing Effects of Nutrition Support on CO2 Production

The caloric and nutrient composition of the diet has a profound effect on gas exchange, especially CO_2 production. The respiratory quotient (RQ) is expressed as the ratio of CO_2 produced to oxygen consumed.

$$RQ = \frac{CO_2 \text{ produced}}{O_2 \text{ consumed}}$$

CO_2 production is greater during carbohydrate metabolism than during fat metabolism. A diet high in carbohydrate thus requires increased ventilation to eliminate the excess CO_2. Because this scenario can make weaning patients from mechanical support more difficult, some enteral nutrition support products have been specifically formulated with higher fat and lower carbohydrate contents for patients who are mechanically ventilated. It is essential to avoid overfeeding these patients because exceeding their caloric requirements will result in excessive CO_2 production and an increased RQ. This, in turn, can make weaning them from mechanical ventilation very difficult.

Cystic Fibrosis

Cystic fibrosis (CF), a life-threatening genetic disorder usually seen in children and young adults, presents with profuse, abnormally thick exocrine gland secretions. These excessive secretions may obstruct the pancreatic and bile ducts, intestines, and bronchi, resulting in coughing, dyspnea, and recurrent respiratory infections. Chronic lung disease and pancreatic insufficiency are the two most common problems in patients with CF. Most patients with CF (80 to 85 percent) have pancreatic insufficiency and consequent malabsorption of fat, protein, carbohydrate, vitamins, and minerals, which, if untreated, leads to malnutrition. Pancreatic enzyme supplements are administered with meals and snacks to assist with the absorption of nutrients. The amount and type of enzyme supplements depend on the degree of malabsorption and the fat content in the diet. Steatorrhea is considered a clinical indicator of fat malabsorption.

Causes of Weight Loss and Malnutrition

Malabsorption

Despite pancreatic enzyme supplementation, the energy and protein needs of CF patients are significantly increased by their loss of nutrients due to malabsorption and by higher than normal protein catabolism and energy expenditure due to frequent infections. Because of this combination of factors, CF patients often are unable to meet their protein and caloric needs. Consequently most suffer from muscle wasting, weakness, and malnutrition, and the associated effects on respiratory muscles and diaphragm strength. (See also Chapter 7 for GI malabsorption.)

Increased Work of Breathing

Patients with CF generally suffer from chronic bronchitis and airway obstruction, both of which increase the work of breathing. This increased work of breathing results in a higher energy expenditure.

Increased Pulmonary and Gastrointestinal Secretions

This common problem can result in coughing and vomiting and thus interfere with eating. Chest percussion, sometimes performed up to four times daily to clear secretions, may also interfere with adequate food intake.

Nutrition Therapy

Because of their increased nutrient needs and losses and often inadequate intake, patients with CF usually are unable to meet their caloric and protein requirements and maintain their weight. CF is usually diagnosed in infancy or early childhood, and monitoring growth and development in these patients is particularly important. Not uncommonly, CF patients remain at or fall below the fifth percentile in both weight and height for their age on the pediatric growth charts. The goals of nutritional therapy for CF patients are to

- supply adequate dietary calories, protein, vitamins, and minerals
- provide high-calorie, high-protein meals with added salt and include nutrient-dense snacks 2 to 3 times daily

- plan a moderate- to high-fat diet (30 to 40 percent of total calories from fat) with pancreatic enzyme replacement adjusted to avoid malabsorption in patients with pancreatic insufficiency
- add milkshakes or nutritional supplements to increase calories and protein
- encourage patients to plan their main meal to coincide with the time of day when their energy level is the highest, because they may find it difficult to eat
- encourage patients to rest before mealtime
- provide high doses of fat-soluble vitamins (A, D, E, and K)

Vitamin K deficiency is observed clinically as an alteration in the prothrombin time (PT) because vitamin K is a cofactor in the clotting cascade. Additional vitamin E also should be prescribed (50 to 400 IU/day depending on the patient's age), along with a multivitamin and mineral supplement equivalent to twice the normal RDAs.

If patients continue to experience weight loss to such an extent that they fall below 85 percent of their ideal body weight, or if they have difficulty maintaining their weight, additional nutrition support may be necessary. Both enteral and parenteral feedings may be employed, as clinically indicated.

Malnourished patients with CF, especially children, may consume a regular diet during the day and receive enteral nutrition support via tube feeding at night while they sleep (nocturnal feedings). If patients still cannot meet their nutritional needs with nocturnal feeding supplements, 24-hour tube feedings may be necessary. Parenteral nutrition is indicated for patients who are malnourished and do not have a functioning gut (e.g., because of bowel obstruction or ileus).

Obstructive Sleep Apnea Syndrome

Obstructive sleep apnea syndrome (OSAS) is defined as recurrent episodes of apnea during sleep caused by occlusion of the upper airway. A primary risk factor for OSAS is obesity. Up to two-thirds of all patients who present with OSAS are obese. However, obesity alone is not sufficient to cause OSAS, because not all obese patients have this disorder. One factor associated with the development of OSAS may be an increased amount of fat surrounding the anatomic structure of the upper airway. Regardless of its exact etiology, symptoms of sleep apnea such as snoring and excessive daytime sleepiness should always be ascertained as part of the medical history in obese patients.

Causes of Weight Gain and Obesity

Fatigue due to chronic sleep disruption, a common complaint of patients with OSAS, may influence their eating behaviors. Often too tired and lacking in motivation to exercise, they tend to lead sedentary lifestyles. In addition, many patients with OSAS report falling asleep often after eating, which further decreases their energy expenditure. Certain overweight patients with OSAS also may be prone to binge eating as a result of depression about their illness and their body image. Whatever the exact causes, a combination of decreased physical activity and increased caloric consumption contributes to weight gain in these patients.

Nutrition Components of the Medical History

The following topics should be covered during the medical history of any obese patient with diagnosed or suspected OSAS.

- weight history and previous dieting experience
- sleep patterns
- frequency of meals and snacks especially after dinner
- binge eating during the day or night
- assessment of nutritional content (e.g., high fat, high sugar) of the diet
- exercise habits
- alcohol intake, including frequency and amount
- other medical problems the patient reports that may respond to dietary modification (e.g., hypertension, diabetes mellitus, cardiovascular disease)

Nutrition Therapy

Weight Loss

Because obesity is a risk factor for OSAS, weight loss is of primary importance. A weight loss as small as ten pounds can improve breathing and sleep patterns dramatically. In addition to weight loss counseling, patients with OSAS are most commonly treated with continuous positive airway pressure therapy (CPAP). Once CPAP treatment has been initiated, many sleep centers refer their patients to a registered dietitian for either individual or group nutritional counseling.

Low-Fat, Low-Calorie Diet

One pound of fat yields 3500 kcal. A net deficit of 500 kcal/day below the patient's maintenance caloric requirements for 7 days thus will result in a weight loss of one pound of fat per week. High-fat foods are the most calorically dense at 9 kcal/g compared to carbohydrate and protein sources, which provide 4 kcal/g. Thus reduction of high-fat food intake (fried foods, cheeses, hot dogs, cream sauces, and so on) significantly decreases calories and helps patients to lose weight. If patients snack in the middle of the night and throughout the day, fruits and pretzels are good choices. Other suggestions for achieving weight loss by reducing total calories include decreasing portion sizes, particularly the main entree, and increasing consumption of fruits, vegetables, and salads.

Increasing Activity

Once patients begin to feel better and have more energy, they should be encouraged to begin a low-intensity exercise program, such as walking 15 minutes once or twice a day.

Lung Transplantation

The nutritional implications for lung transplantation patients vary depending on whether they are awaiting or have received a transplant, and whether they are extubated (breathing on their own) or intubated (mechanically ventilated) following surgery. The following recommendations are listed accordingly.

Nutrition Assessment Prior to Lung Transplantation

Routine nutrition assessment prior to lung transplantation entails the following steps.

- Assess nutritional status using the patient's weight history.
- Assess nutritional status using visceral protein stores such as albumin, transferrin, and prealbumin (half-life: 2 days). If protein stores are depleted, supplement the diet with additional calories and high-protein milkshakes and snacks.
- Assess serum lipid levels. If cholesterol (normal: under 200 mg/dL) and triglyceride (normal: under 150 mg/dL) levels are elevated, appropriate modifications include incorporating foods low in saturated fat and cholesterol into the diet to reduce these levels.
- Monitor the patient's satiety level and gastrointestinal symptoms, such as bloating and gas, that could interfere with adequate dietary intake.

Nutrition Therapy Immediately Following Lung Transplantation

Appropriate nutrition therapy following lung transplantation involves the following measures.

- Increase protein and calories to promote repletion of stores and to assist with wound healing during the catabolic state following surgery.
- Decrease sodium intake if patients develop fluid retention.

Nutrition Therapy Upon Discharge

Patients treated with cyclosporine to prevent rejection of transplanted organs are prone to hyperkalemia (elevated serum potassium). Therefore, their dietary potassium intake must be limited. Cyclosporine also may elevate serum cholesterol and triglyceride levels, increasing the patient's risk of heart disease. Dietary intake of saturated fat and cholesterol should therefore be limited if the patient's lipid levels are elevated.

Patients receiving steroids such as prednisone to prevent organ rejection may experience a significant enough increase in appetite to cause weight gain and ultimately lead to obesity. Calorie and fat intake, as well as weight, should be carefully monitored following lung transplantation. Patients taking prednisone also may experience fluid retention, which requires limiting dietary sodium intake.

Chronic Obstructive Pulmonary Disease (COPD)

Scott Manaker and Frances Burke

Objectives

- To use the medical history and physical examination to identify factors affecting the nutritional status of a patient with pulmonary disease.
- To apply nutrition assessment techniques to the patient with pulmonary disease.
- To identify the causes of chronic weight loss in a patient with chronic obstructive pulmonary disease.
- To develop a nutritional care plan for a patient with chronic obstructive pulmonary disease who suffers from chronic weight loss.

PD, a 53-year-old woman diagnosed with COPD eight years ago, visits her physician complaining of dyspnea (shortness of breath) that has worsened progressively over the last three days since she caught a cold from her grandchildren. She explains that her customary shortness of breath worsens when she is sick or under increased stress, when the humidity is high or the temperature is extremely cold, and whenever she is exposed to certain perfumes. Currently, PD has two-pillow orthopnea (i.e., she experiences difficulty in breathing when lying in a prone position) and bilateral lower extremity edema. She has lost 40 pounds within the last year. Pulmonary function tests from last year confirm severe COPD with a forced expiratory volume (FEV1) of 0.65 L, a forced vital capacity (FVC) of 1.65 L and a ratio of FEV to FVC of 35%. A recent chest x-ray revealed hyperinflation of lung fields, with diminished lung markings in the upper lung fields.

Past Medical History

PD has been under treatment for hypertension for 12 years. She has no previous history of diabetes mellitus, thyroid disease, or liver disease.

Medications

PD is currently taking verapamil (Calan SR), furosemide (Lasix), potassium chloride (K-lyte CL), prednisone, theophylline (Theodur), ipratropium bromide (Atrovent), and albuterol (Ventolin). She is not presently taking a vitamin/mineral supplement. PD has no known food allergies.

Family History

PD's mother died at age 70 of a heart attack. Her father also died of a heart attack at age 73.

Social History

PD lives with her husband in a two-story home. They have four children and fourteen grandchildren. PD worked in a local department store as a saleswoman until last year, when she retired because of her illness. She formerly attended church regularly with her husband, but lately has been too tired to go. PD usually follows a low-salt, low-fat diet at home. Her husband has recently taken over the food shopping. She reports the following substance use.

Alcohol intake: None

Tobacco: 87 pack year smoking history; nonsmoker for one year.

Caffeine: One cup of coffee/day

Diet History

PD provided the following 24-hour dietary recall that reportedly reflects her typical daily intake.

PD's 24-Hour Dietary Recall

Breakfast (Home)	Farina	1 bowl
	White toast	1 slice
	Jelly	2 Tbs.
	Coffee	1 cup
	1% milk	4 oz.
Lunch (Home)	Low-fat yogurt	1 cup
	Apple juice	6 oz.
Dinner (Home)	Chicken breast	4 ounces
	Baked potato	1 medium
	Cooked carrots	1/2 cup
	Diet margarine	1 Tbs.
	Water	1 glass
Snack (Home)	Banana	1 medium

Total calories: 1170 kcal/day
Protein: 64 g/day (21% of calories)
Fat: 15% of calories
Carbohydrate: 64% of calories

Review of Systems

General: Weakness, fatigue, weight loss (40 pounds in the last year)

Mouth: Wears dentures (top and bottom)

GI: Poor appetite; no diarrhea, nausea, or vomiting

Extremities: No joint pain; has difficulty walking without a walker

Physical Examination

Vitals signs

Temperature: 97°F

Heart rate: 94 BPM

Respiration: 20 BPM

Blood pressure: 150/80 mm Hg

Anthropometric data

Height: 5'6"

Current weight: 147 lb (66.8 kg)

Usual weight: 187 lb (85 kg)

Ideal body weight: 130 lb (59 kg)

Percent ideal body weight: 113%

General: Frail woman in no acute distress

Skin: Ecchymoses

Head/neck: Thyroid unenlarged

Mouth: Properly fitting dentures; no sores; symmetrical soft palate and uvula

Cardiac: Regular rate and rhythm; normal first and second heart sounds; a third heart sound is also present as well; jugular venous distention and hepatojugular reflux noted

Lung: Increased A-P diameter, decreased breath sounds; diffuse expiratory wheezing throughout the chest with a prolonged expiratory phase

Abdomen: Nondistended, nontender; enlarged liver 12 cm in span; no splenomegaly; normal bowel sounds

Extremities: Pitting 2+ edema on both ankles

Rectal: Soft, brown stool in vault; test for occult blood negative (heme)

Neurological: Alert; appropriate reactions; good memory; no evidence of sensory loss

Laboratory Data

Patient's Values	Normal Values
Albumin: 4.3 g/dL	3.5–5.8 g/dL
Hemoglobin: 10.8 g/dL	12–15 g/dL
Hematocrit: 38%	40–48%
Cholesterol: 365 mg/dL	<200 mg/dL
Triglycerides: 150 mg/dL	<150 mg/dL

Case Questions

1. Using PD's current weight, calculate her percent weight change. Is this a significant weight loss?
2. What factors have contributed to PD's weight loss?
3. Based on PD's history, what may account for her severe fatigue?
4. How does poor nutritional status compromise pulmonary function?
5. Considering PD's nutritional status, why is her albumin normal?
6. What general conclusions can you draw regarding PD's diet?
7. What are appropriate nutritional goals for this patient?
8. Should a vitamin and mineral supplement be prescribed for this patient?
9. What specific recommendations may improve PD's nutritional and fluid status?

Answers begin on the following page.

Answers to Questions: Case 1

Part 1:   Nutrition Assessment

1. **Using PD's current weight, calculate her percent weight change. Is this a significant weight loss?**

    Applying the percent weight change equation to PD's case, we find

    $$\text{Percent weight change} = \frac{\text{Usual weight} - \text{Current weight}}{\text{Usual weight}} \times 100$$

    $$= \frac{187 \text{ lb} - 147 \text{ lb}}{187 \text{ lb}} \times 100$$

    $$= \frac{40 \text{ lb}}{187 \text{ lb}} \times 100 = 21.4\% \text{ change}$$

    A weight change greater than 15 percent within a one-year period is considered a severe weight loss.

2. **What factors have contributed to PD's weight loss?**

    PD has reduced lung function and therefore requires more energy to breathe. The normal daily intake of calories required to maintain body weight is insufficient to meet the demands of the excessive work of breathing in patients with COPD. Also, patients with pulmonary disease may ingest even fewer calories because they are too tired to prepare food or to eat a meal. Many patients with COPD complain that they become short of breath because chewing and swallowing food prevents them from breathing adequately, reducing the amount of oxygen in their blood (oxygen desaturation). Patients on home oxygen should be advised to use it when preparing and eating meals.

3. **Based on PD's history, what may account for her severe fatigue?**

    COPD, a debilitating condition often characterized by limited airflow in the lungs, can cause high concentrations of carbon dioxide in the blood, reducing oxygen available to the tissues and other organs. Clinical signs of COPD include dyspnea on exertion and fatigue, which together can ultimately interfere with the ability to lead a normal life.

4. **How does poor nutritional status compromise pulmonary function?**

    Weight loss is very common in patients with COPD. Patients who experience progressive weight loss to less than 90 percent of their ideal body weight are considered malnourished. The greater the severity of COPD, the greater the associated malnutrition and weight loss. Poor nutritional status can severely compromise a patient with COPD by adversely affecting pulmonary defense mechanisms and respiratory muscle structure and function. Altered pulmonary defense mechanisms include decreased surfactant production, decreased immunoglobulin levels, and impaired cellular resistance of the tracheobronchial mucosa to bacterial infection. In addition, poor nutritional status can affect pulmonary structure and function by causing a reduction in the diaphragmatic muscle mass. The reduced diaphragm results in loss of muscle strength and contractility, as well as a diminished vital capacity and depressed ventilatory response even to minimal exertion such as walking.

5. **Considering PD's nutritional status, why is her albumin normal?**

    Although PD sustained a chronic weight loss, she was able to maintain her visceral protein status. If acute weight loss recurred, PD's albumin would likely decrease because her visceral protein status would decline.

6. **What general conclusions can you draw regarding PD's diet?**

    An analysis of PD's actual intake indicates that she is consuming under 1200 kcal/day. Her diet is low in calories due to her poor appetite as well as the low-fat diet she has followed since she learned that she has high cholesterol.

Part 2:   Recommendations

7. **What are appropriate nutritional goals for this patient?**

    Providing adequate calories and protein for weight and body protein maintenance is a major goal of nutritional therapy for this patient. Managing PD's fluid balance to avoid dehydration in the future is also an important consideration. The following suggestions (box on p.294) for each meal are intended to increase her calorie and protein intake.

8. **Should a vitamin and mineral supplement be prescribed for this patient?**

    Yes. PD's usual diet is not supplying adequate vitamins and minerals, and she therefore would benefit from a multiple vitamin and mineral supplement. Because her diet is low in calories, achieving an adequate vitamin and mineral intake is difficult. PD is at increased risk for osteoporosis because she is on chronic corticosteroid therapy and her lifestyle is inactive. Therefore, at the minimum she should receive a calcium and vitamin B supplement and increase her dairy intake. Since PD's hemoglobin and hematocrit levels are low, she should be evaluated for iron deficiency anemia. Patients with iron deficiency anemia benefit from foods with higher iron content, such as lean red meat, dark-green leafy vegetables, and dried fruit.

Recommended Intake for PD

Breakfast (Home)	Coffee	1 cup
	Instant oatmeal	1 cup
	2% milk	6 oz.
	Raisins	1/4 cup
	Whole wheat toast	1 slice
	Diet margarine	1 Tbs.
Snack (Home)	Apple juice	6 oz.
Lunch (Home)	Tuna salad	3 oz.
	Whole wheat bread	1 slice
	Tomato soup (low sodium)	1 bowl
Snack (Home)	2% milk	1/2 cup
	Saltines (low sodium)	6
	Peanut butter	1 Tbs.
	Jelly	2 Tbs.
Dinner (Home)	Lean ground beef patty	4 oz.
	Baked potato	1 medium
	Tomatoes	3 slices
	Applesauce	1/2 cup.
	Diet margarine	1 Tbs.
Snack (Home)	Low-fat yogurt	6 oz.
	Total calories: 2237 kcal/day	
	Protein: 92 g/day (16% of calories)	
	Fat: 29% of calories	
	Carbohydrate: 55% of calories	

9. **What specific recommendations may improve PD's nutritional and fluid status?**

   - PD should be encouraged to adopt the following measures to increase her intake and thereby improve her nutritional and fluid status.
   - Rest before mealtime.
   - Eat foods that are easy to chew, such as soft meats and casseroles.
   - Avoid eating in bed; sit upright when eating.
   - Drink Carnation Instant Breakfast, Ensure, Sustacal, or add nonfat powdered milk for additional calories, protein, vitamins, and minerals.
   - Use the microwave oven to prepare convenience foods and decrease cooking time.
   - Consume small, frequent meals consisting of nutrient-dense foods, such as peanut butter and jelly sandwiches.

- Consume the main meal when her energy level is at its highest.
- Avoid foods that may cause gas or bloating and make breathing more difficult.
- Increase intake of fiber-rich foods to enhance gastrointestinal motility.
- Limit fluid intake during meals and salty foods such as canned, smoked, or cured products to avoid fluid retention and bloating. Instead, drink fluids between meals.

Cystic Fibrosis and Tube Feeding

Maria R. Mascarenhas and Natalie McGuigan

Objectives

- To conduct nutritional assessment of patients with cystic fibrosis.
- To understand the nutritional abnormalities commonly observed in patients with cystic fibrosis.
- To develop a nutritional care plan for patients with cystic fibrosis including specialized diets, tube feeding, and enzyme management.
- To monitor appropriately the nutritional status of patients with cystic fibrosis.

FC, a 21-year-old female with cystic fibrosis, presents to the Pulmonary Clinic with a one-week history of increased cough, shortness of breath, and a three-pound weight loss. She reports increased mucous production and a change in its color from yellow to green. She also reports three to four foul-smelling, floating stools daily. On physical exam she manifests tachypnea (elevated respiratory rate) and tachycardia (elevated heart rate). Her chest examination reveals new crackles in the right upper lobe, and her pulmonary function tests have decreased by 20 percent. Because of her worsening symptoms, abnormal physical examination, and decreasing pulmonary function, she is diagnosed with an acute exacerbation of cystic fibrosis and admitted to the hospital.

Past Medical History

FC's cystic fibrosis was diagnosed when she was five years old on the basis of her recurrent upper respiratory tract infections, bulky, foul-smelling stools, and hepatomegaly. She has been hospitalized a number of times for acute cystic fibrosis exacerbations. In addition, she has scoliosis, diagnosed two years ago, and hearing loss secondary to frequent intravenous antibiotic therapy. FC has no known food or drug allergies.

Menstrual History

Menses started late at age 15 years, which is commonly seen in females with cystic fibrosis due to chronic malnutrition.

Medications

FC's current medication regimen includes pancrelipase (Pancrease), MT10 (10 capsules per meal, 5 capsules with snacks), cotrimoxazole (Bactrim), cefaclor (Ceclor), albuterol (Ventolin) and acetylcysteine (Mucomyst) via inhalation, cromolyn sodium (Intal inhalers), triamcinolone acetonide (Azmacort inhaler), rhDNase (Pulmozyme via inhalation), and ranitidine (Zantac). She also receives frequent chest percussion therapy.

Vitamins and Dietary Supplements

FC's current vitamin therapy includes a multivitamin with iron BID, vitamin E (400 IU) QD, and vitamin K (5 mg 3 times per week). She also takes the food supplement Scandishakes twice daily. This high-calorie, high-protein powder supplement mixes with milk and provides 600 kcal, 12 grams of protein, and 30 grams of fat per eight-ounce serving.

Social History

FC, a junior in college, lives at home with her parents. She denies smoking, alcohol, drug use, and sexual activity.

Diet History

FC follows a high-calorie, high-protein, high-fat, extra-salt diet that includes three meals and three snacks daily. She also drinks two servings per day of a liquid supplement (Scandishakes) recommended by the registered dietitian. FC prepares her breakfast and lunch, and her mother prepares dinner.

Review of Systems

Results of the review of systems were unremarkable except in the following regards.

General: Weight loss (3 lb in one week), fatigue

Lung: Shortness of breath, cough, green mucous production

GI: Poor appetite, 3 to 4 foul-smelling stools per day

Physical Examination

Vital signs

Temperature: 101°F

Heart rate: 110 BPM

Respiration: 24 BPM

Blood pressure: 134/74 mm Hg

Anthropometric data

Height: 5'2" (158 cm)

Current weight: 88 lb (40 kg)

Usual weight (UBW): 91 lb (41 kg)

Ideal weight (IBW): 110 lb (50 kg)

Percent IBW: 80%

Percent UBW: 97%

Triceps skinfold (TSF): 13 mm (<25th percentile)

Mid-arm muscle circumference (MAMC): 200 mm (20 cm)
   (<25th percentile)

The patient's physical examination is normal except for the following observations.

General: Thin, ill-appearing female

Skin: Warm to the touch

HEENT: Right nasal polyp

Chest: New rales and rhonchi in right upper lung zone, no dullness
   to percussion or wheezing

Cardiac: Elevated rate, normal rhythm, no murmurs

Laboratory Data

Patient's Values	Normal Values
Albumin: 4.2 g/L	3.5–5.8 g/L
Hemoglobin: 13.4 mg/dL	12–14 mg/dL
Prothrombin time: 14 seconds	0–15 seconds

Treatment

FC has been in the hospital for one week. During that time she has received intravenous antibiotics, respiratory treatments, and vigorous chest percussion to help mobilize her secretions. Since her admission, her appetite has remained poor, and she has lost an additional four pounds. Three-day calorie counts reveal that she is consuming 500 calories and 20 grams of protein per day.

Follow-up

FC was discharged when her weight reached 91 pounds. At that time she was still receiving nasogastric tube feedings, which she was advised to continue for one month. She then returned for her one-month follow-up visit.

Case Questions

1. What is the importance of assessing FC's nutritional status?

2. What factors are most likely contributing to FC's weight loss?

3. What nutritional problems are patients with cystic fibrosis at risk of developing?

4. Is albumin a valid indicator of FC's nutritional status?

5. Are FC's present nutritional status and vitamin therapy appropriate?

6. Is FC's present enzyme therapy appropriate?

7. Assume that FC's intake is significantly below her requirements, she continues to experience weight loss, and tube feedings are initiated to supplement her intake. What are the advantages of nocturnal feedings for patients with cystic fibrosis?

8. Considering FC's admission history and physical examination, what long-term feeding recommendations should be given?

9. What parameters should be monitored during the one-month follow-up visit?

10. Assuming that FC is tolerating her tube feedings well, what are her long-term feeding options?

Answers begin on the following page.

Answers to Questions: Case 2

Part 1:   Nutrition Assessment

1. **What is the importance of assessing FC's nutritional status?**

   The importance of nutritional status in the long-term survival and well-being of patients with cystic fibrosis is well documented. Pancreatic insufficiency occurs in about 80 percent of patients with cystic fibrosis. Analysis of pancreatic secretions in these patients shows a marked decrease in the amounts of water, electrolytes, and the enzymes lipase, protease, and amylase. As a consequence of these deficiencies, inadequate digestion of food results in malabsorption and malnutrition with growth retardation. Protein-energy malnutrition is associated with an impaired immune response and an increased risk of pulmonary infection. Muscle weakness and declining respiratory muscle strength may adversely affect survival.

2. **What factors are most likely contributing to FC's weight loss?**

   A negative calorie balance accounts for FC's weight loss. Anorexia is compounded by ongoing malabsorption and by increased energy needs due to fever and infections. FC's poor appetite is due partly to her current lung infection and partly to her antibiotic therapy. Esophagitis, biliary tract disease, salt depletion, and vitamin and mineral deficiency cause altered taste (dysgeusia) and may contribute to decreased appetite. Psychosocial factors that commonly contribute to anorexia should also be considered. FC's bulky, foul-smelling stools suggest fat malabsorption. In addition, FC has protein losses due to maldigestion caused by pancreatic enzyme insufficiency.

3. **What nutritional problems are patients with cystic fibrosis at risk of developing?**

   Patients with cystic fibrosis are at risk of developing multiple nutrient deficiencies with associated clinical manifestations. Protein and energy deficiencies lead to wasting and growth retardation. Protein deficiency also may lead to hypoalbuminemia and resultant edema.

   The most commonly encountered deficiency involves vitamin K and results in coagulopathy. Vitamin E deficiency can lead to hemolytic anemia in infants and to neuropathy, ophthalmoplegia, ataxia, and diminished vibration sense and proprioception in older children and adults. Vitamin D deficiency causes rickets in young children and osteomalacia in adults. Vitamin A deficiency can lead to elevated intracranial pressure, conjunctival xerosis, and night blindness.

   Deficiencies of the water-soluble vitamins B6 and B12 also occur frequently in CF patients. Vitamin B12 deficiency results in macrocytic anemia and neuropathy. This deficiency occurs as a result of pancreatic insufficiency when patients are not receiving (or are not complying with) enzyme therapy. Although salt depletion is uncommon even in cystic fibrosis patients, its presence leads to lethargy, weakness, dehydration, and metabolic alkalosis. Essential fatty acid deficiency results in desquamation, thrombocytopenia, and poor wound healing.

4. **Is albumin a valid indicator of FC's nutritional status?**

The circulating protein albumin is an indicator of visceral protein stores. Hypoalbuminemia reflects poor protein intake, increased protein losses, and may suggest acute visceral protein depletion. This deficiency may develop in as little as two weeks. Most commonly, patients with cystic fibrosis are malnourished at the time of diagnosis and throughout their lives, but their albumin levels are normal until the terminal stages of their disease because the body preserves protein stores in chronically ill patients. Therefore, the clinical diagnosis of malnutrition should be based on physical exam findings such as temporal and interosseus muscle wasting. Anthropometric results such as diminished triceps skinfold thickness and mid-arm muscle circumference reflect fat and muscle wasting due to chronically inadequate protein and energy intake.

5. **Are FC's present nutritional status and vitamin therapy appropriate?**

Nutrition therapy: A high-calorie, high-fat, and high-protein diet is indicated for patients with cystic fibrosis because of their high caloric, protein, and fat requirements. Extra salt is needed to replace the large amounts of sodium lost in perspiration. Six small meals per day generally are better tolerated than fewer but larger meals by patients with high caloric requirements. According to the Cystic Fibrosis Consensus Report, a patient whose weight is less than 85 percent of ideal body weight should receive enteral supplementation via nasogastric tube or enterostomy. Because oral high-calorie supplements have not been successful in meeting FC's caloric needs, supplemental tube feedings should be implemented.

Vitamin therapy: Most patients with cystic fibrosis suffer from pancreatic insufficiency, which causes malabsorption of protein, carbohydrate, and fat. Even with appropriate enzyme therapy, fat malabsorption and associated fat-soluble vitamin deficiencies may still persist. A daily multivitamin supplement enriched in fat-soluble vitamins is indicated in these patients. Vitamin K is produced by microorganisms in the gut. Antibiotic therapy significantly decreases gut bacteria and, as a result, diminishes vitamin K production. Therefore, vitamin K supplements should be given to all patients receiving chronic antibiotic therapy.

6. **Is FC's present enzyme therapy appropriate?**

Malabsorption should be suspected in any patient with cystic fibrosis who reports an increased incidence of foul-smelling, floating stools. Such patients require higher enzyme dosages to help them digest and absorb fat. Presently, FC is taking 10 capsules per meal and 5 capsules per snack of pancrease MT 10 (10,000 units of lipase per capsule).

Instead of increasing the number of MT 10s, changing the prescription to MT 16s (16,000 units of lipase per capsule) and altering the dosage to 8 capsules per meal and 4 capsules per snack will increase the total units of lipase the patient receives and decrease the number of capsules the patient must ingest with each meal and snack. The usual recommended dose is 1500 to 2000 units of lipase/kg per meal.

Part 2:   Feeding Options

7. Assume that FC's intake is significantly below her requirements, she continues to experience weight loss, and tube feedings are initiated to supplement her intake. What are the advantages of nocturnal feedings for patients with cystic fibrosis?

Nocturnal feedings supplement oral intake and increase caloric intake, but permit patients to lead a normal lifestyle during the day. Night feedings normally do not interfere with usual patterns of daytime eating. However, some patients may feel full in the morning after nocturnal tube feeding and may therefore be inclined to skip breakfast.

8. Considering FC's admission history and physical examination, what long-term feeding recommendations should be given?

FC is clearly malnourished. She has anorexia and needs supplemental nutrition. Because FC tolerated the nocturnal tube feeding regimen and demonstrated improvement in her nutritional status, this modality should be continued. One option for FC is to continue nocturnal naso-gastric feedings after hospital discharge. This requires inserting the naso-gastric tube every night, infusing the formula, and removing the tube in the morning. While enteral feedings are successful in the short term, compliance decreases when they are required for more than 6 to 12 weeks. However, studies have shown that tube feedings for a period of less than three months do not yield long-term benefits. A permanent feeding tube is therefore recommended for patients who need supplemental feedings for an extended period of time. A percutaneous gastrostomy tube is recommended because it can be placed either endoscopically or radiologically with ease. General anesthesia usually is not required for this procedure, and recovery time is short when compared to a surgically placed gastrostomy tube.

Part 3:   Follow-up

9. What parameters should be monitored during the one month follow-up visit?

The following parameters should be followed during FC's one-month follow-up visit.

Nutritional status Weight must be measured and weight change noted. FC's nutritional intake and tube feeding also should be reviewed using a 24-hour diet recall.

Tolerance Assess symptoms such as vomiting, diarrhea, and gastroesophageal reflux to determine continued tolerance of the tube feedings. Also ask FC if she is having problems administering the tube feedings or handling tubing and other apparatus.

Enzymes Review FC's enzyme dosage and ask her about stool characteristics to determine if she still has symptoms of malabsorption.

10. **Assuming that FC is tolerating her tube feedings well, what are her long-term feeding options?**

    Because FC is doing well, placement of a permanent percutaneous gastrostomy tube or gastrostomy button should be discussed. A gastrostomy button is a low-profile device used instead of a gastrostomy tube. The external configuration of the gastrostomy button is at the skin level, making it cosmetically more appealing. Most older children and adults opt for placement of the gastrostomy button. If significant vomiting or gastroesophageal reflux had developed, then a permanent gastrojejunostomy tube might have been considered. This tube, which is placed via the gastrostomy site into the jejunum, permits the infusion of formula directly into the jejunum, thus decreasing vomiting and gastroesophageal reflux.

See Chapter Review Questions, pages A15–A16.

REFERENCES

Aitken ML, Fiel SB. Cystic fibrosis. *Dis Mon* 1993;39(1):1–52.

Cannella PC, Bowser EK, Guyer LK, et al. Feeding practices and nutrition recommendations for infants with cystic fibrosis. *J Am Diet Assoc* 1993;93(3): 297–300.

Chin R, Haponk EF. Nutrition, Respiratory Function, and Disease. In Shils ME, Olson JA, Shike M (eds). *Modern Nutrition in Health and Disease.* 8th ed. Philadelphia: Lea and Febiger, 1994.

Consensus Report. Bethesda, MD: Cystic Fibrosis Foundation. Vol. 1, Section V, April 1990.

Engelen MP, Schols AM, Baken WC, et al. Nutritional depletion in relation to respiratory and peripheral skeletal muscle function in out-patients with COPD. *Eur Respir J* 1994;7(10):1793–1797.

Fiaccadori E, Coffrini E, Ronda N. et al. Hypophosphatemia in course of COPD: prevalence, mechanisms, and relationships with skeletal muscle phosphorus content. *Chest* 1990;97(4):857–868.

Grant JP. Nutrition care of patients with acute and chronic respiratory failure. *Nut Clin Pract* 1994;9(1):11–17.

Heijerman HG. Chronic obstructive lung disease and respiratory muscle function: the role of nutrition and exercise training in cystic fibrosis. *Respir Med* 1993;87 (Suppl B):49–51.

Kersten, Laurel. *Comprehensive Respiratory Nursing: A Decision-Making Approach*. Philadelphia: W.B. Saunders, 1989.

Kryger MH, Roth T, Dement WC. *Principles and Practice of Sleep Medicine*. 2nd ed. Philadelphia: W.B. Saunders, 1994.

Kuo CD, Shiao GM, Lee JD, et al. The effects of high fat and high carbohydrate diet loads on gas exchange and ventilation in COPD patients and normal subjects. *Chest* 1993;104(1):189–196.

Laaban JP, Kouchakji B, Dore MF, et al. Nutritional status of patients with chronic obstructive pulmonary disease and acute respiratory failure. *Chest* 1993; 103(5):1362–1368.

Schols AM, Soeters PB, Dingemans AM, et al. Prevalence and characteristics of nutritional depletion in patients with stable COPD eligible for pulmonary rehabilitation. *Am Rev Respir Dis* 1993;147(5):1151–1156.

Steinkamp G, Von der Hardt H. Improvement of nutritional status and lung function after long-term nocturnal gastrostomy feedings in cystic fibrosis. *J Pediatr* 1994;124(2):244–249.

Talpers S, Romberger DJ, Bunce SB, et al. Nutritionally associated increased carbon dioxide production: excess total calories vs. high proportion of carbohydrate calories. *Chest* 1992;102(2):551–555.

Tizzano EF, Buchwald M. Recent advances in cystic fibrosis research. *J Pediatr* 1993;122(6):985–988.

Weinsier RL, Morgan SL. Nutritional support of medical problems. In *Fundamentals of Clinical Nutrition*. St. Louis: Mosby, 1993.

Wilmott RW, Fiedler MA. Recent advantages in the treatment of cystic fibrosis. *Pediatr Clin North Am* 1994;41(3):431–451.

10

Renal Disease

Gail Morrison, Jean Stover, Nancy Matthews, Eileen Smith, and Lisa K. Diewald

Objectives

- To understand the various stages of renal disease and adjust patients' diets accordingly.
- To recognize the various stages, signs and symptoms, and treatment modalities of renal disease and to regulate a patient's protein intake appropriately.
- To devise diets that provide sufficient caloric intake to prevent catabolism in patients with renal disease.
- To regulate sodium, potassium, and phosphorous intake and maintain normal serum levels of these minerals.
- To balance fluid intake and excretion in patients with renal disease.
- To assess the need for vitamin and mineral supplementation in patients with renal disease.

Acute Renal Failure

Acute renal failure (ARF) is characterized by a sudden decline in the glomerular filtration rate (GFR) of the kidney due to insults such as infection, exogenous nephrotoxins, trauma, dehydration, and shock resulting in ischemia. The goals of nutritional management for patients with ARF are to

- minimize uremia and maintain the chemical composition of the body as close to normal as possible

- preserve body protein stores until renal function returns
- maintain fluid, electrolyte, and acid-base homeostasis

Patients with ARF are at high risk for malnutrition because of underlying illnesses, recent surgical procedures, or trauma, all generally catabolic states. In ARF precipitated by major trauma, critical illness, or sepsis, patients frequently undergo metabolic changes that accelerate degradation of protein and amino acids and result in the loss of lean body mass. The dramatic effects of this catabolic state include poor wound healing and increased infection and mortality rates.

Decisions on implementing aggressive nutrition therapy depend on the patient's nutritional status and catabolic rate, the phase of ARF with or without residual GFR, and clinical indications for initiating dialysis treatments, such as the development of symptoms of uremia. Thus nutrition therapy for the patient with ARF should be highly individualized.

Nutrition Therapy

Protein

Restricting protein intake to 0.6 g/kg/day is indicated for the nonhypercatabolic, nondialyzed patient with ARF whose GFR falls to less than 10 ml/min. The protein intake of patients with ARF who are receiving hemodialysis should be liberalized to 1.1 to 1.4 g/kg/day. Patients receiving peritoneal dialysis are encouraged to ingest 1.2 to 1.5 g/kg of protein each day. Severely catabolic patients with ARF may have even higher protein requirements.

Calories

Caloric requirements for patients with ARF vary depending on the degree of hypermetabolism present. Usual recommendations are 35 kcal/kg/day. Patients who have adequate gastrointestinal tract function but cannot tolerate food because of anorexia, nausea, or poor compliance should receive nourishment by enteral tube feeding. Those with a dysfunctional GI tract require total parenteral nutrition (TPN).

Peripheral insulin resistance may cause hyperglycemia in catabolic patients with ARF, and their blood glucose levels therefore should be closely monitored.

Vitamins and Minerals

Vitamin and mineral requirements for patients with ARF vary depending on their nutritional status and whether they are dialyzed on admission. Serum electrolytes must be closely monitored in all patients with ARF. Initially, serum potassium and phosphate are likely to be elevated and serum sodium lowered in nondialyzed patients who are oliguric. Patients with acute intrinsic renal failure—most often defined as acute tubular necrosis (ATN), the major cause of

ARF—may experience salt and water overload during the oliguric phase and salt and water depletion during the diuretic or recovery phase of the disease. In the recovery phase, sodium, potassium, and fluid usually must be replaced. Oliguric or anuric patients receiving hemodialysis usually still require a sodium restriction of 2 to 3 g/day and a potassium restriction of 1.5 to 3 g/day. Those undergoing peritoneal dialysis or frequent hemodialysis (more than three times per week) usually have more liberal sodium and potassium allowances.

Fluids

Daily fluid intake for oliguric patients should equal urine output plus approximately 500 ml to replace insensible losses, which increase if the patient has a fever. Most anuric patients can tolerate approximately 1000 ml/day with hemodialysis three times per week. These restrictions may be liberalized in patients receiving continuous or daily peritoneal dialysis or hemodialysis more frequently than three times per week.

Intravenous infusions of medications and TPN used to treat acutely ill patients with ARF often involve large volumes of fluid. Complications of such treatment, including fluid overload, edema, and hyponatremia, can be alleviated by initiating continuous arteriovenous hemofiltration (CAVH) to maintain fluid balance. In CAVH, catheters are placed into a large artery and vein (often, the femoral artery and vein). The blood flows through a small filtering device with a large pore membrane where plasma is filtered and albumin and blood products return to the vascular space through the vein. This form of therapy removes large volumes of essentially albumin-free plasmanate, leaving water and electrolytes in a concentration equal to normal serum levels. TPN can be combined with CAVH to provide intravenous nutrition while controlling salt and water balance and removing small amounts of metabolic waste products that accumulate in renal failure. Continuous arteriovenous hemodiafiltration (CAVHD) combines hemodialysis and hemofiltration simultaneously and removes larger amounts of solutes as well as large volumes of fluid.

Chronic Renal Failure (Predialysis)

The objectives of nutrition therapy for patients with chronic renal failure (CRF) prior to dialysis or renal transplantation are:

1. retarding the progression of CRF while providing adequate calories to maintain or achieve ideal body weight

2. preventing or alleviating the symptoms of uremia and restoring biochemical balance while providing adequate calories to maintain or achieve ideal body weight

Nutrition Therapy

Protein

In CRF, as the GFR and excretion of nitrogenous wastes declines, it is necessary to control the level of protein intake while continuing to maintain a positive nitrogen balance. Protein restriction can minimize the symptoms of uremic toxicity by reducing the production of nitrogenous wastes in the blood. A growing body of evidence also suggests that protein restriction early in the course of CRF due to glomerular damage may slow the progression of the disease and delay the need to initiate dialysis therapy. The generally accepted level of protein restriction is 0.6 g/kg/day (using an adjusted body weight if the patient is obese). Approximately 65 percent of high biological value protein should be incorporated to ensure that essential amino acid requirements are met. The biological value of a dietary protein is determined by its constituent amino acids, with the highest value given to proteins that contain all essential amino acids in concentrations that meet nutritional requirements when fed at adequate levels. A more liberal protein intake of 0.8 g/kg/day may be recommended for patients who are malnourished.

When patients exhibit significant proteinuria, as in diabetic nephropathy, the daily urinary protein losses should be added to the daily allowance. Additional increased protein needs due to catabolism from use of corticosteroid therapy or recent surgery may contraindicate limiting dietary protein.

Calories

The daily recommendations for adequate energy intake for individuals with chronic renal insufficiency not yet on dialysis are generally 35 kcals/kg to maintain body weight and allow for effective protein utilization. Calories from complex and simple carbohydrates must be included in the diet to provide adequate energy to prevent weight loss. Adding regular carbonated beverages, hard candy, fruit ices, fruit drinks, sugar, honey, and jelly to the diet accomplishes this goal.

Fat

Additional fat may be needed in the diet to provide adequate calories for patients with CRF. If the patient is not hypertriglyceridemic, fat calories can be increased using mono- and polyunsaturated fat sources. The patient's lipid levels should be monitored, and an effort should be made to keep cholesterol and LDL levels within normal limits. Pharmacological therapy also may be considered to achieve these goals.

Sodium

As renal failure progresses, renal sodium excretion subsequently falls. Serum sodium concentration is a result of the intake of dietary sodium and the amount of water ingested minus the sodium eliminated by the body. Because sodium is essentially eliminated by urinary excretion, sodium intake may have to be limited to prevent sodium retention, generalized edema, hypertension, and/or congestive heart failure, especially in the advanced stages of renal failure when excretion diminishes. Sodium balance can usually be maintained by limiting sodium intake to 2 to 3 grams per day, but occasionally a sodium restriction of 1 gram per day is needed. The typical American diet contains between 4 and 8 grams of sodium per day.

Measuring urinary sodium may be helpful in determining how much sodium is being returned. Urinary sodium is reported in milliequivalents (mEq), making it necessary to convert from milligrams to milliequivalents to determine how many milliequivalents of sodium are associated with any given diet. To convert milligrams of sodium to milliequivalents, divide the number of milligrams by the molecular weight of sodium (23 mg Na = 1 mEq Na). For example, assuming that a low-sodium diet is limited to 2000 mg/day, it contains 87 mEq of sodium (Table 10-1).

Potassium

The kidney usually handles potassium efficiently, and thus a dietary restriction is often unnecessary until the latter stages of CRF. When serum potassium levels are greater than 5.0 mEq/day, a potassium restricted diet of 2 to 3 g/day (51 to 77 mEq/day) should be initiated (Table 10-2). Use of an angiotensin converting enzyme (ACE) inhibitor to control blood pressure in some individuals may require a mild to moderate potassium restriction, even with good urine output. ACE inhibitors suppress the renin-angiotensin system, resulting in decreased aldosterone levels and subsequent elevations in serum potassium levels.

Table 10-1   High sodium foods.

Bacon	Nuts	Canned soups*
Salt pork	Popcorn	Boullion cubes*
Sausages	Processed cheeses	Dried soup mixes
Scrapple	Chinese food, especially soups	Salted crackers*
Ham	Pickles	Pizza
Dried beef	Relish	Delicatessen salads
Tongue, smoked	Sauerkraut	Packaged or prepared
Corned beef	Meat tenderizers	casserole type dishes
Frankfurters	Soy sauce	Frozen dinners
Cold cuts	Barbecue sauces	Olives
Canned or smoked meats or fish	Chili sauce	Worcestershire sauce
Canned seafood	Packaged gravy	Vegetable juice
Potato chips	Tomato juice*	
Pretzels	Canned tomato sauce	

Generally, any labeled food with a sodium content greater than 400 mg per serving is considered high in so-dium.

*These items may be purchased "salt-free" in most grocery stores.

Table 10-2   Foods with high and low potassium content.

High-potassium vegetables and juices	High-potassium fruits and juices
Artichokes	Apricots
Beans (navy, lentil, pinto, kidney)	Avodados
Broccoli	Bananas
Brussels sprouts	Cantaloupes
Carrots, raw	Dates
French fries	Figs
Greens	Honeydew melons
Lima beans	Mangos
Parsnips	Nectarines
Potato, baked	Oranges, orange juice
Pumpkin	Papayas
Spinach	Prunes
Sweet potato	Raisins
Tomato	Rhubarb
Winter squash (butternut, acorn)	Watermelon
Tomato juice	Apricot nectar
Vegetable	Prune juice

Low-potassium vegetables and juices	Low-potassium fruits and juices
Asparagus	Apples, apple juice
Beets	Applesauce
Cabbage	Blueberries
Carrots, cooked	Cherries
Cauliflower	Cranberries, cranberry juice
Celery	Fruit cocktail
Corn	Grapefruits, grapefruit juice (only 4 oz. per day)
Cucumber	Grapes, grape juice
Eggplant	Lemons
Green beans	Limes
Green peppers	Peaches, fresh (small)
Kale	Pears, fresh (small), pear nectar
Lettuce	Pineapples, pineapple juice (only 4 oz. per day)
Okra	Plums
Onions	Raspberries (1 cup)
Peas	Strawberries (1 cup)
Potato (only when presoaked)	Tangerines
Radishes	
Wax beans	
Zucchini	

Calcium and Phosphate

Renal osteodystrophy refers to the complex lesions of bone present in the majority of patients with CRF, including osteitis fibrosa and osteomalacia. Restriction of dietary phosphate has been shown to prevent the development of secondary hyperparathyroidism, which is seen frequently in patients with CRF. Calcium supplementation and phosphate restriction usually are needed when the GFR reaches less than 25 ml/minute due to the decreased absorption of calcium secondary to abnormal vitamin D levels and decreased excretion of phosphate (Table 10-3). At this level of renal function, glomerular filtration is inadequate to excrete a normal dietary phosphate load, and a phosphate restriction of 8 to 12 mg/kg/day is recommended. Because foods rich in phosphate, such as dairy products, also are rich in calcium, calcium supplements are needed when phosphate is restricted. When serum phosphate levels are less than 6.0 mg/dL, calcium carbonate or calcium acetate should be prescribed with meals to interfere with the absorption of phosphate in the small intestine and to provide added dietary calcium.

Table 10-3   High-phosphate foods

Foods	Portion size	Phosphate content (mg)
Dairy		
Cheese, all types	1 oz.	110–220
Half-and-half	1/2 cup	103
Cream pies or desserts	1/8	100
Custard	1/2 cup	155
Frozen custard	1/2 cup	100
Ice cream	1/2 cup	77
Ice milk	1/2 cup	80
Milk, all kinds	1/2 cup	123
Pudding	1/2 cup	123
Yogurt	1/2 cup	110–160
Protein foods		
Braunschweiger	1 oz.	70
Eggs	1 large	103
Liver	1 oz.	152
Peanut butter	2 Tbsp.	122
Salmon	1 oz.	70–80
Sardines	1 oz.	70–141
Tuna	1 oz.	55–70
Vegetables		
Baked beans and pork and beans	1/2 cup	132
Dried beans	1/2 cup	130
Dried peas	1/2 cup	89
Lentils	1/2 cup	90
Mixed vegetables	1/2 cup	58
Soybeans	1/2 cup	161
Bread and cereals		
Barley	1/2 cup	189
Bran	1/2 cup	350
Cornbread (from mix)	2-1/2 x 2-1/2 x 1-3/8 in.	209
Waffles (from mix)	7-in. diameter	257
Whole-grain breads	1 slice	60
Miscellaneous		
Chocolate	1 oz.	65
Nuts	1 oz.	102
Beverages		
Beer	12 oz.	50
Colas	12 oz.	54

Source: Norwood K. Renal osteodystrophy. In Stover J. *A Clinical Guide to Nutrition Care in End-Stage Renal Disease.* Chicago: The American Dietetic Association, 1994.

Water Balance and Fluid Restriction

Fluid intake for individuals with CRF should be balanced by their ability to eliminate fluid. As long as the urine output essentially equals the daily fluid intake, fluid balance is maintained. If edema becomes apparent, prescribing loop diuretics often increases sodium and water excretion sufficiently to maintain balance. In the latter stages of CRF, a fluid limit equal to the volume of urine output plus 500 ml/day for insensible fluid losses may be necessary to prevent edema and hyponatremia.

Vitamins and Iron

Protein and mineral restrictions to manage CRF almost always result in a diet deficient in vitamins. Supplementing folic acid (1 mg/day), pyridoxine (5 mg/day), the RDA for other B-complex vitamins, and ascorbic acid (60 to 100 mg/day) is often necessary. In addition, the kidney's inadequate conversion of vitamin D from 25-hydroxycholecalciferol [25(OH)D3] to its active form, 1,25-dihydroxycholecalciferol [1,25(OH)2D3], often requires supplementation of vitamin D in its active form. Vitamin A, on the other hand, may accumulate as CRF progresses and should not be supplemented. Vitamin preparations designed specifically for individuals with renal failure are available to meet these needs. Iron supplementation is often necessary for patients receiving erythropoietin therapy to correct anemia before initiating dialysis.

Dialysis

The goals of dietary management for patients on maintenance hemodialysis (HD) and maintenance peritoneal dialysis (PD), including both continuous ambulatory peritoneal dialysis (CAPD) and continuous cycling peritoneal dialysis (CCPD) are

1. maintaining protein equilibrium to prevent a negative nitrogen balance

2. maintaining serum potassium and sodium concentrations within an acceptable range and maintaining total body sodium as close to normal as possible

3. maintaining fluid homeostasis by preventing fluid overload or volume depletion

4. maintaining serum phosphate and calcium levels within an acceptable range to prevent renal osteodystrophy and metastatic calcification

Nutrition Therapy

Protein

Protein intake in patients undergoing maintenance dialysis must be controlled in two ways. First, protein intake must at least equal the minimum dietary protein requirements of such patients. Secondly, the maximum allowable protein intake must not significantly worsen the uremic syndrome. The loss of amino acids, and the catabolic stress of dialysis and the level of protein intake in the predialysis period may all contribute to protein malnutrition in the chronic dialysis patient. A daily protein allowance of 1.1 to 1.4 g/kg for HD patients and 1.2 to 1.5 g/kg for PD patients will often minimize the accumulation of excessive nitrogenous wastes, maintain a positive nitrogen balance, and replace the amino acids lost during dialysis. During episodes of peritonitis, patients receiving peritoneal dialysis have increased dietary protein needs due to greater losses of protein across an inflamed peritoneum.

Calories

The caloric intake for maintenance dialysis should be adequate to maintain or achieve ideal body weight. Unless the diet provides sufficient calories from carbohydrate and fat, endogenous protein is used for energy production, and the patient develops a negative nitrogen balance.

With PD, calories gained from glucose absorbed from the dialysate must be considered when determining total caloric needs to prevent excess weight gain and obesity.

Fats

Hyperlipidemia reportedly occurs in patients with CRF at a rate between 30 and 70 percent. These patients present with elevated LDL and triglyceride levels and normal or low HDL. Whether treatment of the hyperlipidemia decreases the incidence of coronary heart disease and prolongs life in these patients is unresolved. Dietary modifications aimed at decreasing cholesterol and triglyceride levels without adversely affecting protein and overall caloric intakes in dialysis patients are advisable if lipid levels are elevated. As in the predialysis phase of CRF, pharmacological therapy for hyperlipidemia may also be considered.

Sodium and Fluid

Daily sodium recommendations are determined by a patient's blood pressure, weight, and level of kidney function. Excessive ingestion of sodium may precipitate pulmonary edema and congestive heart failure. The fluid allowance for maintenance dialysis patients depends largely on their interdialytic weight gain. For patients on HD, sodium intake is generally restricted to 2 to 3 g/day, with a fluid allowance of 1000 ml/day plus the amount of urine output, if any. Sodium and water may be removed more easily with PD because it is performed daily or continuously. Therefore allowing these patients a more liberal sodium and water intake is often possible (see Table 10-1).

Potassium

Potassium intake must be individualized to maintain normal serum potassium levels. Patients on maintenance HD usually can maintain serum potassium levels between 3.5 and 5.5 mEq/L with diets containing 1.5 to 3 g/day (38 to 75 mEq/day). Patients on maintenance PD usually maintain a normal serum potassium level without restricting potassium intake. Occasionally, patients on PD may require potassium supplementation if serum potassium levels fall below normal.

Calcium and Phosphate

As renal function diminishes, phosphate excretion decreases. With a GFR less than 25 ml/min, filtration is inadequate to excrete a normal dietary phosphate load (1000 to 1800 mg). The goal of nutrition therapy is to achieve and maintain a serum phosphate level of approximately 4.0 to 6.0 mg/dL. Phosphate is widely distributed in foods, but is found primarily in muscle tissue (meats, poultry, and fish) and dairy products (see Table 10-3). Therefore reducing dietary phosphate intake often involves a concomitant reduction in total protein intake. For patients on maintenance HD, the usual phosphate restriction is 12 to 17 mg/kg/day. Patients on maintenance PD also may require some degree of phosphate restriction, but their increased protein needs make it difficult to restrict their phosphate intake to less than 15 mg/kg/day.

Controlling serum phosphate by diet alone usually is not possible, and as a consequence, dialysis patients often take phosphate binders to increase their phosphate excretion. Aluminum containing binders are used initially until the calcium × phosphorus product ≤ 70 or the serum phosphate is ≤ 6.0 mg/dL.

Vitamins and Iron

Patients on both PD and HD generally receive supplementation of folic acid (1 mg/day), pyridoxine (10 mg/day), the RDA for other B-complex vitamins, and ascorbic acid (60 to 100 mg/day) due to probable existing dietary deficiencies of these vitamins and losses occurring during dialysis. As in the predialysis phase of CRF, dialysis patients also may require supplements containing the active form of vitamin D, administered either orally or parenterally. Intermittent high doses of oral calcitriol or IV calcitriol given in HD may be used to suppress high levels of parathyroid hormone (PTH). Iron supplements for patients receiving either PD or HD usually are necessary if they also are receiving erythropoietin (EPO) therapy for anemia. Periodic administration of intravenous iron may be required if oral therapy cannot sustain a serum transferrin saturation greater than 20–30 percent or ferritin greater than 200–300 ng/ml (normal: 3 to 1321 ng/ml).

Renal Transplantation

The goal of nutritional management of patients who have undergone renal transplant surgery is to provide optimal nutrition without exacerbating the metabolic side effects of immunosuppressive drugs and other medical therapy. During acute tubular necrosis (ATN) and/or organ rejection, nutrient modifications may be necessary to prevent uremia and hyperkalemia, and to control hypertension and circulating blood volume.

Nutrition Therapy

Protein

Protein catabolism may occur in the postoperative period secondary to the stress of surgery and high doses of corticosteroids. The recommended daily protein intake for these patients is 1.3 to 2.0 g/kg, depending on graft function, stress, and metabolic needs. However, unless carbohydrate intake is markedly decreased, this high protein intake may cause excessive weight gain. Therefore a daily protein intake of 1.2 to 1.5 g/kg is a realistic goal that may be adjusted postoperatively as the patient's overall nutritional status changes.

Calories

Adequate calories along with protein are necessary in the postoperative period to promote wound healing and to withstand rejection, infection, and other complications. The recommended daily calorie intake for these patients is 30 to 35 kcal/kg, based on dry weight or usual body weight (UBW). Because increased appetite is a common side effect of corticosteroid therapy, the long-range goal is weight maintenance with controlled caloric intake, once a reasonable weight is achieved.

Carbohydrate

Hyperglycemia also may occur as a consequence of high-dose corticosteroid therapy and requires a diet limited in concentrated sweets. Patients who develop glucose intolerance or diabetes require a long-term, calorie-controlled diet to help achieve or maintain a reasonable body weight.

Fat

Hyperlipidemia frequently occurs after renal transplantation due to immunosuppressive and antihypertensive therapy, as well as obesity. Consequently, total dietary fat may need to be limited with emphasis on mono- and polyunsaturated fat intake in the long-term, chronic posttransplant period.

Sodium, Fluid, and Potassium

If corticosteroid therapy results in sodium and fluid retention, a reduced sodium intake is encouraged (see Table 10-1). In the absence of edema and hypertension, a more liberal sodium intake is acceptable. Fluid generally is not restricted unless ATN or rejection of the transplanted kidney is present. A higher incidence of hyperkalemia with the use of cyclosporine may indicate periodic potassium restriction, even in patients with a good functioning kidney. Rejection or ATN may also require potassium restriction (see Table 10-2).

Calcium and Phosphate

Generally neither dietary phosphate restriction nor phosphate binding medication is needed when the transplanted kidney is functioning well. In fact, hypophosphatemia due to increased phosphate excretion and bone uptake sometimes develops in the acute posttransplant period and may require a high-phosphate diet (see Table 10-3) and/or phosphate supplementation. Calcium supplementation may be required in the chronic post-transplant period because corticosteroid therapy interferes with calcium absorption.

Vitamins and Iron

Renal vitamin preparations may be continued temporarily in the posttransplant patient, especially if dietary restrictions are needed to treat ATN or rejection. Iron therapy may also continue if EPO administration is necessary to treat anemia.

Nephrotic Syndrome

Nephrotic syndrome, a kidney disorder with many etiologies, is characterized by large quantities of protein (greater than 3.0 to 3.5 g/day) in the urine. In all cases, this proteinuria is a consequence of damage to the glomerular basement membrane resulting in its increased permeability to protein. Patients often exhibit poor appetite, muscle wasting, and protein malnutrition secondary to these large protein losses. Nephrotic syndrome is also characterized by edema when it is associated with a decrease in serum albumin resulting in decreased plasma oncotic pressure. Hyperlipidemia, with elevations either in serum cholesterol and/or triglycerides, also occurs in nephrotic syndrome. The goals of nutrition therapy for patients with nephrotic syndrome are to

- reduce proteinuria
- prevent negative nitrogen balance
- control hyperlipidemia
- minimize edema

Nutrition Therapy

Protein

A high-protein diet may exacerbate albumin excretion through the damaged glomerular membrane. Therefore, a moderate protein restriction is recommended early in the diagnosis of nephrotic syndrome. A moderate protein restriction also may reduce the amino acid load to the glomerulus, subsequently diminishing the quantity of albumin crossing the damaged glomerular membrane. The currently recommended daily amount of protein for patients on a moderate restriction is 0.8 to 1.0 g/kg, but this amount may need to be adjusted based on their nutritional status, clinical condition, and degree of proteinuria. Protein restriction may not be warranted in patients with the following clinical signs:

- severe muscle wasting or malnutrition
- no quantitative improvement of proteinuria with protein restriction
- worsening serum albumin levels

Calories

Adequate calories from nonprotein sources are needed to utilize protein and promote weight maintenance or weight gain in patients with nephrotic syndrome. Caloric needs for weight maintenance are estimated to be 35 kcal/kg/day. Because these patients are often edematous, dry weight should be used for this calculation.

Fats

Hyperlipidemia due to increased hepatic protein synthesis and reduced lipoprotein clearance from the blood by lipoprotein lipase is common in patients with nephrotic syndrome. Elevated VLDL, LDL, cholesterol, and triglyceride levels, along with normal or decreased HDL levels, may warrant a dietary fat restriction to less than 30 percent of total calories with an equal balance among saturated, monounsaturated, and polyunsaturated fats. Dietary cholesterol should be limited to less than 300 mg/day. Pharmacological therapy may be necessary if diet has no effect on hyperlipidemia.

Sodium and Fluid

Controlling edema through sodium restriction and appropriate use of diuretics is essential in the management of nephrotic syndrome. Because edema is commonly associated with nephrotic syndrome, restricting daily sodium intake to approximately 2 grams may be necessary. The exact level of restriction must be individualized based on the degree of edema (see Table 10-1). Fluid restriction is not generally recommended.

Potassium

Hyper- or hypokalemia may occur in patients with nephrotic syndrome depending on the diuretic prescribed to control their edema. Monitoring their serum potassium levels is essential to determine whether alterations require a low- or high-potassium diet in response (see Table 10-2).

Calcium

Hypocalcemia frequently occurs in individuals with nephrotic syndrome if they are hypoalbuminemic. Serum calcium measurements include both free calcium and calcium bound to serum albumin. When attempting to determine if a calcium deficiency is present, it is therefore essential to correct the patient's serum calcium level to reflect the degree of hypoalbuminemia.

A concurrent vitamin D deficiency may lead to inadequate calcium absorption from the GI tract in a number of these patients. In such cases, if the serum calcium level still falls below normal levels after correcting for the degree of hypoalbuminemia, a calcium deficiency is likely. Thus vitamin D supplementation may be recommended for individuals who are persistently hypocalcemic after their serum calcium value has been corrected for the level of hypoalbuminemia they exhibit.

Vitamins and Minerals

Because certain vitamins and most minerals are bound to albumin, patients with nephrotic syndrome are at particular risk for developing vitamin deficiencies. Supplemental B vitamins, including niacin, riboflavin, and thiamin, are recommended for those patients on a protein-restricted diet of less than 60 g/day.

Nephrolithiasis

The goal of nutrition therapy for patients with nephrolithiasis (kidney stones) is to eliminate the diet-related risk factors for stone formation and prevent the growth of existing stones. The influence of specific nutrients such as calcium, oxalate, protein, refined carbohydrates, and sodium on the risk factors for calcium stone formation are discussed in the following section.

Nutrition Therapy

Fluids

First and most importantly, a high fluid intake is the essential component of diet therapy for patients with nephrolithiasis. An increase in daily urine volume to two liters or more is needed to maintain a dilute urine and reduce the concentration of stone-forming substances. Producing this volume of urine requires a daily fluid intake of approximately 2.5 to 3 liters.

Calcium

Hypercalciuria is the most common metabolic abnormality in persons who form calcium stones. Although much attention is directed toward the effect of dietary calcium on urinary calcium excretion, in reality most cases of calcium urolithiasis are not attributed to variations in dietary calcium. In fact, a very low-calcium diet may increase the absorption and subsequent excretion of oxalate, which promotes formation of calcium oxalate stones in susceptible individuals. Maintaining a calcium intake in the range of 600 to 800 mg/day should prevent hyperoxaluria and long-term negative calcium balance. Specified amounts of milk or milk products can be added to the diet to achieve the desired level of calcium intake.

Oxalate

Changes in oxalate excretion are more important than calcium excretion in altering the probability of developing calcium oxalate stones. Oxalate has a greater relative effect than calcium on urine supersaturation of calcium oxalate. Normally, the quantity of oxalic acid excreted in urine does not exceed 10 to 40 mg/day. Only 10 percent of this amount comes from the diet (Table 10-4); the remainder is a product of endogenous metabolism.

Gastrointestinal disorders that cause malabsorption are the most common cause of enteric hyperoxaluria. Oxalate absorption tends to be excessive when malabsorbed fat forms soaps and binds calcium in the gut. Free oxalate is then

Table 10-4   High-Oxalate foods

Beans	Fruitcake
String, wax	Eggplant
Legume types	Gooseberries
(including baked beans	Grits (white corn)
canned in tomato sauce)	Instant coffee (more than 8 oz/day)
Beets	Leeks
Blackberries	Nuts, nut butters
Carob powder	Okra
Celery	Peel: lemon, lime, orange
Chocolate/cocoa and	Raspberries (black)
other chocolate drink mixes	Red currants
Concord grapes	Rhubarb
Dark-leafy greens	Soy products (tofu)
Spinach	Strawberries
Swiss chard	Summer squash
Beet greens	Sweet potatoes
Endive, escarole	Tea
Parsley	Wheat germ
Draft beer	

Source: Kasidas GP, Rose GA. Oxalate content of some common foods: Determination by enzymatic method. *J Human Nutr* 1980;34:255.

easily absorbed in the intraluminal intestine. Small increases in urinary oxalate concentration greatly increase the potential for crystal formation. Control of dietary oxalate therefore may benefit those susceptible to oxalate stones, because large fluctuations in urinary oxalate are attributable to variations in diet. Oxalate in the urine can be decreased by reducing oxalate in the diet while maintaining enough calcium to achieve a proper balance between these two elements. Thus eliminating all calcium-containing foods is not advisable for patients with calcium oxalate stones.

Protein

A high intake of animal protein, with its acid load, increases urinary calcium excretion. In addition, the binding effect of sulfate in dietary protein decreases renal tubular calcium reabsorption. Therefore, limiting intake of foods such as meat, fish, poultry, and eggs is recommended in patients with nephrolithiasis.

Sodium

A high sodium intake increases calcium excretion by expanding extracellular fluid volume, increasing the GFR, and decreasing renal tubular calcium reabsorption. These alterations result in an increased quantity of calcium-containing crystals in the urine. A moderate reduction of high sodium foods therefore is recommended (see Table 10-1).

Carbohydrate

Simple carbohydrates (concentrated sweets) promote calcium and oxalate excretion, induce calciuria, and promote calcium absorption from the intestine. Evidence exists that a subgroup of individuals prone to idiopathic calcium stone formation has a high, sustained insulin response to glucose following meals. Because insulin is calciuretic in such individuals, urinary calcium excretion increases when they ingest large amounts of refined carbohydrates.

	CALORIES	PROTEIN	SODIUM	POTASSIUM	CALCIUM/PHOSPHATE	VITAMINS/OTHER MINERALS	FLUID
Acute Renal Failure	~35 kcal/kg/day. 20–50% higher for stressed patients. Monitor glucose due to potential for hyperglycemia with catabolism.	0.6 gm/kg IBW/day for non-hyper catabolic, non-dialyzed patient. 1.1–1.4 gm/kg IBW-HD. 1.2–1.5 gm/kg IBW-PD. >1.5 gm/kg IBW—very catabolic.	2–3 gm per day - oliguric with or without 3x/wk HD. >3 gm/day—with more frequent HD/daily PD. Liberalize and possibly replete during diuretic recovery phase.	1.5–3.0 gm per day—oliguric with or without 3x/wk HD. >3 gm/day with more frequent HD/daily PD. Liberalize and possibly replete during diuretic recovery phase.	Supplement calcium and restrict phosphorus as needed to keep serum calcium 8.5–10.5 mg/dL and phosphorus 4.0–6.0 mg/dL.	Supplement B – complex + C vitamins if malnourished or being dialyzed ("renal" vitamin). May need to use standard MVI with TPN (due to practicality).	Oliguric – 500 ml (insensible) + urine output – non dialyzed. 3x/wk HD – 1000 ml/dl + urine output. Liberalize with more frequent HD/daily PD/CAVH. May need to be encouraged with diuresis.
Chronic Renal Failure Pre-Dialysis	30–35 kcal/IBW/d (maintenance). 35–50 kcal/kg/IBW/d (repletion). 20–30 kcal/kg/IBW/day (wt. reduction). May need to increase fat/carbohydrate to increase calories. May need to modify fat/chol if hyperlipidemic.	0.6 gm/kg IBW or adjusted IBW/day (non-catabolic). 0.8 gm/kg/IBW/day (malnourished). Add daily protein losses to restrictions if significant proteinuria 65% high biological value protein.	2–3 gm/day may want to measure urinary sodium for better estimate of needs. Occasionally <2gm/day needed.	2–3 gm per day when serum levels consistently >5.0 mEq/L. Restrictions usually not necessary until later stages of CRF unless on ACE inhibitor.	Calcium supplementation and phosphorus restriction usually needed when GFR ≤ 25 ml/min. 8–12 mg/kg IBW/day + phosphate binders. Use AlOH3 binders only until phosphate < 6.0 mg/dL or calcium and phosphate product >70.	Supplementation B complex plus vitamin C if malnourished or diet restrictive ("renal" vitamin). Active form Vit D (calcitriol) if PTH increases or calcium decreases. May need iron if on EPO.	Unrestricted if good fluid balance with or without diuretics. 500 ml + urine output may be needed in later stages of CRF.

Chapter Summary Table (continued)

	CALORIES	PROTEIN	SODIUM	POTASSIUM	CALCIUM/PHOSPHATE	VITAMINS/OTHER MINERALS	FLUID
Hemo Dialysis (HD)	Same as predialysis (CRF). Limit cholesterol—modify fat intake if hyperlipidemic and this does not jeopardize total calorie intake.	1.1–1.4 gm/kg IBW/day. May be greater with malnutrition.	2–3 gm/day.	Generally 1.5–3.0 gm/day.	Supplement calcium as needed to keep serum levels at least 8.5–10.5 mg/dL. 12–17 mg/kg IBW phosphorus. Use binders as in pre-dialysis to keep serum levels 4.0–6.0 mg/dL.	"Renal" vitamin as in ARF. Active vitamin D (calcitriol) either p.o. or IV (on HD) as needed. Iron usually needed with EPO (may need IV if ferrin <200 ng/ml or transferrin saturation <20%.	Same as in ARF.
Peritoneal Dialysis (PD)	25–30 kcal/kg/IBW/day (maintenance). 35–50 kcal/kg IBW/day (repletion). 20/25 kcal/kg IBW/day (Wt. reduction). Consider glucose absorption with PD. Limit chol/modify fat as needed (see HD).	1.2–1.5 gm/kg IBW/day. May be greater with malnutrition and peritonitis.	Generally 2–3 gm/day but may be liberalized to >3 gm/day if no edema or increased BP.	May be unrestricted due to daily removal of potassium. May even need to encourage or give supplements if serum levels <nl values.	As in HD with at least 15 mg/kg IBW phosphorus to allow sufficient protein intake.	"Renal" vitamin oral calcitriol as needed. Iron often needed with EPO as in HD.	May be able to liberalize >1000 ml + urine output if no edema increased BP.

	Calories/Energy	Protein	Sodium	Potassium	Calcium/Phosphorus	Vitamins	Fluid
Renal Transplant	Generally 35 kcal/kg IBW/day. Repletion/reduction as in CRF (pre-dialysis). Decrease conc. sweets with hyperglycemia. Modify chol/fat in long-term post-transplant period if hyperlipidemia.	1.3–2.0 gm/kg IBW/day post-op ideal. 1.2–1.5 gm/kg IBW/day—most practical.	2–3 gm per day initially (or with rejection). Liberalize when no edema or increased BP when transplant functioning well.	Limit at 2–3 gm/day if hyperkalemic with cyclosporine Rx or ATN/rejection.	Calcium supplements may be needed if ATN/rejection or malnutrition pre-transplant. Phos restrictions not needed with well-functioning kidney — may need repletion, may need restriction and binders with ATN/rejection.	May continue "renal" vitamin if ATN/rejection or malnutrition pre-transplant. May need iron with EPO if needed.	Not usually restricted unless ATN/rejection.
Nephrotic Syndrome	Generally 35 kcal/kg IBW/day. May need to restrict fat (30% total cal) and chol (300 mg) if hyperlipidemia.	0.8–1.0 gm/kg IBW/day. Protein restriction may not be warranted if severe muscle wasting/malnutrition/worsening serum albumin or no improvement in proteinuria.	2 gm/day.	May need to encourage or restrict; monitor serum potassium levels.	Probably do not need to supplement calcium (see vitamins) or restrict phosphate.	Supplement B vitamins if on a diet <60 gm protein/day. Vitamin D supplementation if continued hypocalcemia after correction for low albumin.	Restriction not usually recommended.

Case 1

Chronic Renal Failure Advancing to Dialysis

Gail Morrison and Jean Stover

Objectives

- To use the medical history, physical exam, and laboratory data to identify factors that affect the nutritional status of an adult with chronic renal failure.
- To adjust nutritional recommendations for individuals with chronic renal failure to the specific phase of the disorder or the current treatment modality.
- To evaluate the appropriateness of the diet of an individual whose chronic renal failure requires dialysis.

AB, a 22-year-old college student, presented to the emergency room with headaches and shortness of breath. Earlier, he had gone to the Student Health Service at the university he attends complaining of shortness of breath and frequent headaches. He was admitted to the hospital for evaluation when he was found to have a blood pressure of 200/120 mm Hg and mild congestive heart failure (CHF) by chest X-ray. AB reports that over the past year, his weight has increased about 10 pounds, although his diet has remained unchanged. He attributed this weight gain to decreased exercise and a busy class schedule.

Past Medical History

AB has had no recent viral illness, sore throat, or upper respiratory infection. He has never had rheumatologic complaints, and has no family history of renal disease. He had a history of multiple streptococcal infections of the throat as a child, some of which were treated with antibiotics. He is not taking any medications and has no known drug or food allergies.

Social History

AB shares a dormitory room with a fellow student who is in good health. He reports the following information concerning substance abuse.

AB's Usual Dietary Intake

Breakfast	Coffee	8 oz.
	Whole milk	2 Tbs.
Lunch	Cheeseburger on bun	1 each
	French fries	large
	Iced tea	16 oz.
Dinner	2 slices of chicken breast	6 oz.
	Baked potato	1 medium
	Butter	2 Tbs.
	Vegetable (broccoli, spinach)	1/2 cup
	Chocolate cake	1 slice
	Cola soda	16 oz.
Snack	Salted nuts	small bag
	Cola soda	16 oz.

Total calories: 2547 kcal/day
Protein: 108 g/day (17% of calories)
Fat: 40% of calories
Carbohydrate: 43% of calories
Potassium: 3442 mg/day
Sodium: 1940 mg/day

Alcohol intake: none

Tobacco: none

IV drug abuse: none

Review of Systems

General: Fatigue, weakness, shortness of breath
GI: Anorexia

Physical Examination

Vital signs

Temperature: Afebrile
Heart rate: 96 BPM
Respiration: 24 BPM
Blood pressure: 210/124 mm Hg

Anthropometric data

Height: 5'9" (175.3 cm)
Current weight: 170 lb (77.3 kg) [usual weight = 155 lb (70.5 kg)
6 months ago]

General: Well developed male
Lungs: Decreased breath sounds with faint crackles at the right base
Cardiac: Regular rate and rhythm, systolic murmur at the apex, S3 gallop
Abdomen: Soft, non-tender, no hepatomegaly
Extremities: 3+ peripheral edema on both legs, ring tight on finger
Skin: Warm to touch
Neurological: Intact, mild asterixis

Laboratory Data #1

Patient's Values	Normal Values
Sodium: 135 mEq/L	133–143 mEq/L
Potassium: 4.4 mEq/L	3.5–5.3 mEq/L
Chloride: 111 mEq/L	97–107 mEq/L
CO2: 15 mEq/L	24–32 mEq/L
Calcium: 7.5 mg/dL	8.5–10.5 mg/dL
Phosphate: 10.2 mg/dL	2.5–5.0 mg/dL
BUN: 108 mg/dL	10–20 mg/dL
Creatinine: 14.0 mg/dL	0.8–1.3 mg/dL
Albumin: 3.2 g/dL	3.5–5.8 g/dL
Hemoglobin: 8.3 g/L	13.5–17.5 g/L
Hematocrit: 24.3%	40–52%
MCV: 70 fl	80–100 fl
WBC: 8.7 cells/uL	4–11 cells/uL

EKG: Normal sinus rhythm at 100, no ischemic changes
Chest X-ray: Cardiomegaly, CHF
Urinalysis: 3+ heme by dipstick, 1+ protein by dipstick
Sediment: 15–20 RBC/HPF, 3–5 WBC/HPF
2–4 red blood cell casts and broad waxy casts/HPF--

Dialysis Treatment Plans

AB received a Tenckoff catheter a week after hospital discharge and began training for CAPD two weeks later. At the end of the training period a new diet plan was developed. He would now be receiving four 2-liter PD exchanges daily. The following data was available:

Laboratory Data #2: (changes from initial)

Patient's Values	Normal Values
Sodium: 136 mEq/L	133–143 mEq/L
Potassium: 4.5 mEq/L	3.5–5.3 mEq/L
Chloride: 102 mEq/L	97–107 mEq/L
CO_2: 18 mEq/L	24–32 mEq/L
Calcium: 8.8 mg/dL	8.5–10.5 mg/dL
Phosphate: 6.0 mg/dL	2.5–5.0 mg/dL
BUN: 70 mg/dL	10–20 mg/dL
Creatinine: 9.2 mg/dL	0.8–1.3 mg/dL
Albumin: 3.3 g/dL	3.5–5.8 g/dL

AB did fairly well on CAPD for 3 months until he began to have difficulty with the drainage of PD fluid through the Tenckoff catheter. He had repeated doses of urokinase infused into the catheter in an attempt to dissolve the proteinaceous material with only minimal success. He eventually had a new catheter inserted which only worked temporarily before the same problem developed. He was subsequently readmitted to the hospital for a hemodialysis (HD) catheter and started regular outpatient hemodialysis treatments. At this time his urine output had declined to less than 200 ml/24 hours.

Case Questions

1. Based on AB's history, physical exam, and laboratory data, what is the most likely diagnosis?

2. What additional laboratory tests or studies help confirm your diagnosis?

3. What medications are indicated to manage his clinical condition at this time?

4. Based on AB's physical exam, should his current body weight be used to estimate his caloric and protein needs?

5. How can AB's caloric and protein requirements be estimated?

6. What dietary recommendations are indicated before dialysis based on his current lab values and what fluid and electrolyte management does AB require?

7. Using AB's lab values that estimate renal function and his vital signs and chest x-ray results to determine his hemodynamic status, what are the immediate and long-term treatment modalities you would recommend?

8. What modifications in phosphate binding medication should be made once AB's phosphate level becomes acceptable?

9. What dietary modifications are indicated once AB begins receiving CAPD?

10. When AB's dialysis modality changes to hemodialysis, what dietary modifications are appropriate based on his weight and current laboratory data?

     Predialysis weight: 74 kg

     Estimated dry weight: 70.5 kg

     Laboratory Data #3:   (changes from initial)

Patient's Values	Normal Values
Sodium: 138 mEq/L	133–143 mEq/L
Potassium: 4.8 mEq/L	3.5–5.0 mEq/L
Chloride: 106 mEq/L	96–105 mEq/L
CO_2: 22 mEq/L	24–28 mEq/L
Calcium: 8.8 mg/dL	8.5–10.5 mg/dL
Phosphate: 8.4 mg/dL	2.5–5.0 mg/dL
Albumin: 3.4 g/dL	3.5–5.8 g/dL
Hemoglobin: 8.3 g/L	13.5–17.5 g/L
Hematocrit: 25%	40–52%

Answers begin on the following page.

Answers to Questions: Case 1

Part 1:   Diagnosis and Medications

1. **Based on AB's history, physical exam, and laboratory data, what is the most likely diagnosis?**

   AB has a history of recurrent streptococcal infections in childhood, which most likely increased his risk of developing acute post-strepto-coccal glomerulonephritis. Approximately 5 to 10 percent of patients with a history of streptococcal infections and acute glomerulonephritis (AGN) develop chronic glomerulonephritis (CGN) 15 to 20 years following the acute infections. CGN results in a markedly decreased glomerular filtration rate (GFR), which prevents sodium and water excretion and causes increased sodium and water retention. The result is volume-induced high blood pressure, and with significant sodium and water retention, eventually CHF.

2. **What additional laboratory tests or studies help confirm your diagnosis?**

   Urinalysis The urinalysis having blood and protein by dipstick indicate renal glomerular damage. Red blood cell casts are highly suggestive of glomerulonephritis and broad waxy casts suggest dilated renal tubules associated with CGN.

   24-hour urine collection This procedure reveals the quantity of protein and creatinine excreted over 24 hours. Knowing the amount of urinary creatinine excreted allows calculating creatinine clearance.

   Protein excretion 2.2 g/24 hours

   Creatinine excretion 900 mg/24 hours

   Renal ultrasound Renal ultrasound revealed small kidneys bilaterally which indicates irreversible renal disease (9 and 10 cm—right and left respectively). Only a renal biopsy could actually confirm the diagnosis of CGN, but it is not done once small kidneys are identified since no treatment can reverse the kidney damage. AB's significantly increased serum phosphate and a decreased serum calcium suggests that the GFR is less than 30 ml/min, indicating significant renal dysfunction. Tests to eliminate other possible causes of CGN include:

   > *Compliment levels* CH5O, C3, and C4 within normal limits (makes the diagnosis of membranoproliferative disease, SBE, and acute post-streptococcal glomerulonephritis highly unlikely).

   > *24-hour protein collection* Eliminates the diagnosis of nephrotic syndrome. AB's history and physical examination eliminate other causes of CGN such as Alport's syndrome.

3. **What medications are indicated to manage his clinical condition at this time?**

   In cases like AB's, management normally consists of diet modifications and medications until the patient begins CAPD. AB should be discharged on the following medications:

   Diuretic Use to control sodium and H2O balance (as long as he has urine output).

   Phosphate binder Use aluminum hydroxide (AlOH3), since serum calcium and phosphate product is greater than 70.

   Antihypertensive medication Use as necessary to achieve blood pressure less than 140/90 mm Hg.

   Renal multivitamin A supplement to correct dietary deficiencies.

   Iron supplement Use for anemia.

Part 2: Nutrition Assessment

4. **Based on AB's physical exam, should his current body weight be used to estimate his caloric and protein needs?**

   This patient's total body water is elevated, as evidenced by 3+ peripheral edema of his legs and CHF; his current weight therefore does not reflect his "dry" weight. To estimate "dry" weight, first ascertain the patient's usual weight. AB's usual body weight six months ago was 155 lb (70.5 kg), and this is the value that should be used to estimate his protein and caloric requirements since he is also close to his ideal body weight.

5. **How can AB's caloric and protein requirements be estimated?**

   The normal estimated total daily caloric requirement is 35 kcal/kg. In AB's case, this amounts to

   > 35 kcal x 70.5 kg = 2468 kcal

   Daily protein requirements for acute or chronic renal failure (not catabolic) without dialysis are 0.6 g/kg. If significant proteinuria is present, the urinary protein losses should be added to the daily protein allowance. The 24-hour urine collection indicated a protein loss of 2.2 g in AB's case. His daily protein intake therefore should be:

   > 0.6 g x 70.5 kg = 42 g/day

6. **What dietary recommendations are indicated before dialysis based on his current lab values and what fluid and electrolyte management does AB require?**

   Protein AB's current meal plan contains 2547 kcals and 108 grams of protein. To achieve a protein restriction of 45 grams per day, the following modifications are recommended:

- Limit milk in coffee to 1 to 2 oz/cup.
- Substitute a plain hamburger on a bun or an equivalent such as two ounces of roast beef, turkey, chicken, or rinsed, water-packed tuna on 2 slices bread for a cheeseburger at lunch time.
- Limit the amount of chicken at dinner to 2 ounces.
- Omit all cheese and nuts because they are high in protein, phosphorus, and sodium; and substitute unsalted pretzels or chips as a night snack.

Electrolytes AB's total body water and sodium are elevated, as evidenced by 3+ peripheral edema and mild CHF on his chest X-ray. Therefore, a low-sodium diet (2 to 3 g/day) is indicated at this time, which AB is already following. AB's potassium level is within the normal range; thus, no potassium restriction is indicated at this time.

The serum calcium and phosphate levels of 7.5 and 10.2 mg/dL, respectively, are a result of decreased GI calcium absorption and phosphate retention. Lowering serum phosphate levels by dietary restriction and phosphate binding medication will improve serum calcium initially without calcium supplementation. Foods high in calcium are also high in phosphate content, so supplementing the diet with calcium-rich foods is not feasible at the present time. Restricting the daily allowance of dietary phosphate to 8 to 12 mg/kg (600 to 900 mg/day) is indicated (see Table 10-3). Aluminum hydroxide was added to AB's medication regimen to reduce serum phosphate levels to less than or equal to 6.0 mg/dL.

Fluid Given that AB's 24-hour urine output was 700 ml in the hospital, a total fluid intake of 1200 ml/day or 40 ounces (700 ml + 500 ml for insensible fluid losses) should be recommended.

To stay within the fluid restriction of 1200 ml/day, limit morning coffee to 8 ounces, the lunch beverage to 12 ounces, the dinner beverage to 8 ounces, and the beverage with the snack to 8 ounces. Allowing for an additional 4 ounces of juice with medications is acceptable.

7. **Using AB's lab values that estimate renal function and his vital signs and chest x-ray results to determine his hemodynamic status, what are the immediate and long-term treatment modalities you would recommend?**

From these data, AB has a creatinine of 14 mg/dL, blood pressure of 210/124 mm Hg and CHF. Therefore, AB underwent a single acute hemodialysis treatment which effectively removes sodium and water as well as the buildup of uremic products secondary to CGN. He chooses continuous ambulatory peritoneal dialysis (CAPD) instead of HD for his long-term treatment because CAPD allows him to perform dialysis exchanges himself in his dormitory room rather than receiving HD treatments in an outpatient dialysis unit and have more freedom during the day. A Tenckoff catheter (used to instill peritoneal dialysis solution into the peritoneal cavity) was placed during AB's hospitalization. CAPD usually is started two weeks after a Tenckoff catheter is inserted to allow for adequate wound healing.

8. **What modifications in phosphate binding medication should be made once AB's phosphate level becomes acceptable?**

   AB's phosphate level at the outset of PD is now more satisfactory at 6.0 mg/dL. Given the potential for aluminum toxicity with long-term use of aluminum containing medications, his phosphate-binding medication should be changed to calcium carbonate or calcium acetate preparation, with a starting dose of 2 Oscal tablets three times per day (tid) with meals. This supplement provides a total of 3000 mg of elemental calcium daily.

9. **What dietary modifications are indicated once AB begins receiving CAPD?**

   The protein allowance "must" increase because AB's laboratory values at the start of CAPD exhibit a mildly depleted albumin level, and CAPD will remove significant amounts of albumin. A protein intake of 1.2 to 1.5 g/kg/day (based on UBW or "dry" weight) is 85 to 105 g/day. To reach that goal, the meat, fish, or poultry portions at lunch and dinner need to be increased to 4 ounces, and AB should be encouraged to eat a sandwich with at least 1.5 ounces of meat as his nightly snack.

   Since AB's weight is still 166 pounds (170 pounds minus the 4 pounds of PD fluid indwelling), he remains at least 11 pounds over his previous usual body weight of 155 pounds. Thus, until a regular schedule of PD exchanges can be performed, the same sodium (2 to 3 g/day) and fluid restrictions (1200 cc/day) are indicated. A potassium restriction is still unnecessary because AB's serum potassium level is normal and may drop as a result of continuous removal of potassium with daily PD.

   Phosphate should still be restricted to maintain phosphate levels below 6.0 mg/dL, but the restriction can be liberalized somewhat to allow a greater protein intake (animal protein sources are the foods highest in phosphate). By continuing to limit milk to no more than 4 ounces per day, and limiting cheese and cola sodas to two times per week, AB can achieve the new daily phosphate allowance of 15 mg/kg or 1100 mg/day. An extra Oscal tablet may be prescribed with the night sandwich as well.

10. **When AB's dialysis modality changes to hemodialysis, what dietary modifications are appropriate based on his weight and currrent laboratory data?**

    AB has the potential to gain fluid weight between HD treatments, because he receives them only three times per week (his pre-dialysis weight is 3.5 kg greater than his dry weight). In addition, AB's urine output is diminished because of his renal dysfunction. Thus his fluid intake should be decreased to 1 liter/day, and he should be encouraged to maintain a sodium restriction of 2 to 3 g/day. The recommended daily protein allowance is now 1.1 to 1.4 g/kg for a total of 75 to 100 grams, which does not much differ significantly from his previous recommendations.

Because HD is intermittent, and AB reports that his urine output is minimal, he should be advised to limit his potassium intake to approximately 85 mEq/day or 1 mEq/g of protein prescribed. AB can accomplish this goal by eliminating fruits and vegetables high in potassium such as bananas, orange juice, potatoes, and dark-green, leafy vegetables. Phosphate restrictions for HD are similar to those for PD because no significant change is recommended in the protein content of AB's diet. However, because his phosphate level is now greater than 6.0 mg/dL, AB is advised to avoid dairy products completely except for 4 ounces of milk per day.

See Chapter Review Questions, pages A16–A18.

REFERENCES

Ahmed K, Kopple JD. Nutritional management of renal disease. In Greenberg A. *Primer on Kidney Diseases*. New York: Academic, 1994.

Anderson SA, Fedje L, Pulliam JP. Slowing the process of renal failure. *Patient Care* 1993:114–115.

Camel SP. Nutrition management of the adult renal transplant patient. In Stover J. *A Clinical Guide to Nutrition Care in End Stage Renal Disease*. 2nd ed. Vol. 2. Chicago: American Dietetic Association, 1994:57–67.

Cheung AK. Hemodialysis and hemofiltration. In Greenberg A. *Primer on Kidney Diseases*. New York: Academic, 1994.

Drum I. Nutritional support in the patient with acute renal failure. In Mitch WE, Klahr S (eds), *Nutrition and the Kidney*. 2nd ed. Boston: Little, Brown, 1993.

Harum P. Nutrition management of the adult hemodialysis patient. In Stover J. *A Clinical Guide to Nutrition Care in End Stage Renal Disease*. 2nd ed. Chicago: American Dietetic Association, 1994.

Hood S, Liftman C. Parenteral nutrition for the patient with renal failure. In Stover J. *A Clinical Guide to Nutrition Care in End Stage Renal Disease*. 2nd ed. Chicago: American Dietetic Association, 1994.

Hutchison FN. Management of acute renal failure. In Greenberg A. *Primer on Kidney Diseases*. New York: Academic, 1994.

Kaufman CE. Fluid and electrolyte abnormalities in the nephrotic syndrome. *Postgrad Med* 1984;76:135.

Kaysen GA. Nephrotic syndrome: nutritional consequences and dietary management. In Mitch WE, Klahr S. *Nutrition and the Kidney*. 2nd ed. Boston: Little, Brown, 1993.

Kaysen GA. Nutritional management of nephrotic syndrome. *J Renal Nutr* 1992; 2(2):50.

Keane WF, Mulcahy WS, Kasiske BL, et al. Hyperlipidemia and progressive renal disease. *Kidney Int* 1991;(Suppl.)31:S41–S48.

Kopple JD. Nutrition, diet and the kidney. In Shils ME (ed). *Modern Nutrition in Heath and Disease*. Philadelphia: Lea and Febiger, 1993.

Makoff R. Water-soluble vitamin status in patients with renal disease treated with hemodialysis or peritoneal dialysis. *J Renal Nutr* 1991;1(2):56.

Massry SG, Kopple JD. Requirements for calcium, phosphorus and vitamin D. In Mitch WE, Klahr S (eds). *Nutrition and the Kidney* Boston: Little, Brown, 1993.

McCann L. Nutrition management of the adult peritoneal dialysis patient. In Stover, J. *A Clinical Guide to Nutrition Care in End Stage Renal Disease*. 2nd ed. Chicago: American Dietetic Association, 1994:37–55.

Mitch WE. Restricting diets and slowing the progression of chronic renal insufficiency. In Mitch WE, Klahr S (eds). *Nutrition and the Kidney*. Boston: Little, Brown, 1993.

Pruchno CJ, Hunsicker LG. Nutritional requirements on renal transplant patients. In Mitch WE, Klahr S (eds). *Nutrition and the Kidney*. 2nd ed. Boston: Little, Brown, 1993.

Roberts C, Stover J. Conservative management—dietary treatment of early stages of CRF. In Stover J. *A Clinical Guide to Nutrition Care in End Stage Renal Disease*. 2nd ed. Chicago: American Dietetic Association, 1994.

Wasserstein AG. Nephrolithiasis. In Greenberg A. *Primer on Kidney Diseases*. New York: Academic, 1994.

Wendland BE. Nutrition management of the patient with urolithiasis. In Stover J. *A Clinical Guide to Nutrition Care in End Stage Renal Disease*. 2nd ed. Chicago: American Dietetic Association, 1994.

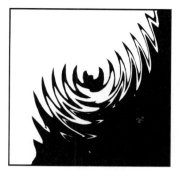

PART IV

Fundamentals of
Nutrition Support

Enteral and Parenteral
Nutrition Support

Scott Stuart, Melanie Stuart, and Lisa D. Unger

Objectives

- To understand the indications and contraindications of enteral and parenteral nutrition.
- To determine appropriate administration and monitoring of enteral and parenteral modalities.
- To understand the benefits and complications of enteral and parenteral nutrition support.

Enteral Nutrition Support

Enteral nutrition (EN) is a nutrition support consisting of a liquid formula administered via a tube into the gastrointestinal (GI) tract, where the nutrients are absorbed via normal GI processes. When the gut is functional, enteral nutrition is the preferred approach to nutrition support because it offers major advantages over parenteral nutrition (PN).

Advantages

Gut Integrity

Research has demonstrated that enteral nutrition maintains the integrity of the gut. When patients do not receive enteral alimentation for an extended period, the gut mucosa atrophies, which may increase the risk of sepsis from gut bacteria and reduce tolerance of oral feedings.

Safety

Compared with parenteral nutrition, enteral nutrition is associated with fewer metabolic abnormalities and infectious complications.

Cost

Enteral formulas are much less expensive than parenteral formulas. Furthermore, enteral nutrition costs less to set up, administer, and monitor than PN, and its complications are generally less costly to diagnose and treat.

Indications

Enteral nutrition is indicated in patients with a functioning GI tract who are unable to eat enough food to maintain or restore their nutritional status (Table 11-1). The status of gut function is the key guide to the use of enteral versus parenteral nutrition support.

Contraindications

Enteral nutrition is contraindicated in the following situations:

- complete gastric or intestinal obstruction if access cannot be placed distal to obstruction
- ileus
- high-output enteric fistulas (>500 ml/day)
- acute pancreatitis (moderate to severe)
- refusal of nutrition support by the patient or the patient's legal guardian
- severe diarrhea or vomiting

Enteral Formulas

Selecting the appropriate formula for enteral feeding is very important and depends on several factors, including physical properties, ingredients, and nutrient content of the formula.

Physical Properties

Osmolality Osmolality affects the patient's ability to tolerate the formula. However, most enteral formulas are well-tolerated and range from 300 to 700 mOsm/kg. Hypertonic medications greater than 2000 mOsm/kg can be administered via the tube but should be diluted to prevent diarrhea.

Table 11-1   Indications for use of enteral feeding.

Inability to ingest food normally
     Prolonged NPO (nothing by mouth) status
     Postoperative period (abdominal or upper GI surgery)
     Stupor, unconsciousness, coma
     Stroke
     Fracture of mandible
     Oropharyngeal neoplasms
     Head and neck surgery
     Dysphagia
     Irradiation of head or neck
     Chemotherapy
     Multiple sclerosis
     Amyotrophic lateral sclerosis
     Guillain-Barré syndrome

Obstruction of GI tract (if access is below obstruction)
     Esophageal stricture or neoplasm
     Pyloric obstruction
     Neoplasm, foreign body, or other obstruction of stomach or intestine

Impairment of digestion and/or absorption
     Pancreatic insufficiency; chronic pancreatitis
     Crohn's disease
     Enteric fistulas if feeding access is distal to fistula

Physiological deterrents to food intake
     Hyperemesis gravidarum
     Drug reactions
     Radiation
     Chemotherapy
     Diabetic gastroparesis

Protein-energy malnutrition
     Hypermetabolic state (burns, trauma, infection)

Psychiatric illness
     Anorexia nervosa
     Depression causing inadequate food intake

Renal Solute Load   If the renal solute load (RSL) of a formula is too high, a large quantity of water must be administered to allow the patient to excrete it. Patients receiving formulas with a high RSL must be carefully monitored for dehydration.

Viscosity Formulas containing larger molecules and formulas with a higher caloric content per unit volume tend to be more viscous. Viscous formulas may require larger tubes for administration.

Nutrient Content and Ingredients

Caloric Density Caloric density is the amount of energy per unit volume of food, expressed as kcal/ml. Most tube feeding formulas contain 1 kcal/ml, but some are more concentrated with 1.5 to 2.0 kcal/ml. These hypercaloric formulas are appropriate for patients with increased caloric needs or patients with fluid restrictions.

Protein Density Protein density is the amount of protein per unit volume of formula. The protein needs of each patient vary depending on their nutritional status and disease state, and protein content is thus a useful criterion in selecting enteral formulas.

Fluid Balance The fluid requirements for a healthy adult are about 1 ml for each calorie ingested, or 30 to 40 ml/kg. Patients' fluid balance is an important consideration, particularly when enteral nutrition is the sole source of fluid intake. Because the amount of water in tube feeding formulas varies, additional water is usually necessary to meet the patient's hydration needs. It is therefore important to monitor fluid input and output in all patients receiving tube feedings to prevent dehydration.

Polymeric Formulas Polymeric formulas are composed of intact proteins, sugars, and starches. Their fat content varies. Usually they are lactose-free and they may include fiber. Polymeric formulas require the ability to digest nutrient polymers.

- *Lactose-free formulas* Some patients require lactose-free formulas because of lactose intolerance. Lactose intolerance is common in older adults and in patients with AIDS and malabsorption.
- *High-fiber formulas* Formulas high in fiber have been found to help normalize bowel function in tube-fed patients. Generally, fiber increases formula viscosity, and care must be taken to infuse these formulas via a tube of adequate size to prevent clogging.

Elemental Formulas Also called defined, monomeric, or predigested formulas, elemental formulas require less digestive and absorptive capacity. Protein is provided as short-chain peptides and amino acids. Carbohydrates come from oligosaccharides, fragments of starch with only 2 to 8 molecules of glucose. The fat content is low and usually contains small amounts of long-chain triglycerides, some of which supply essential fatty acids. These formulas often have a high osmolarity, and patients' GI function therefore must be monitored closely. Patients with pancreatic insufficiency, malabsorption, or massive bowel resection may require an elemental formula.

Specialized Formulas Some patients may benefit from specialized or disease-specific formulas that are specifically designed to meet their needs. Specialized formulas have been developed for patients with renal, hepatic, and respiratory diseases, glucose intolerance, and trauma.

Modular Supplements In the event that the patient has an increased need for a single nutrient category, modular supplements can be added to the formula. These supplements can supply carbohydrate, protein, fat (MCT oil), fiber, or vitamins and minerals. Modular components can supplement other enteral feedings or be combined to provide individualized total nutrition.

Routes of Administration

Which route to choose for enteral feeding depends on the anticipated duration of tube feeding support and the patient's risk for aspiration. Short-term feedings usually are administered via nasogastric (NGT), nasoduodenal (NDT), or nasojejunal (NJT) tubes. The nasoduodenal and nasojejunal (postpyloric) routes are chosen over the nasogastric route if the patient is at risk for aspiration. For long-term feedings, a gastrostomy or jejunostomy is usually indicated. Jejunostomy is the preferred approach when the patient is at risk for aspiration.

Short-Term Feedings

By definition, the duration of short-term enteral nutrition support is expected to be less than 3 to 4 weeks.

Nasogastric Tube (NGT) The nasogastric tube extends from the nose and empties into the stomach. NGTs are chosen when the stomach is intact and empties normally. The patient must have a normal gag reflex with good mental status to prevent aspiration.

Advantages

The stomach normally accepts high osmotic loads without cramping, distention, vomiting, diarrhea, or fluid and electrolyte shifts.

The stomach has a large reservoir capacity and readily accepts intermittent or bolus feedings.

It is easier to position a tube into the stomach than into the jejunum.

The presence of hydrochloric acid in the stomach may help prevent infection.

Nasoduodenal Tube (NDT) The nasoduodenal tube extends from the nose through the pylorus and into the duodenum.

Indications

Patients at risk for aspiration: debilitated, demented, stuporous, or unconscious; those with poor gag reflexes (stroke, Guillain-Barré syndrome, amyotrophic lateral sclerosis)

Patients with gastroparesis or delayed gastric emptying

Long-Term Feedings

Enteral nutrition support for a period anticipated to be greater than 3 to 4 weeks is considered long term.

Tube Enterostomies For long-term feedings, enterostomies are the preferred access route. The tube may be placed in the GI tract either surgically during another intervention or endoscopically. Surgical placement of the tube into the stomach is called gastrostomy. Alternatively, a percutaneous endoscopic gastrostomy (PEG) tube may also be placed into the stomach. In patients at risk for aspiration the tube is placed in the small intestine either surgically via a jejunostomy or nonsurgically via a percutaneous jejunostomy tube.

Feeding Rates

Continuous Feeding

Continuous infusions are controlled by a pump over a 24-hour period or less. Duodenal or jejunal feedings necessitate continuous delivery because the small intestine does not tolerate sudden changes in volume well. Continuous feeding also may be used with gastric feedings.

Advantages

Decreased risk of distention, bloating, aspiration, and osmotic diarrhea

Improved tolerance, especially with hyperosmolar formulas

Disadvantages

Requires the patient to be physically connected to the apparatus during infusion

Expense associated with the purchase of volumetric infusion pumps

Intermittent or Bolus Feeding

Intermittent or bolus feedings are rapid infusions of 200 to 500 ml of formula administered over a 20- to 40-minute period on an intermittent basis (every 3 to 6 hours). This procedure is used only with gastric feedings, because the stomach can tolerate sudden changes in volume, whereas the intestine cannot.

Advantages

Convenient and inexpensive

May be more physiologic than continuous feeding as it closely simulates the normal feeding pattern and the distention may stimulate digestion

Disadvantages

Increased risk of aspiration if gastric emptying is delayed

May result in nausea, vomiting, diarrhea, distention, or cramps

Cycled Feeding

When freedom, mobility, and ease of care are desired, continuous feedings can be consolidated into 10- to 12-hour cycled infusions. Cycled infusions are beneficial for patients who will progress to home enteral nutrition and during the transition to oral feeding. The patient can eat meals during the day and use cycled enteral support at night. Once the patient meets two-thirds of his or her caloric needs by mouth, enteral feeding can be stopped.

Starter Regimen and Progression

When enteral nutrition is initiated, it is usually best to start with a slow rate to prevent complications and assess tolerance. The delivery rate can then be systematically increased by 30 to 50 ml/hour increments every 24 hours. Diluting enteral formula on initiation is not recommended because doing so delays achievement of the nutritional goals. For gastric feedings, tolerance to the rate and volume of formula administration is checked periodically by aspirating the stomach contents, or checking gastric residuals. If the volume of gastric residuals exceeds half the amount of formula given in the previous feeding, or a minimum of 100 cc, further gastric feedings should be withheld until the residuals have decreased. When restarting the enteral feeding, the volume of the feeding may be reduced. The final infusion rate depends on the patient's total caloric and protein requirements and tolerance.

Complications

Enteral feeding complications can be divided into three categories: gastrointestinal, metabolic, and mechanical. Table 11-2 lists some of the common complications, their possible causes, and suggested corrective measures.

Monitoring

It is very important to monitor patients for signs of formula intolerance, hydration and electrolyte status, and nutritional status. Physical indicators that should be monitored include incidence of vomiting, stool frequency, diarrhea, abdominal cramps, bloating, signs of edema or dehydration, and weight changes. In addition, the following laboratory parameters should be monitored daily when the patient begins receiving enteral nutrition support:

- Serum electrolytes (sodium, potassium, chloride, bicarbonate, calcium, magnesium, phosphorus)
- Blood urea nitrogen (BUN) and creatinine

Table 11-2   **Common nutrition-related complications in the tube-fed patient.**

PROBLEMS	POSSIBLE CAUSES	SUGGESTED CORRECTIVE MEASURES
Gastrointestinal		
Nausea and vomiting	Improper location of tube tip	Replace or reposition tube
	Excessive rate or volume of feeding	Decrease volume or rate of feeding
Diarrhea	Very cold formula	Give formula near room temperature
	Too rapid infusion	Give formula more slowly
	High osmolality or high concentration of feeding	Change formula
	Lactose intolerance	Use lactose-free formula
Vomiting and diarrhea	Contamination	Check sanitation of formula and equipment; consult with bacteriologist
Constipation	Lack of fiber	Use high-fiber formula or add stool softener
	Inadequate fluid intake	Increase fluid intake
Aspiration or gastric retention	Altered gastric motility, altered gag reflex, altered mental status	Change route of administration to postpyloric feedings
	Head of bed not at 30 degrees	Elevate head of bed
	Displaced feeding tube	Check feeding tube placement
Metabolic		
Dehydration	Osmotic diarrhea caused by rapid infusion	Administer tube feeding slowly
	Excessive protein or electrolytes or both	Reduce protein, electrolytes, or increase fluid intake
	Inadequate fluid intake	Increase fluid intake
Elevated or depressed serum electrolytes	Excessive or inadequate electrolytes in formula	Change formula
	Inadequate or excessive fluid intake	Modify fluid intake
Hyperglycemia	Metabolic stress	Treat origin of stress and cover with insulin as needed
	Diabetes	Give appropriate insulin dose
Gradual weight loss	Inadequate calories	Check if patient is receiving prescribed amount of feeding by comparing actual intake versus calculated
		Increase volume of formula or change to a different formula
Visceral protein depletion	Protein content of formula inadequate for needs	Change to high-protein formula or add high-protein supplements
Excessive weight gain	Excess calories	Change formula or decrease volume/day
Mechanical		
Obstructed tube	Formula viscosity excessive for feeding tube	Use less viscous formula or larger tube Flush tube before and after feeding
	Obstruction from crushed meds administered through tube	Give meds as elixir or crush medications thoroughly
		Flush tube before and after infusing medications

- Blood glucose
- Hemoglobin and hematocrit

Once the patient is stable, the frequency with which these parameters are monitored can be decreased as appropriate. Other parameters that should be monitored initially and weekly if abnormal include the following.

- Liver function tests (ALT, AST, bilirubin, alkaline phosphatase) and triglycerides
- Albumin and prealbumin (weekly)

Parenteral Nutrition Support

In parenteral nutrition a sterile, nutrient-dense solution is infused intravenously by a peripheral or a central venous access, entirely bypassing the digestive tract.

Peripheral Parenteral Nutrition

Peripheral parenteral nutrition (PPN) is a means of nutrition support in which the parenteral solution is administered directly into a peripheral vein. PPN is indicated for anticipated short-term use (less than 10 days) because PPN usually does not meet all the nutritional needs of the patient. This approach provides a limited amount of calories (generally 1000 to 1500 kcal/day), protein, and nutrient supplementation for patients who are unable to meet their needs via oral or enteral means. The osmolarity of PPN solutions must be less than 900 mOsm/L to avoid phlebitis.

Total Parenteral Nutrition

Total parenteral nutrition (TPN) is a means of nutrition support in which a parenteral solution is administered directly into a central vein (usually the superior vena cava). TPN is indicated for anticipated long-term use (greater than 7 to 10 days). TPN provides total caloric, protein, and nutrient supplementation for patients who cannot tolerate oral or enteral feedings. Osmolarity of the TPN solutions is often greater than 1000 mOsm/L because concentrations this great can be administered into the central veins due to the high flow rate of the blood returning through them to the heart.

Indications

Enteral nutrition should always be considered first if the gastrointestinal tract is functional. TPN is considered for patients who are unable to receive adequate calories, protein, and nutrients via the enteral route for a period greater than 5 to 7 days, or less if the patient is malnourished. The ultimate goal of TPN is to prevent or correct malnutrition. The following conditions may warrant the use of TPN:

- Mechanical intestinal obstruction or pseudo-obstruction
- Severe malabsorption (short bowel syndrome, celiac sprue disease)
- Active inflammatory bowel disease (Crohn's disease, ulcerative colitis)
- Small bowel fistula
- Pancreatitis
- Bone marrow transplant
- Intractable diarrhea
- Radiation enteritis
- Gastrointestinal malignancy
- Prolonged ileus
- Hyperemesis gravidarum
- Severe malnutrition and/or catabolic states in which the GI tract will not be functional within 5 to 7 days
- Preoperative feeding in severely malnourished patients with a dysfunctional GI tract
- Excessive nutritional needs that cannot be met by enteral feedings because of intolerance (for example, burn or trauma victims and patients who have undergone extensive surgery)

Because enteral nutrition support must be initiated gradually over a period of time, TPN can be used along with tube feeding in the initial stages to meet patients' increased calorie, protein, mineral, and vitamin needs. As tube feeding advances, TPN administration is decreased until enteral feeding meet 100 percent of the patient's nutritional requirements.

Factors to Consider

During the medical and nutrition assessment, a number of factors enter into the decision to use TPN, including

- anticipated duration of therapy
- caloric and protein requirements
- fluid requirements or limitations
- venous access

Contraindications

TPN is contraindicated in the following situations.

- The gastrointestinal tract is functional, and enteral nutrition support can be used safely to meet the patient's nutritional needs.
- Nutrition support is refused by the patient or the patient's legal guardian.

Macronutrient Requirements

Glucose

The maximum rate of glucose oxidation in adults is 5 mg/kg/min. Thus, for example, a man weighing 70 kg oxidizes approximately 500 grams of glucose every 24 hours (70 kg) (1440 min/day) (5 mg/kg/min), whereas a woman weighing 50 kg oxidizes 360 grams of glucose during the same period (50 kg) (1440 min/day) (5 mg/kg/min). D-Glucose (dextrose monohydrate) used in TPN provides 3.4 kcal/gram.

Careful consideration of the amounts of glucose administered during TPN is important for several reasons If glucose is infused at rates greater than the patient's maximal glucose oxidation capacity, fat synthesis will occur. Converting glucose to fat requires energy and also generates excess CO_2, which may contribute to CO_2 retention in patients with respiratory disease. Excessive glucose delivery may also contribute to hepatic steatosis, or fat deposition in the liver.

Protein

Parenteral protein in the form of synthetic amino acids contains a mixture of essential and nonessential amino acids. The recommended protein intake for a given patient is based on grams of protein/kg. Protein requirements vary depending on the patient's disease state, degree of stress, and unusual nitrogenous losses. TPN should provide adequate energy to allow for optimal utilization of protein. Estimated daily protein requirements for patients on TPN under the following conditions are:

Mild to moderate stress: 1.5 g/kg
Severe stress: 2.0 g/kg

Lipids

The principal indications for using parenteral lipid emulsions are to provide essential fatty acids and a concentrated source of calories. In adult patients, two percent of total calories from fat provides adequate essential fatty acids (EFA) to prevent deficiency. When lipid emulsions cannot be infused for a period greater than 14 days, the patient may be at risk for EFA deficiency.

The maximum daily rate of lipid oxidation for adults is 2.5 g/kg. Under normal circumstances, lipid emulsions provide 30 percent of total calories. Generally, parenteral lipid emulsions provide 9 kcal/gram. A 10-percent lipid emulsion provides 1.1 kcal/ml, while a 20-percent lipid emulsion provides 2 kcal/ml.

To assure lipid clearance, it is important to obtain a baseline triglyceride level prior to the first lipid dose and repeat testing after TPN infusion has begun. If lipid clearance is impaired and the serum triglyceride level is greater than 500 mg/dL, the patient may be at risk for pancreatitis. Therefore parenteral lipids should not be infused in patients with

- fasting triglycerides greater than 500 mg/dL
- pancreatitis accompanied by hyperlipidemia with triglycerides greater than 500 mg/L
- nephrotic syndrome with hypertriglyceridemia
- fat emulsion hypersensitivity (rare)

Basic Formulation of Standard TPN Solutions

Caloric, protein, fluid, electrolyte, mineral, and vitamin requirements are all critical parameters when determining TPN orders. Dextrose solutions are available in varying concentrations. For example, D50 contains 500 grams of dextrose per liter, whereas D70 has 700 grams of dextrose per liter. The selected dextrose solution is added to the TPN and diluted by the volume of other additives.

Amino acid solutions come in a variety of concentrations: 5.2 percent (52 grams of amino acids per liter) to 15 percent (150 grams of amino acids per liter). Amino acid solutions also are added to TPN and diluted by the volume of other additives.

Lipid emulsion solutions are available in concentrations of 10 percent (100 grams of fat per liter) or 20 percent (200 grams of fat per liter). They can be mixed directly with the combined dextrose and amino acid solution (resulting in a 3-in-1 solution) or infused separately.

Vitamins, minerals, and trace elements, in amounts equivalent to 100 percent of the daily requirements, are routinely added to TPN to prevent deficiencies. Although vitamin K is not found in the standard solution, 1 mg of vitamin K may be administered daily via the TPN. In the event that vitamin, mineral, or trace element deficiencies or unusual losses occur, they can be supplemented above the amount normally added to the TPN solution.

Electrolytes are routinely added to the TPN solutions in amounts sufficient to provide for daily needs. Increased or decreased amounts of electrolytes can be specially ordered.

Infusing Parenteral Nutrition

Access to the Venous System TPN infusions are delivered through the venous system via one of the following access routes:

- *Central access:* Subclavian, jugular, femoral, or peripherally inserted central catheter (PICC) via the cephalic or basilic veins.
- *Peripheral access:* Peripheral catheters are generally standard IV catheters.

Administering TPN Infusion When using a continuous TPN regimen, it is important to determine the desired volume to be delivered and the rate of infusion to fulfill the patient's caloric and protein needs over a 24-hour period.

Patients on continuous TPN over 24 hours who are clinically or metaboli-cally stable and exhibit no complications may benefit from cycled TPN to increase their freedom, mobility, and ease of care. Cycled TPN generally is infused over a 10- to 16-hour period.

Monitoring

The following parameters should be monitored in patients on TPN:

Metabolic parameters The following values should be monitored daily initially, then three times weekly once they are stable: sodium, potassium, chloride, CO2, BUN, creatinine, glucose, hematocrit, hemoglobin, WBC, calcium, magnesium, phosphorus, and platelets. Other values that also should be evaluated daily initially and then weekly (once they are stable) are: PT/PTT, triglycerides, bilirubin, alkaline phosphatase, ALT, and AST.

Nutrition parameters Daily weight evaluations should include estimated dry weight and weight change. Albumin and prealbumin levels should be moni-tored weekly.

Fluid status To determine if the patient is dehydrated or at risk for fluid overload, monitor input and output volumes closely.

Infection If the WBC count is increasing or the patient is febrile (tempera-ture above 100°F), a blood culture from the catheter and peripheral site should be obtained. Evidence of an infection requires instituting appropriate antibiotic therapy. An infected central line may need to be replaced.

Complications of Parenteral Nutrition

Complications of Catheterization Mechanical complications of catheter insertion include pneumothorax, hydrothorax, and great vessel injury. To minimize mor-bidity, obtaining a chest x-ray before using a new central line for TPN is impor-tant to ensure that the line was correctly placed and that no internal injuries occurred during its insertion.

Venous thrombosis increases these patients' risk for pulmonary embolism. To minimize this risk, heparin (3000 units per liter) may be added to the TPN if it is not otherwise contraindicated by the patient's medical conditions.

Catheter related sepsis usually is caused by staphylococcal, fungal (*Candida*), and gram-negative organism infections. The occurrence of these infections can be minimized with meticulous catheter insertion and good maintenance catheter care.

Metabolic Complications Hyperglycemia may be associated with glucosuria, osmotic diuresis, hyperosmolar nonketotic dehydration and diabetic ketoaci-dosis. A fingerstick blood glucose should be performed four times daily in patients found to be hyperglycemic. Insulin administered on a sliding scale is

used to bring blood glucose to acceptable levels. Once a stable insulin requirement is established, regular doses of insulin can be added to the TPN.

Hypoglycemia may be seen in patients after abrupt discontinuation of TPN
infusion with a high glucose load. To avoid this problem, infusions can be
tapered down over a period of two to three hours to allow for serum insulin
adaptation, however, this approach is rarely necessary.

Electrolyte imbalances are common in severely stressed patients both before
and after TPN infusions are begun. Furthermore, serum electrolyte levels may
fluctuate significantly as TPN infusions begin. Close monitoring of electrolytes,
magnesium, calcium, and phosphorus during the first few days of TPN is
important. Corrections for electrolyte imbalances must be made promptly to
avoid serious complications such as seizures, arrhythmias, or even death.

Fluid imbalances Dehydration and fluid overload are two major concerns when
TPN administration is the primary route of fluid infusion. In cases where fluid
restriction is not indicated, fluid requirements for maintenance are generally
calculated at 30 to 35 ml/kg. Clinically dehydrated patients may have fluid
requirements as high as 40 to 50 ml/kg, which should be met as long as no contraindications are present. Fluid overload or edema is seen in patients with
renal failure, liver failure, congestive heart failure, and hypoalbuminemia.
Excessive TPN volume infusion can significantly exacerbate diseases that are
known to cause fluid retention. Under these circumstances, a concentrated TPN
solution may be used.

Refeeding syndrome occurs in victims of prolonged starvation with severe
imbalances of serum phosphorus, potassium, and/or magnesium as well as
fluid and glucose. Once nutrition support begins, increased cellular uptake of
electrolytes may cause extremely low serum electrolyte levels. This dramatic
shift can lead to cardiac dysfunction and potentially death. Phosphorus, potassium, magnesium, glucose, and fluid status must be monitored closely in these
patients when nutrition support is initiated. The initial TPN infusion should
aim to meet 75 to 100 percent of BEE (not total energy needs). Subsequent
infusions should advance slowly toward the goal of meeting total energy
needs, with repletion of electrolytes and minerals as needed (see Chapter 3,
Case 3).

Biliary disease is common in patients receiving long-term TPN, and particularly in those who are also NPO. The incidence of cholelithiasis and biliary sludge
increases with the duration of TPN. Bile stasis may be minimized by oral feedings when feasible.

Hepatic steatosis is the most frequent liver abnormality in adult patients receiving long-term TPN. Biochemically, hepatic steatosis is marked by increases in
transaminases, alkaline phosphatase, and bilirubin. The presence of hepatic fat
is often due to excessive carbohydrate infusion. In rare cases, this generally
benign condition can lead to liver failure.

Abdominal Trauma

Scott Stuart, Melanie Stuart, and Lisa D. Unger

Objectives

- To assess the nutritional status of a patient with abdominal trauma resulting in small bowel resection.
- To identify the indications for TPN in a patient with short bowel syndrome.
- To calculate calorie, protein, and fluid requirements for a patient receiving TPN.
- To understand the clinical and laboratory parameters that must be monitored in a patient receiving TPN.

HP, a 26-year-old man, presents to the emergency room by ambulance with multiple stab wounds to the abdomen. On arrival, HP was taken to the operating room for an exploratory laparotomy, and a large section of the small bowel was removed.

Past Medical History

HP has no significant past medical history.

Medications

HP takes a multivitamin with minerals daily. He has no known drug allergies.

Social History

HP is single and shares an apartment with two roommates. He reports the following information regarding substance use.

Alcohol: 6 beers per week
Smoking: None
Illicit drug use: None
Diet: Not following any special diet

Review of Systems

Findings from the review of systems were deemed noncontributory.

Physical Examination

Vital signs

Temperature: 102.1°F

Heart rate: 93 BPM

Respiratory rate: 23 BPM

Blood pressure: 109/54 mm Hg

Anthropometric data

Height: 6'3" (190.5 cm)

Current weight: 195 lb (88.6 kg)

IBW: 196 lb (89.1 kg)

General: Well-developed man lying in bed with moderate abdominal discomfort

Skin: Warm

HEENT: Normocephalic, EOMI, PERRLA, hearing intact bilaterally, nasogastric tube in place to drain gastric secretions; carotid pulses +2 bilaterally with no jugular venous distention·

Chest: Clear to auscultation

Cardiac: Regular rate and rhythm; normal S1 and S2; no rubs, gallops, or murmurs appreciated

Abdomen: Distended and tender; no bowel sounds noted. Twenty-centimeter midline incision noted with multiple staple stitches and two drainage tubes in place; impalpable liver and spleen

Extremities:

No edema noted

All peripheral pulses +2

Hep-lock in place on right arm with an infusion of normal saline at 75 ml/hour

Neurological:

Alert and oriented ×3

Cranial nerves II–XII intact

Gross vibration, light touch, and proprioception intact bilaterally

Laboratory Data

Patient's Values (Admission)	Normal Values
Albumin: 3.0 g/dL	3.5–5.8 g/dL
Sodium: 135 mEq/L	133–143 mEq/L
Potassium: 3.5 mEq/L	3.5–5.3 mEq/L
Chloride: 106 mEq/L	97–107 mEq/L
CO2: 25 mEq/L	24–32 mEq/L
BUN: 35 mg/dL	10–20 mg/dL
Creatinine: 1.3 mg/dL	0.8–1.3 mg/dL
Magnesium: 1.8 mg/dL	1.8–2.9 mg/dL
Phosphorus: 3.1 mg/dL	2.5–5.0 mg/dL
Glucose: 142 mg/dL	70–110 mg/dL
Calcium: 9.1 mg/dL	8.5–10.5 mg/dL

Case Questions

1. Is this patient a candidate for enteral or parenteral nutrition support? What additional information is needed to make this determination?

2. A double lumen catheter is placed into the subclavian vein for TPN. Before the catheter is used, what should be done to ensure that it was positioned appropriately?

3. What baseline anthropometric and laboratory data are important to obtain?

4. Calculate HP's caloric, protein, and fluid requirements.

5. What are the maximum amounts of calories from glucose and lipids that should be administered to this patient via TPN?

6. What clinical and laboratory parameters should be monitored in patients receiving TPN?

Answers begin on the following page.

Answers to Questions: Case 1

Part 1:   Nutrition Assessment

1. Is this patient a candidate for enteral or parenteral nutrition support? What additional information is needed to make this determination?

    HP is one day postoperative from an extensive small bowel resection. The attending surgeon reports that HP's duodenum is still intact, but the entire jejunum and proximal three-fourths of the ileum were resected, leaving about 21 inches of small bowel. Consequently, HP has short bowel syndrome, which can lead to malabsorption of nutrients as well as excessive losses of fluid and electrolytes because the jejunum and ileum play a major role in nutrient absorption and maintaining fluid and electrolyte balance. HP is therefore at significant risk for developing malnutrition, dehydration, and electrolyte abnormalities, and requires total parenteral nutrition (TPN) support to meet his current calorie, protein, fluid, and electrolyte requirements.

Part 2:   Nutrition Therapy and Plan

2. A double lumen catheter is placed into the subclavian vein for TPN. Before the catheter is used, what should be done to ensure that it was positioned appropriately?

    The position of the catheter must be verified with a chest x-ray and a pneumothorax must be ruled out before initiating TPN infusion. Injury to the lung during catheter insertion may result in pneumothorax, the presence of air in the pleural cavity.

3. What baseline anthropometric and laboratory data are important to obtain?

    Current weight, estimated dry weight, sodium, potassium, chloride, CO_2, BUN, creatinine, glucose, calcium, magnesium, phosphorus, hematocrit, hemoglobin, WBC, platelets, PT/PTT, bilirubin, alkaline phosphatase, ALT, AST, triglycerides, albumin, and prealbumin.

4. Calculate HP's caloric, protein, and fluid requirements.

    Calories: HP is currently hypermetabolic and hypercatabolic secondary to his stab wounds, fever, and extensive surgery, and has therefore increased energy, protein, mineral, and vitamin needs. His energy requirements, based on the Harris-Benedict equation, are as follows.

    For men,

    $$BEE = 66 + 13.7 \text{ (Weight in kg)} + 5.0 \text{ (Height in cm)} - 6.8 \text{ (Age)}$$

In HP's case,

BEE = 66 + 13.7 (88.6 kg) + 5.0 (190.5 cm) – 6.8 (26) = 2054 kcal

Adjusting this figure by a factor of 1.3 to account for weight mainte-nance, hospitalization, and confinement to bed gives

Total energy requirements = 2054 kcal x 1.3 = 2670 kcal/day

Since lipid emulsions generally provide 30 percent of calories, HP should receive 800 lipid kcals and 1900 glucose kcals.

Protein Protein requirements for patients who have undergone surgery and are under severe stress are estimated at 2.0 g/kg/day.

(88.6 kg) (2.0 g/kg/day) = 177 g/day

Fluid Fluid needs are 35 ml/kg/day. In HP's case, this amounts to 3100 ml/day. Because of his high fluid needs, this patient would benefit from receiving 3 liters of a 3-in-1 TPN mixture daily, with the appropriate decrease in IV fluids. Patients with short bowel syndrome will also have fluid losses through the nasogastric tube and through the GI tract with diarrhea. These losses must be replaced with IV fluids to avoid dehy-dration.

5. **What are the maximum amounts of calories from glucose and lipids that should be administered to this patient via TPN?**

   Dextrose The maximum rate of glucose oxidation in adults is 5 mg/kg/min. Thus, in HP's case,

   (5.0 mg/kg/min) (88.6 kg) (1440 min/day) = 638 grams of dextrose per day

   Dextrose provides 3.4 kcal of energy per gram. Therefore HP should receive no more than the following number of calories daily from glu-cose.

   3.4 kcal/g x 638 g/day = 2169 kcal/day

   Lipids The maximum recommended daily lipid dose is 2.5 g/kg. In HP's case this amounts to

   (2.5 g/kg/day) (88.6 kg) = 221.5 g/day

   (221.5 g/day) (9 kcal/g) = 1993 kcal/day from lipids

6. **What clinical and laboratory parameters should be monitored in patients receiving TPN?**

   Multiple parameters must be monitored on a regular basis in patients receiving TPN.

   1. Fluid input and output should be monitored daily, particularly during the first week, to prevent dehydration or fluid overload. Vital signs such as blood pressure and heart rate and physical exam changes (e.g., edema, ascites) also offer evidence of fluid status.

   2. Daily weights should be measured. If the rate of weight loss or gain

is greater than 4 pounds in one week, consider fluid changes before adjusting caloric infusion.

3. The following metabolic parameters should initially be monitored daily, then three times per week when values are stable: sodium, potassium, chloride, CO_2, BUN, creatinine, glucose, hematocrit, hemoglobin, WBC, calcium, magnesium, phosphorus, and platelets. In addition, these values should be monitored weekly: PT/PTT, triglycerides, bilirubin, alkaline phosphatase, ALT, and AST.

4. Infections are a potential complication during TPN. If the WBC count is increasing or the patient is febrile, blood from the catheter and peripheral site should be cultured. When an infection is present, appropriate antibiotic therapy should be instituted, and catheter removal may be required.

Case 2

Pancreatitis

Myhanh E. T. Bosse and Anita Guevera

Objectives

- To utilize clinical, anthropometric, and laboratory data to assess the nutritional status of a patient with pancreatitis.
- To evaluate the use of Total Parenteral Nutrition (TPN) as part of the nutritional management plan for a patient with pancreatitis.

MG, a 45-year-old female, presents to the Emergency Room with sudden onset abdominal pain of increasing intensity, worse than she has previously experienced. She describes her pain as radiating through the mid-back and notes some improvement when she sits up and leans forward. She also complains of nausea and vomiting. MG reports similar episodes of abdominal pain over the past three years that resolved spontaneously within several days. However, this time the pain was severe enough for her to seek medical attention.

Past Medical History

MG's past medical history is unremarkable. It is negative for diabetes. She presently takes no medications on a regular basis, but reports taking Tylenol (acetaminophen) occasionally. She has no known drug or food allergies.

Social History

MG, a stockbroker, works 70 to 80 hours per week including the time she spends socializing nightly with clients from the office. She is recently divorced and has two teenage children. MG states that she has drunk several glasses of Scotch with dinner for the past 20 years. Her alcohol intake has increased over the past 5 years due to her hectic lifestyle and the recent stresses surrounding her marriage and her job. She does not smoke.

MG provided the dietitian with the following 24-hour recall, which she feels is typical of her usual intake at home.

MG's Usual Dietary Intake

Breakfast (Coffee Shop) 7:30 A.M.

Coffee	8 oz.
Half-and-half	2 Tbs.
Bagel	1 whole
Cream cheese	2 Tbs.

Lunch (Deli) 12:30 P.M.

Chicken salad sandwich	1
Potato chips	1 bag
Coconut custard pie	1/8 of pie
Coffee	8 oz.
Creamers	4

Dinner (Restaurant) 8:00 P.M.

Vodka on the rocks	3 oz.
Tossed salad	1/2 cup
Russian dressing	2 Tbs.
Baked salmon	4 oz.
Baked potato	1 medium
Sour cream	3 Tbs.

Total calories: 2369 kcal/day

Protein: 13% of calories

Fat: 45% of calories

Carbohydrate: 42% of calories

Review of Systems

The review of systems was unremarkable except for nausea, abdominal pain, and weight loss.

Physical Examination

Vital signs

Temperature: 100.1°F

Heart rate: 120 BPM

Respiration: 22 BPM

Blood pressure: 100/60 mm Hg

Anthropometric data

Height: 5'6" (168 cm)

Current weight: 105 lb (48 kg)

Usual weight: 139 lb (63 kg) one year ago

Ideal weight: 130 lb (59 kg)

Percent ideal weight: 81%

Triceps skinfold (TSF): 10 mm (<5th percentile)

Mid-arm muscle circumference (MAMC): 18 cm (180 mm) (<5th percentile)

General: Thin female who appears in moderate distress

Skin: Normal color, warm and dry

HEENT: Anicteric

Cardiac: Normal rate and rhythm

Abdomen: Marked abdominal tenderness, particularly in the epigastrium with guarding but no rebound; hypoactive bowel sounds

Extremities: No cyanosis or edema

Neurological: A + O × 3, non-focal

Clinical Studies

An obstruction series showed a mildly distended loop of the small bowel in left upper quadrant (sentinel loop) and calcifications of the pancreas. An abdominal ultrasound revealed a slightly enlarged pancreas, but no pseudocyst. There was no evidence of cholelithiasis (gallstones). Bile ducts appeared normal.

Laboratory Data

Patient's Values	Normal Values
Sodium: 138 mEq/L	133–143 mEq/L
Potassium: 3.5 mEq/L	3.5–5.3 mEq/L
Hemoglobin: 13.7 g/dL	13.5–17.5 g/dL
Hematocrit: 40%	40–52%
Albumin: 3.2 g/dL	3.5–5.2 g/dL
Calcium: 8.0 mg/dL	9–11 mg/dL
WBC: 10 tho/uL	4.0–11.0 tho/uL
BUN: 10 mg/dL	10–20 mg/dL
Glucose: 250 mg/dL	80–120 mg/dL
Amylase: 632 U/dL	60–180 U/dL
Lipase: 600 U/L	<150 U/L
Bilirubin: 1.0 mg/dL	0.2–1.2 mg/dL
Alkaline phosphatase: 122 U/L	60–220 U/L
AST: 22 U/L	0–40 U/L

ALT: 23 U/L	0–36 U/L
PT: 10 seconds	<12 seconds
Triglycerides: 57 mg/dL	<150 mg/dL

Hospital Course and Therapy

Upon admission to the hospital, MG was designated NPO (nothing to eat or drink) in an effort to promote bowel rest and allow for resolution of her abdominal pain, nausea, and vomiting. At the same time, she was rehydrated with IV fluids. However, seven days after admission she continued to experience abdominal pain, intermittent nausea, and vomiting despite bowel rest and the use of medications to treat her symptoms.

Case Questions

1. List MG's medical problems in the context of her overall clinical picture.

2. What are the possible etiologies of MG's abdominal pain, nausea, and vomiting?

3. Explain why amylase, lipase, calcium, and glucose are abnormal in patients with pancreatitis.

4. Using MG's current weight, calculate the percentage change from her usual weight over the past year.

5. What additional evidence from MG's physical exam should be used to assess her nutritional status prior to initiating TPN?

6. What is the primary concern with regard to MG's nutritional status at this time?

7. Why is TPN the most appropriate form of nutritional intervention at this point in MG's clinical course?

8. Using the Harris-Benedict equation, calculate MG's resting energy expenditure (REE). Then calculate her estimated daily calorie and protein needs for weight gain and anabolism.

9. What other nutrients should be added to the TPN in addition to protein, fat, and carbohydrates?

10. What biochemical and laboratory data should be used to monitor MG's TPN?

11. After MG's pancreatitis began to resolve and her bowel sounds showed increased activity, her physician decided that she should begin an oral diet. How should MG's feeding begin and what recommendations are appropriate upon discharge?

Answers begin on the following page.

Answers to Questions: Case 2

Part 1:   Clinical Assessment

1.   **List MG's medical problems in the context of her overall clinical picture.**

   - Acute pancreatitis given the clinical picture and elevated amylase and lipase
   - Chronic pancreatitis as evidenced by prior bouts of abdominal pain and calcification of the pancreas
   - Glucose intolerance secondary to acute pancreatitis in addition to chronic pancreatitis
   - Weight loss
   - Moderate to severe malnutrition

2.   **What are the possible etiologies of MG's abdominal pain, nausea, and vomiting?**

   Inflammation of the pancreas secondary to alcoholism is one possibility. Alcohol abuse is one of the most common causes of pancreatitis. Though the exact mechanism whereby alcoholism leads to pancreatitis is not clear, one theory is autodigestion, an excessive accumulation of pancreatic enzymes in the pancreas that overcomes the trypsin inhibitor. Trypsin is then activated within the pancreas and "digests" the pancreas itself. The major symptom of pancreatic autodigestion is abdominal pain; nausea, vomiting, fever, and abdominal distention are also common. The loss of 90 percent of pancreatic tissue causes pancreatic insufficiency, resulting in the loss of digestive enzymes, and ultimately leads to malabsorption of multiple nutrients, diarrhea, and weight loss.

Part 2:   Assessment of Laboratory Data

3.   **Explain why amylase, lipase, calcium, and glucose are abnormal in patients with pancreatitis.**

   Amylase is elevated because of secretion of digestive enzymes from the pancreas into neighboring tissues and the bloodstream. Lipase also is elevated because of secretion of lipase from the pancreas into the bloodstream, which splits fat into glycerol and fatty acids. Calcium is decreased because of the combination of fatty acids released by lipolysis in the abdomen with calcium in the gut to form soaps (saponification), which depletes plasma levels of this ion. Glucose is elevated because of impaired insulin secretion in response to glucose and inflammatory destruction of islets of Langerhans. Glucagon released from alpha cells may contribute to the elevation of blood glucose. This phenomenon occurs in severe pancreatitis or chronic pancreatitis.

Part 3:   Nutrition Assessment

4. Using MG's current weight, calculate the percentage change from her usual weight.

$$\text{Percent weight change} = \frac{\text{Usual weight} - \text{current weight}}{\text{Usual weight}} \times 100$$

$$= \frac{139 \text{ lb} - 105 \text{ lb}}{139 \text{ lb}} \times 100 = 24.5\%$$

This represents a severe weight loss because it is greater than 20 percent in one year.

5. **What additional evidence from MG's physical exam should be used to assess her nutritional status prior to initiating TPN?**

To complete an overall assessment of her nutritional status, take into consideration her percent weight change and anthropometric data. Using these data, MG is moderately to severely malnourished. She has experienced a 24-percent weight change, is currently 81 percent of ideal body weight, and has anthropometric measurements below the fifth percentile.

6. **What is the primary concern with regard to MG's nutritional status at this time?**

The primary nutritional concern is the possibility of a continued downward trend in MG's nutritional status in the face of increased calorie and protein needs during this episode of acute pancreatitis. The goals of nutrition therapy are to stop her weight loss and maintain her protein stores.

7. **Why is TPN the most appropriate form of nutritional intervention at this point in MG's clinical course?**

Enteral nutrition support is the first option for feeding patients with mild to moderate pancreatitis, especially through a jejunostomy if access is available. However, with severe pancreatitis, or if symptoms worsen because the enteral feeding stimulates pancreatic secretions and exacerbate the pancreatitis, TPN should be initiated. Since MG does not have an enteral jejunal access available for feeding and she has continued to have nausea and vomiting seven days into her admission, TPN is the most appropriate nutritional intervention. It was decided that she would benefit from total parenteral nutrition (TPN). A central line was placed on day 8, and TPN was initiated.

Part 4:   Hospital Course and Therapy

8. Using the Harris-Benedict equation, calculate MG's resting energy expenditure (REE). Then calculate her estimated daily calorie and protein needs for weight gain and anabolism.

> To calculate MG's daily calorie and protein needs for weight gain and anabolism,
>
> REE = 655 + 9.6 (Weight in kg) + 1.8 (Height in cm) − 4.7 (Age)
>
> = 655 + 9.6 (48 kg) + 1.8 (168 cm) − 4.7 (45)
>
> = 655 + 460.8 + 302.4 − 211.5
>
> = 1206 kcal/day
>
> Calorie needs = REE x 1.5 = 1800 kcal/day
>
> Protein needs = Current weight x 2.0 g/kg
>
> = 48 kg x 2.0 g/kg = 96 g/day

9. What other nutrients should be added to the TPN in addition to protein, fat, and carbohydrates?

> *Electrolytes* Sodium, potassium, calcium, magnesium, phosphorus, chloride
>
> *Water-soluble vitamins* Thiamin, riboflavin, niacin, vitamin C, vitamin B6, vitamin B12, folic acid, pantothenic acid, biotin
>
> *Fat-soluble vitamins* Vitamin E, vitamin D, vitamin A
>
> *Minerals and trace elements* Zinc, copper, selenium, chromium, manganese

10. What biochemical and laboratory data should be used to monitor MG's TPN?

> - Sodium, potassium, chloride, CO_2, hematocrit, hemoglobin, WBC, platelets, electrolytes, BUN, creatinine, calcium, magnesium, phosphorus, and glucose daily
> - Liver function tests every week
> - Albumin, transferrin, triglycerides, and prealbumin weekly

11. After MG's pancreatitis began to resolve and her bowel sounds showed increased activity, her physician decided that she should begin an oral diet. How should MG's feeding begin and what recommendations are appropriate upon discharge?

> Oral feedings should begin with a clear liquid diet. The diet should be advanced as tolerated to a low-fat, high-protein diet. MG's usual alcohol intake is too high given that her pancreatitis in most likely secondary

to her excessive alcohol intake. She should be advised to avoid alcohol and encouraged to join a support group to help her abstain.

MG's usual fat intake also is too high and will be difficult for her to tolerate given her chronic pancreatitis with decreased digestive enzymes. She should be advised to reduce her fat intake to less than 30 percent by using low-fat or fat-free cream cheese and margarine, substituting skim milk for the half-and-half in her coffee, and selecting fruits and pretzels instead of sweets and chips for snacks.

See Chapter Review Questions, pages A18–A19.

REFERENCES

American Dietetic Association. Enteral feeding by tube. In *The American Dietetic Association Handbook of Clinical Dietetics*. 2nd ed. New Haven, CT: Yale, 1992.

Bickston SJ. Nutritional therapy. In Ewald GA, McKenzie CR (eds). *The Washington Manual of Medical Therapeutics*. Boston: Little, Brown, 1995. 34–42.

Cavallini G, Vaona B, Bovo P, et al. Diabetes in chronic alcoholic pancreatitis. Role of residual beta cell function and insulin resistance. *Dig Dis Sci* 1993;38(3):497–501.

Fischer JE (ed). *Total Parenteral Nutrition*. 2nd ed. Boston: Little, Brown, 1991.

Ideno KT. Enteral nutrition. In Gottschlich MM, Matarese LE, Shronts EP (eds). *Nutrition Support Dietetics: Core Curriculum*. Silver Springs, MD: American Society for Parenteral and Enteral Nutrition, 1993:71–104.

Kinney JM, Jeejeebhoy KN, Hill G, et al. *Nutrition and Metabolism in Patient Care*. Philadelphia: WB Saunders, 1988.

Lowenfels AB, Maisonneuve P, Cavallini G. Prognosis of chronic pancreatitis: an international multicenter study. International Pancreatitis Study Group. *Am J Gastroenterol* 1994;89(9):1467–71.

Marotta F, Labadarios D, Frazer L, et al. Fat-soluble vitamin concentration in chronic alcohol-induced pancreatitis. Relationship with steatorrhea. *Dig Dis Sci* 1994;39(5):993–8.

Noel-Jorand MC, Bras J. A journal comparison of nutritional profiles of patients with alcohol-related pancreatitis and cirrhosis. 1994;29(1):65–74.

Robin AP, Campbell R., Palani CK, et al. Total parental nutrition during acute pancreatitis: clinical experience with 156 patients. *World J Surg* 1990;14(5): 572–579.

Rombeau JL, Caldwell MD (eds). *Enteral and Tube Feeding*. 2nd ed. Philadelphia: W.B. Saunders, 1990.

Rombeau JL, Caldwell MD (eds). *Parenteral nutrition*. Volume 2. 2nd ed. Philadelphia: WB Saunders, 1993.

Rombeau JL, Caldwell MD, Forlaw L, et al. *Atlas of Nutrition Support Techniques*. Boston: Little,Brown, 1989.

Shils ME, Olson JA, Shike M (eds). *Modern Nutrition in Health and Disease*. 8th ed. Philadelphia: Lea and Febiger, 1994.

Skipper A, Marian MJ. Parenteral nutrition. In Gottschlich MM, Matarese LE, and Shronts EP (eds). *Nutrition Support Dietetics*. Silver Spring, MD: American Society for Parenteral and Enteral Nutrition, 1992:105–124.

Torosian MH (ed). *Nutrition for the Hospitalized Patient*. New York: Marcel Dekker 1995.

Weinsier RL, Heimburger DC, Butterworth CE (eds). *Handbook of Clinical Nutrition*. 2nd ed. Baltimore: C.V. Mosby, 1989:221–242.

Zeman FJ. Methods of nutrition support. In *Clinical Nutrition and Dietetics*. 3rd ed. New York: MacMillan, 1994.

Appendix: Nutrition Food Pyramid

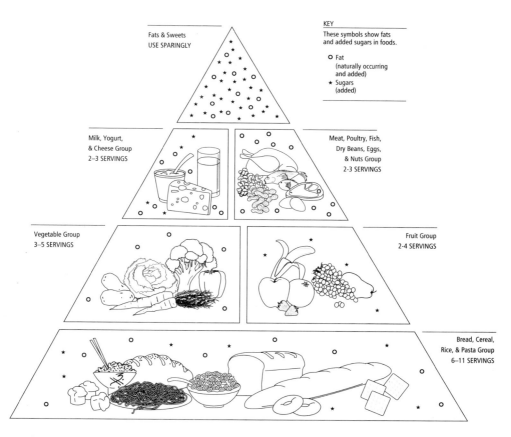

Fats & Sweets
USE SPARINGLY

KEY
These symbols show fats
and added sugars in foods.

○ Fat
(naturally occurring
and added)
★ Sugars
(added)

Milk, Yogurt,
& Cheese Group
2–3 SERVINGS

Meat, Poultry, Fish,
Dry Beans, Eggs,
& Nuts Group
2-3 SERVINGS

Vegetable Group
3–5 SERVINGS

Fruit Group
2-4 SERVINGS

Bread, Cereal,
Rice, & Pasta Group
6–11 SERVINGS

The Pyramid is an outline of what to eat each day. It's not a rigid prescription, but a general guide that lets you choose a healthful diet that's right for you. The Pyramid calls for eating a variety of foods to get the nutrients you need and at the same time the right amount of calories to maintain a healthy weight.

The food guide pyramid emphasizes foods from the five food groups shown in the three lower sections of the Pyramid.

Each of these food groups provides some, but not all, of the nutrients you need. Foods in one group can't replace those in another. No one food group is more important than another—for good health, you need them all.

Source: U.S. Department of Agriculture and the U.S. Department of Health and Human Services.

A closer look at fat and added sugars

The small tip of the Pyramid shows fats and sweets. These are foods such as salad dressing, cream, butter, margarine, sugars, soft drinks, candies, and sweet desserts. Alcoholic beverages are also part of this group. These foods provide calories but few vitamins and minerals. Most people should go easy on foods from this group.

Some fat or sugar symbols are shown in the other food groups. That's to remind you that some foods in these groups can also be high in fat and added sugars. When choosing foods for a healthful diet, consider the fat and added sugars in your choices from all the food groups, not just fats and sweets from the Pyramid tip.

How many servings do you need each day?

Calorie levels*	Women & some older adults about 1600	Children, teen girls, active women, most men about 2200	Teen boys & active men about 2800
Bread group	6	9	11
Vegetable group	3	4	5
Fruit group	2	3	4
Milk group	2–3**	2–3**	2–3**
Meat group	2	2	3
	for a total of 5 ounces	for a total of 6 ounces	for a total of 7 ounces

*These are the calorie levels if you choose lowfat, lean foods from the 5 major food groups and use foods from the fats and sweets group sparingly.

**Women who are pregnant or breastfeeding, teenagers, and young adults to age 24 need 3 servings.

What counts as a serving? The amount you eat may be more than one serving. For example, a dinner portion of spaghetti would count as 2 or 3 servings.

Bread, Cereal, Rice, Pasta Group	1 slice of bread
	1/2 cup of cooked rice or pasta
	1/2 cup of cooked cereal
	1 ounce of ready-to-eat cereal
Vegetable Group	1/2 cup of chopped raw or cooked vegetables
	1 cup of leafy raw vegetables
Fruit Group	1 piece of fruit or melon wedge
	3/4 cup of juice
	3/4 cup of canned fruit
	1/4 cup of dried fruit
Milk, Yogurt & Cheese Group	1 cup of milk or yogurt
	1 1/2 ounces of natural cheese
	2 ounces of process cheese
Dry Beans, Eggs & Nuts Group	2 1/2 to 3 ounces of cooked lean meat, poultry, or fish
	Count 1/2 cup of cooked beans, or 1 egg, or 2 tablespoons of peanut butter as 1 ounce of lean meat
Fats & Sweets Group	LIMIT CALORIES FROM THESE especially if you need to lose weight

Source: U.S. Department of Agriculture and the U.S. Department of Health and Human Services.

Review Questions

Chapter 1

1. Nutritional information may be integrated into the medical history, review of systems, and physical examination. Column A lists topics that should be addressed when working up a patient. Match each issue with the appropriate part of the medical workup in Column B.

Column A		Column B
Alcohol intake	_____	a. Past Medical History
Vitamin intake	_____	b. Social History
Food intake	_____	c. Review of Systems
Appetite	_____	d. Physical Exam
Weight change	_____	
Height/Weight	_____	
Triceps skinfold	_____	

2. SD is a 50-year-old obese woman who wants to reduce her calorie intake sufficiently to lose one pound per week. By how many calories must she reduce her intake each week to achieve her goal (that is, how many calories are in one pound of fat)?

   a. 500 calories
   b. 1000 calories
   c. 2000 calories
   d. 3500 calories

3. TF, a 30-year-old man, was diagnosed as HIV+ one year ago. Admitted to the hospital complaining of severe pain on swallowing solid food, he reports a good appetite and stable weight until ten days prior to admission when he began to experience the pain. Which of the following laboratory test(s) are good initial indicators of his recent change in appetite and in dietary intake?

    a. cholesterol
    b. transferrin
    c. prealbumin
    d. albumin

4. What percentage of hospitalized patients in the United States is estimated to be malnourished?

    a. 5–10%
    b. 30–35%
    c. 50–60%
    d. >75%

5. CT, a 68-year-old woman, was found unconscious in her apartment by her landlord. She was admitted to the hospital for dehydration and malnutrition. The diagnosis of malnutrition was based on evidence from CT's review of systems and physical exam. Which of the following clinical manifestations and physiological adaptations are related to the progression of malnutrition and could have offered evidence to support the diagnosis?

    a. weakness
    b. temporal muscle wasting
    c. bradycardia, hypotension
    d. all of the above

6. Energy is provided by the oxidation of dietary protein, fat, carbohydrate, and alcohol. Match the nutrient in Column A with the amount of calories in Column B that are produced during oxidation

Column A		Column B
Protein	_____	a. 4 calories per gram
Fat	_____	b. 7 calories per gram
Carbohydrate	_____	c. 9 calories per gram
Alcohol	_____	

Chapter 2

1. What vitamin or mineral is routinely given to alcoholics to decrease the neurological complications associated with alcohol abuse?

    a. vitamin C
    b. zinc
    c. thiamin
    d. vitamin A

2. Which of the following individuals is most likely to be consuming an adequate diet and therefore not require an additional vitamin and mineral supplement?

    a. a strict vegetarian (vegan)
    b. an adolescent with anorexia nervosa

    c. a homeless person with alcoholism

    d. none of the above

3. The following diseases may result in malabsorption of fat-soluble vitamins except

    a. multiple sclerosis

    b. chronic pancreatitis

    c. short bowel syndrome

    d. cystic fibrosis

4. All of the following exhibit antioxidant properties except

    a. vitamin K

    b. vitamin A / beta-carotene

    c. vitamin C

    d. vitamin E

5. Patients with increased metabolic needs due to physical stress may have increased vitamin and mineral needs. Which of the following physical stresses increase a patient's vitamin and mineral requirements?

    a. burns

    b. infection/fever

    c. surgery

    d. all of the above

6. WS is a 55-year-old man with pellagra, characterized by dementia, diarrhea, and dermatitis. Which of the following vitamin deficiencies results in pellagra?

    a. niacin

    b. riboflavin

    c. vitamin B_{12}

    d. vitamin E

7. What vitamin deficiency is associated with an elevated prothrombin time (PT)?

    a. vitamin B_{12}

    b. vitamin C

    c. vitamin K

    d. vitamin A

Chapter 3

1. AB, a 24-year-old woman in the eighth week of gestation. Considering that AB's prepregnancy BMI was 21.2 (normal range), what is the total amount of weight she should gain during her pregnancy according to the National Academy of Sciences?

    a. at least 10 pounds

    b. 15–25 pounds

    c. 25–35 pounds

    d. 28–40 pounds

2. AB also complains of frequent morning sickness that has worsened gradually over the past few weeks. What is the most likely cause of AB's nausea and vomiting at this time in her pregnancy (8 weeks gestation)?

    a. increased levels of estrogen

    b. increased levels of human chorionic gonadotropin (HCG)

    c. frequent fluctuations (increases and decreases) of HCG, estrogen, and progesterone

    d. increased levels of growth hormone

3. LH, a 32-year-old woman planning her second pregnancy, has already delivered an infant with a neural tube defect (spina bifida) and asks if there is anything she can do to prevent a recurrence. Which vitamin supplement has been shown to decrease the incidence of neural tube defects in newborns when given to pregnant women who have previously delivered a child with such a defect?

    a. vitamin B12

    b. folic acid

    c. thiamin

    d. all of the above

4. LH likes to drink one glass of wine when she goes out to dinner on the weekends. Which statement is true concerning alcohol intake during pregnancy?

    a. Alcohol during pregnancy always causes fetal alcohol syndrome and birth defects.

    b. Alcohol during the first trimester of pregnancy is safe in moderation.

    c. Alcohol during the third trimester of pregnancy is safe in moderation.

    d. Alcohol is not recommended for pregnant women, as no known safe threshold for alcohol intake in pregnancy exists.

5. CB, a 30-year-old woman, is in week 35 of gestation. When questioned by her obstetrician, CB is unsure whether or not she will breast-feed her baby. All of the following are benefits of breast-feeding *except*

    a. Breast-feeding reduces the incidence of ear infections and gastrointestinal problems in babies.

    b. Exclusive breast-feeding through the first four months of life is the optimal form of nutrition for babies.

    c. Breast-feeding is convenient and economical. Breast milk is always at the proper temperature and ready to serve.

    d. Breast-feeding causes the nursing mother to lose postpartum weight quickly, therefore she should consume a high fat, high calorie diet (or an extra 800 calories per day).

6. CB begins successfully to breast-feed her new baby after speaking to a lactation consultant in the hospital. Which of the following statements regarding maternal milk production is true?

a. Breast-milk production is dependent on maternal nutritional status.
b. Breast-milk production is independent of the weight of the infant.
c. Breast-milk production is unaffected by the frequency of nursing.
d. Breast-milk production is unaffected by smoking as none of the circulating components of cigarette smoke pass into breast milk.

7. CB asks what vitamins, if any, are lacking in breast milk. Excluding vitamin K, which is routinely given to all infants, what vitamin(s) are most likely to be present only in low levels in breast milk, depending on the mother's diet and genetic makeup?
   a. vitamin A
   b. vitamin D
   c. both (a) and (b)
   d. neither (a) nor (b) because breast milk contains all vitamins

8. NM, a 15-year-old girl, comes to the OB/GYN clinic for her first prenatal visit. She reports having begun menstruation at age 13. NM is 5' 7" tall, and her prepregnancy weight was 115 pounds (BMI <19.8). Based on NM's prepregnancy weight status, how much weight should she gain during her pregnancy?
   a. 15–20 pounds
   b. 20–25 pounds
   c. 25–30 pounds
   d. 30–45 pounds

Chapter 4

Betty Smith gives birth prematurely at 35 weeks gestation (40 weeks is full-term gestation) to triplets: Jennifer, Tiffany, and Fred. They weigh 2.05 kg, 2.10 kg, and 2.15 kg, respectively, at birth. At one month of age, each child weighs 2.4 kg.

1. Ms. Smith is concerned about the children's small size and wants to introduce solid foods to help "fatten them up." Should small infants be given solid foods at one month of age to stimulate more rapid growth?
   a. No, the children do not have the proper head control or oropharyngeal coordination to accept solid food.
   b. Yes, most solid foods are more dense in calories than breast milk or formula.
   c. No. The early introduction of solid food may contribute to the development of food allergies.
   d. Both (a) and (c) are correct.

At six months of age the children are seen again by their pediatrician. Ms. Smith is concerned because her friend's triplets, who are the same age as Jennifer, Tiffany, and Fred, are much bigger. To determine whether the children are growing appropriately, the pediatrician plots their measurements on growth charts. (Remember that premature children's growth measurement must be adjusted for their prematurity until they are two years old. Therefore, these six-month-old children are assessed as if they were five months old.) The following growth measurements and percentiles were obtained.

	Jennifer	Tiffany	Fred
Weight	6.0 kg (10th %ile)	5.8 kg (5-10th %ile)	6.0 kg (25th %ile)
Height	62 cm (10th %ile)	64 cm (25th %ile)	62 cm (25th %ile)
Head circumference	40 cm (10th %ile)	40.5 cm (10-25th %ile)	40.5 cm (10-25th %ile)

2. Are the children's growth measurements within the normal range?

   a. Yes.

   b. No.

   c. The answer cannot be determined without evaluating the children's dietary intake.

3. Because of financial problems, Mr. Smith asks about changing the children from formula to regular cow's milk (whole milk) when they are six months old. Which of the following is the best response?

   a. The introduction of cow's milk before one year of age may induce a low-grade loss of blood from the GI tract.

   b. Although cow's milk is relatively low in iron, the iron is very bioavailable, and milk can be introduced before one year of age.

   c. The high renal solute load of cow's milk helps stimulate the development of an infant's kidneys.

   d. Cow's milk is high in the vitamins and minerals that infants need at six months of age.

4. When the children are 12 months old, Mr. Smith has a severe myocardial infarction (heart attack) and is advised to adhere to a low-fat diet. Based on this history, is it appropriate to recommend that the children follow a low-fat diet at the age of 12 months? Which of the following is the best response?

   a. Because the children have a positive family history of early heart disease, their cholesterol levels should be measured. If the levels are high, they should be put on a low-fat diet.

   b. The children should be placed on a low-fat diet immediately.

   c. Children should not be put on low-fat diets until the age of two years.

   d. None of the preceding answer is correct.

5. The children are found to be anemic and iron-deficient at one year of age. Could this anemia have been prevented?

   a. Because the children were premature, they should have received iron supplements.

   b. All one-year-old children are mildly anemic as a result of normal development.

   c. No. iron supplements are not recommended for young children because they cause severe constipation.

   d. None of the above.

6. Jodie was born on the day Bosnian civil war broke out in her country and was orphaned shortly thereafter. A full-term baby, she weighed 2.9 kg and was 48 cm long (10th percentile). Jodie was delivered to a local orphanage in an area of heavy fighting and fed a low-calorie diet because of food shortages. At six months of age, Jodie weighed 4.0 kg and was 52 cm long (< 5th percentile). Jodie is now one year old, a truce has been reached in her country, and food shipments are delivered regularly to the area. Jodie weighs 5.0 kg, is 55 cm long (both parameters < 5th percentile), and is hypotensive and bradycardic. At this time Jodie is allowed free access to food and within a few days develops heart failure. Why?

   a. Jodie drank too much fluid and is fluid overloaded.
   b. Jodie is severely malnourished and was not refed slowly.
   c. Jodie is protein deficient and was not given protein when the truce was declared.
   d. All of the preceding answers are correct.

7. Mrs. Jones brings Jane, her 15-year-old daughter, to see her pediatrician. Jane's grandmother, who has severe osteoporosis, fell last week and broke her hip. Mrs. Jones and Jane are in the midst of a fight because Jane refuses to drink milk. Mrs. Jones wants Jane to drink milk to prevent her from developing osteoporosis later in life. Which of the following statements is correct?

   a. A large intake of dairy products is not recommended for adolescents because so many of them are lactose intolerant.
   b. Large amounts of dairy products are not recommended because they are a significant source of saturated fat, which promotes atherosclerosis and diabetes.
   c. Dairy products, an efficient source of calcium that promotes proper bone mineralization are required by children and adolescents.
   d. Dairy products are not important for adolescents because bone mineralization ends before puberty starts.

Chapter 5

1. Assessing the functional status of older adults is an important component of the medical history because limited functional capacity may increase the risk of malnutrition. All of the following are activities of daily living (ADLs) except

   a. toileting/bathing
   b. feeding
   c. transferring from bed to chair
   d. shopping

2. All of the following are instrumental activities of daily living (IADLs) except

   a. cooking

  b. dressing
  c. handling money
  d. using the telephone

3. How can medications affect the nutritional status of older adults?
    a. alter food intake, absorption of nutrients, and excretion
    b. decrease appetite, taste, and smell
    c. cause gastrointestinal disturbances, such as constipation
    d. all of the above

4. CT is an 87-year-old nursing home resident who has a permanent jejunostomy feeding tube. His physician recently prescribed phenytoin to control CT's seizure disorder. What is the most appropriate time to administer this medication?
    a. During the morning tube feeding.
    b. During the evening tube feeding.
    c. Two hours before or after the patient receives tube feedings.
    d. Anytime; absorption of the medication is not affected by tube feeding.

5. MF is a 59-year-old, postmenopausal woman. Her gynecologist has prescribed estrogen and progesterone hormonal replacement therapy for her. According to the National Institutes of Health Consensus Development Conference on optimal calcium intake, what is her recommended calcium intake?
    a. 400 mg/day
    b. 800 mg/day
    c. 1000 mg/day
    d. 1500 mg/day

6. TK, a 65-year-old woman who was involved in a motor vehicle accident, has been hospitalized for two weeks and has an altered mental status. A feeding tube was inserted on day 7 to supply her nutritional requirements. To minimize her risk for aspiration, a nasoenteric tube should be placed in which position?
    a. The placement of the tube does not matter.
    b. The tube should empty into the esophagus.
    c. The tube should empty into the stomach.
    d. The tube should empty into the duodenum or jejunum (postpyloric position).

7. All of the following are risk factors for osteoporosis. Place a (P) next to the primary factors and an (S) next to the secondary factors.

	Answers
Smoking	_____
Short stature	_____
Kidney disease	_____
Hyperthyroidism	_____
Family history of osteoporosis	_____
COPD	_____

Early menopause   _____
Sedentary lifestyle   _____

Chapter 6

1. Column A is a list of nutrients from the American Heart Association Step I diet designed to lower serum cholesterol. Match each nutrient with the appropriate recommendation in Column B, assuming a 2000 calorie diet. Answers in Column B may be used more than once.

    Column A   **Column B**
    Total fat   _____   a. Up to 60% of total calories
    Saturated fat   _____   b. <300 mg/day
    Polyunsaturated fat   _____   c. <30% of total calories
    Monounsaturated fat   _____   d. Up to 15% of total calories
    Cholesterol   _____   e. Up to 10% of total calories
    Carbohydrates   _____   f. Up to 20% of total calories
    Protein   _____

2. RJ is a 50-year-old woman with one risk factor for heart disease. At what LDL cholesterol level should dietary therapy be initiated?
    a. 100 mg/dL
    b. 130 mg/dL
    c. 160 mg/dL
    d. 190 mg/dL

3. All of the following diseases or disorders may contribute to secondary hyper-lipidemia except
    a. diabetes mellitus
    b. hypothyroidism
    c. dumping syndrome
    d. nephrotic syndrome

4. According to the National Cholesterol Education Program, in addition to an elevated serum LDL cholesterol, which of the following are risk factors for heart disease?
    a. age: (males: >45 years; females: > 55 years)
    b. family history
    c. smoking
    d. diabetes
    e. HDL: <35 mg/dL
    f. hypertension

5. Monounsaturated fat has fewer calories than saturated fat. Circle the correct answer.

    True   False

6. NJ is a 77-year-old woman with congestive heart failure (CHF). On physical exam she has 2+ edema bilaterally. Her weight appears within normal limits (100% IBW) and she has not experienced a recent weight loss. Laboratory tests reveal an albumin of 2.8 mg/dL (normal: 3.5–5.0 mg/dL). Based on this patient's physical exam findings, what does the abnormal albumin indicate?

    a. It is falsely elevated.
    b. It is falsely reduced.
    c. It is correct and NJ is not consuming enough calories.
    d. It is correct and NJ is not consuming enough protein.

7. PL is a 58-year-old man with a family history of premature heart disease and hyperlipidemia. He has a cholesterol level of 300 mg/dL, LDL level of 190 mg/dL, triglyceride level of 400 mg/dL, and HDL level of 30 mg/dL. What type of hyperlipidemia do these values suggest? Select only one answer.

    a. familial hypercholesterolemia
    b. familial combined hyperlipidemia
    c. familial hypertriglyceridemia
    d. familial chylomicronemia syndrome

8. Patients with significantly elevated triglyceride levels (>1000 mg/dL) are at increased risk of developing which of the following medical conditions?

    a. heart disease
    b. pancreatitis
    c. colon cancer
    d. renal failure

Chapter 7

1. ST is a 27-year-old man admitted to the hospital with severe Crohn's disease and an unintentional weight loss of 20 pounds over the past two months despite a good appetite. Assuming that ST has steatorrhea, what is the most likely cause of his weight loss?

    a. obstruction
    b. malabsorption
    c. cancer
    d. AIDS

2. RF, a 62-year-old woman hospitalized with gastric cancer, undergoes gastric surgery (subtotal gastrectomy with gastrojejunostomy). Postoperatively she complains of diarrhea, cramping, flushing after eating, and early satiety. What is the most likely diagnosis?

    a. gastritis
    b. gastroparesis
    c. dumping syndrome
    d. lactose intolerance

3. RP, a 75-year-old man, presents to the Veterans Administration Medical Center with significant peripheral neuropathy. His past medical history is significant for a total gastrectomy performed when he was in his forties, after which he was never placed on vitamin supplements. He rarely drinks alcohol. RP's neuropathy is most likely secondary to malabsorption of which of the following vitamins?

    a. folate
    b. vitamin A
    c. pyridoxine (B6)
    d. vitamin B12

4. PR, a 50-year-old woman with chronic pancreatitis, is hospitalized for surgical evaluation. Assuming that PR takes pancreatic enzymes and can tolerate food, what diet order should be prescribed at this time?(Only 1 answer)

    a. low-sodium diet
    b. low-protein diet
    c. low-fat diet
    d. low-fiber diet

5. TI is a 65-year-old man with chronic liver disease and ascites. What dietary recommendation is appropriate for this patient? (Only 1 answer)

    a. low-sodium diet
    b. high-protein diet
    c. low-fat diet
    d. low-fiber diet

6. FG, a 31-year-old, moderately obese woman, complains of gastroesophageal reflux that occurs most often when she is sleeping. All of the following recommendations may help alleviate this condition except

    a. reducing alcohol and caffeine intake
    b. slightly elevating the head when sleeping
    c. waiting at least two hours after eating to lie down
    d. increasing consumption of fatty foods

7. TY, a 45-year-old alcoholic, presents to the ER with pain in his stomach. Laboratory tests reveal the following results.

Patient's Value	Normal Value
Hemoglobin: 10 mg/dL	14–16 mg/dL
Mean corpuscular volume: 110 cuu	84–95 cuu

    Using this information, what type of anemia should be suspected in this patient?

    a. iron deficiency anemia
    b. macrocytic anemia
    c. hemolytic anemia
    d. sickle cell anemia

8. Based on your answer to question 1, what other clinical manifestations of this type of anemia would you expect to encounter during TY's physical exam? (Circle the two best answers.)

  a. angular stomatitis
  b. pallor
  c. arthralgia
  d. peripheral neuropathy

Chapter 8

1. Results of the Diabetes Control and Complications Trial (DCCT) concluded that intensive therapy does delay the onset and slow the progression of diabetic retinopathy, nephropathy, and neuropathy in patients with diabetes mellitus. Which of the following was a major adverse effect of this intensive therapy?

  a. weight loss
  b. hypertension
  c. polyuria
  d. hypoglycemia

2. TR is a 60-year-old woman with NIDDM. She is 5'3" (135 cm) tall and weighs 155 pounds (70 kg). Her IBW is 115 pounds (52 kg). TR questions her doctor about the benefits of exercise for diabetics. All of the following are benefits of exercise in individuals with NIDDM *except*

  a. improved blood glucose levels due to decreased hepatic glucose output
  b. improved blood glucose levels due to decreased insulin sensitivity
  c. improved blood glucose levels due to increased peripheral utilization of glucose
  d. improved cardiovascular fitness and lipid levels

3. Diabetic control is optimal when which of the following blood tests are normal?

  a. HgbA1C
  b. albumin
  c. cholesterol
  d. fructose

4. Moderate amounts of alcohol may be included in the diabetic diet but may increase the risk of hypoglycemia in patients with IDDM. Which of the following statements is true concerning alcohol consumption in patients with IDDM?

  a. Insulin is required to metabolize alcohol.
  b. Alcohol may be consumed without food to prevent hyperglycemia.
  c. Alcohol is metabolized in a manner similar to carbohydrates.
  d. Alcohol inhibits gluconeogenesis in the liver.

5. SK, a 68-year-old man of Italian descent with a five year history of NIDDM is presently being treated by diet alone. He is 5' 7" tall and weighs 180 pounds. Current laboratory data reveal a fasting blood glucose of 183 mg/dL. SK loves olive oil and asks the doctor whether he may use it as much as he wants because it is high in monounsaturated fats. Considering his current status, which of the following responses is the best?

 a. Olive oil may be consumed in unlimited amounts.

 b. Olive oil should be limited because SK is overweight.

 c. Olive oil should be avoided because SK has diabetes.

 d. None of the responses is correct.

6. Approximately what percentage of patients with NIDDM are overweight?

 a. 10 percent

 b. 30 percent

 c. 50 percent

 d. 80 percent

7. TK, a 20-year-old student, presented to the Student Health Center four weeks ago complaining of polyuria and polydipsia during the preceding several weeks. His laboratory data indicated hyperglycemia, and he was diagnosed with diabetes mellitus. TK is 5'10" tall and weighs 210 pounds. Based on this patient's newly diagnosed diabetes, what dietary recommendations are indicated at this time? Circle the three best answers.

 a. low-fat

 b. high-fat

 c. no concentrated sweets

 d. low-salt

 e. unlimited calories

 f. calorie reduction

 g. low complex carbohydrates

Chapter 9

1. TF is an 86-year-old man with COPD. His FEV1 has fallen from 700 ml to 500 ml over the past two years. In addition, he has experienced a 25-pound weight loss over the same period and is considered malnourished. All of the following consequences of malnutrition are likely to occur in this patient *except*

 a. decreased respiratory muscle strength

 b. increased respiratory muscle mass

 c. decreased cell-mediated immunity

 d. increased risk for infections, especially pneumonia and bronchitis

2. Potential side effects of medications used to treat COPD, such as bronchodialators, include all of the following *except*

 a. increased energy level

    b. nausea and vomiting

    c. gastric irritation

    d. dysgeusia and dry mouth

3.   DP, an 8-year-old girl with cystic fibrosis (CF), is brought to her pediatrician complaining of weakness and lethargy. She presents with increased stool output, a recent weight loss of 8 pounds, and an abnormal prothrombin time (PT). Based on the chief complaint, the physical exam, and the laboratory information, what is the most likely cause of this patient's weight loss?

    a. heart failure

    b. liver disease

    c. anemia

    d. malabsorption

4.   Patients with obstructive sleep apnea syndrome (OSAS) represent 2 to 4 percent of the population. Which of the following medical conditions occurs in approximately two-thirds of patients with OSAS?

    a. respiratory failure

    b. bronchitis

    c. hypertension

    d. obesity

5.   QA undergoes a successful lung transplant and is prescribed cyclosporine on discharge from the hospital. What two laboratory abnormalities related to nutrition are frequently associated with long-term cyclosporine treatment?

    a. hypokalemia

    b. hyperkalemia

    c. hyperglycemia

    d. hyperlipidemia

6.   QA is also placed on long-term prednisone treatment. What two complications of high-dose prednisone therapy require nutritional intervention?

    a. weight gain that may lead to obesity

    b. anorexia that may lead to weight loss

    c. hyperglycemia

    d. hypoglycemia

Chapter 10

1.   The glomerular filtration rate (GFR) is used to determine whether protein restriction should be initiated in patients with Acute renal failure (ARF). At what GFR level should an ARF patient be prescribed a low-protein diet?

    a. GFR > 60 ml/min.

    b. GFR > 30 ml/min.

    c. GFR < 20 ml/min.

    d. GFR < 10 ml/min.

2. RI is a 65-year-old woman with chronic renal failure. Her 24-hour urinary sodium is 400 mEq. To determine RI's dietary sodium intake, convert the urinary sodium level to milligrams and select from the answers below. (Molecular weight of sodium = 23)

    a. 400 mg
    b. 1740 mg
    c. 4000 mg
    d. 9200 mg

3. Based on your calculation, do you think that RI is complying with her low-sodium diet?

    a. yes
    b. no
    c. not enough information to determine

4. The kidney plays an essential role in vitamin D metabolism. Vitamin D supplementation is usually required for patients with chronic renal failure because of the kidney's inability to convert which of the following? (D3 = cholecalciferol)

    a. 1,25 (OH)2-D3 → 25-(OH)-D3
    b. 25-(OH)-D3 → 1,25-(OH)2-D3
    c. 1,25-(OH)-D3 → 25-(OH)2-D3
    d. 25-(OH)2-D3 → 1,25-(OH)-D3

5. RI's serum potassium level is 5.9 mg/dL. Is a low-potassium diet indicated for RI at this time?

    a. yes
    b. no
    c. not enough information to determine

6. PF, a 50-year-old woman with nephrotic syndrome, has significantly elevated lipid levels. Which of the following mechanisms explains the elevated lipid levels found in patients with nephrotic syndrome?

    a. a defect in the LDL receptor, resulting in increased LDL levels
    b. increased lipoprotein clearance from the blood by lipoprotein lipase
    c. decreased hepatic protein synthesis
    d. decreased lipoprotein clearance from the blood by lipoprotein lipase

7. A low-calcium diet (< 500 mg/day) is indicated for patients with calcium oxalate stones. Circle the correct answer.

    True   False

8. All of the following foods have a high sodium content except

    a. potato chips
    b. canned soup
    c. Chinese food
    d. baked fish

9. Hyperlipidemia frequently occurs following renal transplantation. Which of the following factors is the cause?

    a. immunosuppressive therapy

    b. antihypertensive therapy

    c. weight gain

    d. all of the above

Chapter 11

1. DE, a 78-year-old woman, is being treated for severe depression and anorexia. A nasogastric tube was placed for nutritional support. One reason the nasogastric tube was chosen over other routes of intestinal access in this patient is that

    a. long-term tube feeding was expected

    b. risk of aspiration was high

    c. the stomach was emptying normally

    d. short bowel syndrome was present

2. In which of the following conditions is enteral nutrition contraindicated for a patient with chronic inflammatory bowel disease?

    a. presence of a high-output, enterocutaneous fistula

    b. severe anorexia

    c. a small bowel that is less than 100 percent functional

    d. absent gag reflex

3. ES, an 81-year-old man, recently had a mild stroke that left him unable to swallow without aspirating. He is currently malnourished at 87 percent of his ideal body weight. What type of access should be placed for feeding?

    a. nasogastric tube

    b. heplock for PPN

    c. nasojejunal tube

    d. subclavian catheter for TPN

4. JL, a 32-year-old man with AIDS, was hospitalized for severe diarrhea caused by fat malabsorption. His appetite was poor, so a nasogastric tube was placed to provide nutritional support. Which formula is most appropriate for this patient?

    a. lactose-free polymeric formula

    b. hypercaloric polymeric formula

    c. high-fiber polymeric formula

    d. elemental formula

5. MB, a 52-year-old woman, underwent an uncomplicated cholecystectomy 24 hours ago. Her abdominal exam reveals distention, and no bowel sounds are audible. This patient was well-nourished prior to admission and has lost 5

pounds since the surgery. What type of nutrition support should she receive?

    a. PPN until there are bowel sounds and the patient begins eating

    b. nasogastric feedings until there are bowel sounds and the patient begins eating

    c. TPN until there are bowel sounds and the patient begins eating

    d. no nutrition support unless distention persists and no bowel sounds are heard on reevaluation three days after surgery

6. AF, a 43-year-old woman with a history of chronic pancreatitis, has been receiving a 3-in-1 TPN mixture for the past six months. Which of the following is an indication to discontinue adding lipid emulsions to the daily TPN regimen?

    a. serum triglyceride greater than 800 mg/dL

    b. an acute bout of pancreatitis with a serum triglyceride less than 300 mg/dL

    c. blood glucose greater than 300 mg/dL

    d. loss of 15 pounds in one month

7. AM is a 35-year-old woman hospitalized for a mild bout of alcoholic pancreatitis is placed on NPO (nothing by mouth) status and PPN. PPN is a good choice for her nutritional support because

    a. short-term use of PPN is anticipated

    b. PPN allows for concentrated delivery of nutrients, thereby providing fluid restriction

    c. PPN catheters present low risk for phlebitis

    d. PPN provides patients with total nutritional supplementation

Review Answers

Chapter 1

1. b, a, b, c, c, d, d.
2. d.
3. b, c.
4. c.
5. d.
6. a, c, a, b.

Chapter 2

1. c.
2. d.
3. a.
4. a.
5. d.
6. a.
7. c.

Chapter 3

1. c.
2. b.
3. b.
4. d.
5. d.
6. a.
7. c.
8. d.

Chapter 4

1. d.
2. a.
3. a.
4. c.
5. a.
6. b.
7. c.

Chapter 5

1. d.
2. b.
3. d.
4. c.
5. c.
6. d.
7. Smoking: P
   Short stature: P
   Kidney disease: S
   Hyperthyroidism: S
   Family history of osteoporosis: P
   COPD: S
   Early menopause: P
   Sedentary lifestyle: P

Chapter 6

1. c, e, e, d, b, a, f.
2. c.
3. c.
4. a, b, c, d, e, f.
5. False
6. b.
7. b.
8. b.

Chapter 7

1. b.
2. c.
3. d.
4. c.
5. a.
6. d.
7. b.
8. b, d.

Chapter 8

1. d.
2. b.
3. a.
4. d.
5. b.
6. d.
7. a, c, f.

Chapter 9

1. b.
2. a.
3. d.
4. d.
5. b, d.
6. a, c.

Chapter 10

1. d.
2. d.
3. b.
4. b.
5. a.
6. d.
7. False
8. d.
9. a.

Chapter 11

1. c.
2. a.
3. c.
4. d.
5. d.
6. a.
7. a.

Glossary

Acanthosis nigricans: Skin hyperpigmentation changes on the neck and under the arms. Associated with obesity and endocrine disorders.

Acromion: The lateral extension of the spine of the scapula, forming the highest point of the shoulder. Anatomic landmark for measuring the mid-arm circumference.

Alopecia: Hair loss. Absence of hair from skin where it is normally present. Associated with protein malnutrition or zinc, essential fatty acid, or biotin deficiency.

Anabolism: The constructive process of metabolism, in which a cell converts simple substances from the blood that are required for repair and growth, into more complex compounds, especially into living matter.

Angular stomatitis: Superficial erosions and fissuring at the angles of the mouth. Associated with thiamin (B1), riboflavin (B2), niacin (B3), pyridoxine (B6), and iron deficiencies.

Arthralgia: Pain in a joint, possibly associated with vitamin C deficiency.

Ascites: Fluid accumulation in the peritoneal cavity. Associated with liver disease and hypoalbuminemia.

Asterixis: A motor disturbance marked by intermittent lapses of an assumed posture. Associated with end-stage liver disease and hepatic encephalopathy.

Atrophic lingual papillae: Wasting or diminished size of the cells of the tongue. Associated with severe riboflavin (B2), niacin (B3), or iron deficiency, or protein-energy malnutrition.

Bitot's spots: Squamous, epithelial thickening of the conjunctiva. Associated with vitamin A deficiency.

Bradycardia: Slowness of the heartbeat, evidenced by slowing of the pulse rate to under 60 BPM. Associated with protein-energy malnutrition and hypothyroidism as well as cardiac abnormalities.

Cachexia: Profound, marked state of ill health and/or malnutrition frequently seen in patients with cancer and AIDS.

Caput medusae: A condition resulting from dilation due to stasis of the cutaneous veins around the navel, occurring most commonly in newborns and patients with cirrhosis of the liver.

Catabolism: The opposite of anabolism. Includes those processes concerned with breaking down complex substances into simpler constituents for energy. Commonly seen in patients following trauma or surgery or patients with cancer or AIDS.

Cheilosis: Fissuring/thinning of the lips. Associated with protein malnutrition and pyridoxine (B6), riboflavin (B2), or iron deficiency.

Desquamation: The shedding of skin in sheets or scales. Associated with protein-energy malnutrition.

Dysgeusia/Hypogeusia: Impaired taste acuity. May be associated with zinc deficiency.

Ecchymosis: Excessive bruising of the skin. Associated with vitamin K or C deficiency and liver disease.

Eczema: An inflammation of the skin, with vesiculation, infiltration, watery discharge, and the development of scales and crusts. Associated with allergies.

Epiphyses: Growth plate composed of cartilage at the end of long bones. Present in infants and children prior to completion of skeletal maturation. Abnormalities in growth seen in vitamin D deficiency and lead toxicity.

Follicular hyperkeratosis: Hypertrophy of the corneous layer of the skin. Associated with vitamin A or essential fatty acid deficiency.

Glossitis: Inflammation of the tongue. Associated with pyridoxine (B6), folic acid, iron, or vitamin B12 deficiency.

Hyperglycemia: Elevated blood sugar associated with diabetes and disorders of carbohydrate metabolism.

Hyperkeratosis: Hypertrophy of the skin associated with vitamin A deficiency.

Hypoalbuminemia: Abnormally low serum levels of albumin. Associated with malnutrition, liver disease, and nephrotic syndrome.

Hypokalemia: Low serum potassium levels.

Hyponatremia: Low serum sodium levels.

Interosseous muscles: Muscles between the bones. Those on the hand are helpful indicators of muscle wasting associated with protein-energy malnutrition.

Iron deficiency: Characterized by low or absent iron stores. Diagnosed on the basis of low serum iron concentration, transferrin saturation, hemoglobin, and ferritin levels and elevated transferrin levels.

Keratomalacia: Softening or necrosis of the cornea associated with vitamin A deficiency.

Kwashiorkor: A nutritional disease due to a diet deficient in protein though adequate in calories. Manifested by hypoalbuminemia, resulting in edema of the hands, feet, and face.

Macrocytic anemia: Large, nucleated, immature, abnormal erythrocytes. Marked by an increased mean corpuscular volume (MCV) and mean corpuscular hemoglobin concentration (MCHC). Associated with folate or vitamin B_{12} deficiency. Frequently seen with decreased dietary intake, methotrexate therapy, or ileal and gastric resection.

Marasmus: A form of protein-energy malnutrition characterized by growth retardation and wasting of subcutaneous fat and muscle.

Megaloblastic anemia: (See Macrocytic anemia.)

Microcytic anemia: Marked by decreases in the size of the red blood cells, mean corpuscular volume (MCV), and mean corpuscular hemoglobin concentration (MCHC). Often associated with iron deficiency.

Neuropathy: Functional disturbance or pathological changes of the peripheral nervous system. May be associated with thiamin (B_1), pyridoxine (B_6), or vitamin B_{12} deficiency.

Nystagmus: Involuntary, rapid movement of the eyeball. Associated with Wernicke's encephalopathy secondary to excessive and prolonged alcohol abuse and thiamin deficiency.

Ophthalmoplegia: Paralysis of the eye muscles. May be associated with thiamin (B_1) deficiency.

Orthopnea: Difficulty breathing except in an upright position.

Pallor: Paleness, absence of the normal skin coloration. Associated with folic acid, iron, vitamin B12, copper, or biotin deficiency.

Paresthesia: Abnormal sensation, such as burning or prickling. Associated with thiamin (B1), pyroxidine (B6), or vitamin B12 deficiency.

Parotid enlargement: Enlargement of the parotid gland situated at or occurring near the ear. May be seen in patients with bulimia and protein malnutrition.

Pernicious anemia: Macrocytic anemia due to the failure of the gastric mucosa to secrete adequate potent intrinsic factor, resulting in malabsorption of vitamin B12 (cells are also megaloblastic).

Petechiae: Pinhead size hemorrhagic spots. Associated with vitamin A toxicity and vitamin A, C, or K deficiency.

Protein energy malnutrition (PEM): Disorder that occurs when the diet is deficient in both protein and calories. Results in severe tissue wasting, loss of lean body mass and subcutaneous fat, and usually dehydration. May also be referred to as protein calorie malnutrition.

Purpura: A condition in which confluent petechiae or confluent ecchymoses are present over any part of the body. May be associated with vitamin C or K deficiency.

Rickets: Disturbances of normal ossification marked by bending and distortion of the bones, nodular enlargements of the ends and sides of bones, delayed closure of the fontanels, and muscle pain. Due to vitamin D deficiency in infancy and childhood and poor ultraviolet light exposure in individuals of any age. Rachitic means pertaining to or affected with rickets.

Sclera anicteric: Normal white outer coating of the eyeball, without jaundice.

Steatorrhea: Oily, foul-smelling stools due to the presence of excess fat secondary to pancreatic insufficiency or GI malabsorption. Often seen in Crohn's disease and cystic fibrosis.

Stomatitis: Generalized inflammation of the oral mucosa. Associated with thiamin (B1), riboflavin (B2), niacin (B3), or iron deficiency. (See also angular stomatitis.)

Striae: Stretch marks on the skin associated with obesity.

Tachycardia: Rapid heart rate. Associated with thiamin (B1) deficiency, hyperthyroidism, and iron deficiency anemia. Typically seen in alcoholics.

Temporal muscle: Located in the lateral region on either side of the head just behind the eyes. Depletion or wasting of the temporal muscles is often seen in malnourished patients.

Visceral protein: Protein associated with the major organs of the body.

Xerosis: Abnormal dryness of the skin or the eyes (scleral). Associated with vitamin A or essential fatty acid deficiency.

Index